FOOD ALLERGY

FOOD ALLERGY

New Perspectives

Edited By

JOHN W. GERRARD, D.M.

Professor of Pediatrics
University of Saskatchewan
Saskatoon, Saskatchewan, Canada

CHARLES C THOMAS • PUBLISHER
Springfield • Illinois • U.S.A.

Published and Distributed Throughout the World by

CHARLES C THOMAS • PUBLISHER
BANNERSTONE HOUSE
301-327 East Lawrence Avenue, Springfield, Illinois, U.S.A.

ISBN 0-398-04038-9 cloth
ISBN 0-398-04041-9 paper
Library of Congress Catalog Card Number: 79-26639

With THOMAS BOOKS *careful attention is given to all details of manufacturing and design. It is the Publisher's desire to present books that are satisfactory as to their physical qualities and artistic possibilities and appropriate for their particular use.* THOMAS BOOKS *will be true to those laws of quality that assure a good name and good will.*

Printed in the United States of America
N-11

Library of Congress Cataloging in Publication Data

Gerrard, John W.
Food allergy.

Includes bibliographies and index.
1. Food allergy. I. Title.
RC596.G47 616.9'75 79-26639
ISBN 0-398-04038-9
ISBN 0-398-04041-9 pbk.

to the many patients whom we are trying to help

CONTRIBUTORS

Chaim Brautbar, Ph.D. Senior Lecturer in Immunology, Director of Tissue Typing Laboratory, Hadassah Hebrew University Medical Centre, Jerusalem, Israel.

Tirzah Cohen, M.D. Associate Professor, Department of Human Genetics, Hadassah Hebrew University Medical Centre, Jerusalem, Israel.

Moshe Finelt, M.D. Chief Resident, Shaare Zedek Hospital, Jerusalem, Israel.

Serem Freier, M.B., D.C.H. Head, Department of Pediatrics and Director of Research, The Institute of Gastroenterology, Shaare Zedek Hospital, Jerusalem, Israel.

John W. Gerrard, D.M. Professor of Pediatrics, University of Saskatchewan, Saskatoon, Saskatchewan, Canada.

Vida H. Gordon, M.D. Professor Emeritus, Department of Pediatrics and Associate Professor Emeritus, Department of Microbiology and Immunology, University of Arkansas College of Medicine, Little Rock, Arkansas, U.S.A.

Hsi-Yen Liu, M.D. Associate Professor of Pediatrics, Department of Pediatrics, University of Michigan Medical School, Ann Arbor, Michigan, U.S.A.

Thomas F. McLeod, M.D. Assistant Professor of Pediatrics, University of Miami School of Medicine, Miami, Florida, U.S.A.

Joseph B. Miller, M.D. Clinical Associate Professor, Department of Pediatrics, University of Alabama Medical Center, Birmingham, Alabama, and Consultant, Department of Pediatrics, University of South Alabama Medical Center, Mobile, Alabama, U.S.A.

Doris J. Rapp, M.D. Clinical Assistant Professor of Pediatrics, State University of New York at Buffalo, New York, U.S.A.

William J. Rea, M.D. Clinical Associate Professor of Thoracic and Cardiovascular Surgery, University of Texas Southwestern Medical School, Dallas, and Director, Brookhaven Environmental Unit, Dallas, Texas, U.S.A.

Douglas H. Sandberg, M.D. Professor of Pediatrics, University of Miami School of Medicine, Miami, Florida, U.S.A.

Andre Seban, M.D. Misgab Ledach Hospital, Jerusalem, Israel.

Jose Strauss, M.D. Professor of Pediatrics, University of Miami School of Medicine, Miami, Florida, U.S.A.

Charles W. Suits, B.S. Research Assistant, Human Ecology, Research Foundation of the South West Inc., Brookhaven Environmental Unit, Dallas, Texas, U.S.A.

PREFACE

In the natural state of affairs, man has four major hazards: the first, famine and natural disasters, such as earthquakes and tornados; the second, cancer; the third, the world of viruses, bacteria, and parasites; and the fourth, the animal world—this includes man himself, for he is, unfortunately, his own worst enemy. This book is indirectly related to his battle with the world of viruses and bacteria, for these are detected and destroyed by his immune system, and the latter plays a key role in the development of allergies.

The grosser hazards of the visible world are detected by the senses, and the information received is channelled to the brain where the data are processed and action initiated. The action taken is determined by past experience and present contingencies. If, for example, a burglar were to enter the house and you were defenceless, you would probably lie low and pretend to be asleep, but if you were to have a gun under your pillow, you might well hold him prisoner and phone the police. Your responses would not be automatic and predetermined. The immune response, dealing with organisms, does not have a centre in which policies and programs can be determined. Its actions therefore depend on a series of automatic responses and, in this respect, resemble the well-programmed computer. The system, like the computer, has memory capability, and when an organism is encountered for the second or third time, the defences are marshalled quickly so that the organism does not have the chance to multiply and cause disease. The programmed response has the advantage of being immediate—the host cannot be caught offguard or asleep—but it has the disadvantage that the immune system cannot distinguish between the living and the dead, and that it responds as readily to animal danders, house dust, cow's milk, and egg as it does to viruses and bacteria. In its response to these dead antigens, it seems to get wildly excited in some individuals and, like Don Quixote, finds itself tilting at windmills. We know how to recognize and handle the more obvious of these reactions—hay fever and asthma—because the relationship between the allergens and the reaction of the patient usually is obvious, and because sensitivities can readily be confirmed by prick test and RAST. However, we have been less ready to recognize other reactions in which the relationship between the allergen and the reaction is not so obvious and cannot readily be confirmed by prick test or RAST. This group of reactions often is thought to be psychosomatic in origin rather than allergic, as was once the case with asthma.

Contributors to this volume include those who have become very much aware of the part played by foods and chemicals in foods and in the environment in causing disease, and of the difficulty in identifying these foods and chemicals and in helping patients. Several have suffered from disabling allergies and have gained insight, learning the hard way through bitter experience. For this, and other reasons, their approaches are not uniform.

The diseases under study are triggered by the three elements on which we depend for our survival—air, water, and food. Our air is most highly polluted where it should be most pure—where the population is thickest—and though our city waters are bacteriologically safe, they are far removed from their original source and certainly are no longer "pure." Our foods, although much safer bacteriologically than in the past, are no longer the simple products they used to be. It would seem likely that our various immune systems, which had adapted over many generations to their own local environments, have been jolted and thrown off balance. The recent substitution of cow's milk for the breast certainly is the greatest single change in our dietary habits for the whole of our evolutionary history and has undoubtedly been responsible for more disease than is generally realized. The processing of foods and the rapid transport of foods and populations have also led to tremendous changes in dietary habits, so it is not surprising that diseases related to foods and to the chemicals added to them, and being added daily to our environment, should be triggering our immune systems and leading to disease. We hope that this volume, while raising eyebrows in some quarters, will also shed a little light on what is still a very perplexing problem.

J. W. GERRARD

CONTENTS

FOOD ALLERGY

Chapter 1

GENETIC FACTORS IN FOOD ALLERGY OF EARLY CHILDHOOD*

SEREM FREIER, MOSHE FINELT, ANDRE SEBAN, TIRZAH COHEN, AND CHAIM BRAUTBAR

INTRODUCTION

THE STUDY of food allergy dates back to the beginning of the century, when Finkelstein[11] reported a child who died after ingestion of milk. Recognition of the diagnosis of food allergy was slow: it was first mentioned in the American literature in 1916,[32] and in the English literature in 1958.[8]

The relationship of food allergy to other allergic conditions and its hereditary nature were mentioned thirty years ago by Tufts.[34] He stated that the influence of heredity is equally important in food allergy as in allergy due to other allergens, particularly so in such clinical manifestations as asthma, eczema, and migraine. Withers and Hale reported families where allergy to milk was transmitted through four generations[36]. Doctors who treat infants with food protein allergy realize that this is a familial condition. We recall, for instance, one family where three out of five infants invariably developed periorbital edema within half an hour of drinking cow's milk. Not only may the symptom pattern repeat itself in a single family but also the identical allergens may be responsible for producing disease in siblings.[6] The most thorough family study is from Gerrard et al.,[12] who observed milk allergy in first degree relatives of 60 percent of their affected

*This research was supported in part by a grant from the office of the Chief Scientist, Ministry of Health, Jerusalem, and in part by a grant donated by Mr. and Mrs. Forrest Shaklee.

children. In their 10-year follow up of 150 children,[14] they report that 17 percent of the mothers had adverse reactions on provocation tests with milk, although they had been unaware of this sensitivity. Families who have one infant affected with milk allergy have a 1:2 chance that a subsequent infant will be similarly affected.[9,31]

IS FOOD ALLERGY AN ATOPIC CONDITION?

To establish the relationship between food allergy and other allergies, we reviewed a group of forty-one patients who had been under our care in the past for milk allergy (R. Peleg and S. Freier, unpublished). Detailed information on family history was obtained from one of the patient's parents. This was supplemented by information culled from the patient's case notes. The same details were obtained from parents of sixty-one control children. The latter were patients consecutively seen in a well baby clinic. These patients consisted of Ashkenazi Jews originating from Central and Eastern Europe and non-Ashkenazi Jews of Mediterranean and Middle Eastern origin.

Milk allergy was diagnosed after three challenges with each of the following five isolated milk proteins: bovine gamma globulin, bovine serum albumin, casein (all from Armour Pharmaceutical Co.), beta-lactoglobulin, and alpha-lactalbumin (both from Pentex, Inc.). When two positive reactions were obtained with the same protein the diagnosis was established. In our patients gastrointestinal symptoms and failure to gain weight predominated, but these symptoms were accompanied by rashes in 20 percent and by wheezing in 10 percent. Gastrointestinal allergy to other food proteins, particularly soy protein, was present in many of the patients.

Among our forty-one patients, there was a definite preponderance of males, the sex ratio being 2:1 (27 males, 14 females). The frequency of Ashkenazi and non-Ashkenazi Jews was approximately equal (Ashkenazi 18, non-Ashkenazi 14, mixed 9). Table 1-I shows that various conditions with an allergic etiology were commoner in first degree relatives of patients with milk allergy than in those of controls. The conditions included milk allergy, asthma, chronic sinusitis, hay fever, chronic rhinitis, and eczema.

TABLE 1-I

Frequency of allergic conditions among first degree relatives of probands with milk allergy and of controls.

Diagnosis	*Probands with an affected 1st degree relative* (n=41) No.	%	*1st degree relatives of controls* (n=61) No.	%
Milk allergy	10	24	7	11
Asthma	5	12	2	3
Chronic sinusitis	9	22	6	10
Hay Fever	10	24	5	8
Chronic rhinitis	16	39	4	7
Eczema	10	24	8	13
Celiac Disease	0	0	0	0
Diabetes mellitus	0	0	1	1

A study highlighting the relationship between gastrointestinal and respiratory allergy was recently described by May.[27] This study was performed on children suffering from chronic severe asthma. They were selected from the patient population since in the past they had been observed to react to certain foods. May eliminated those foods suspected of causing symptoms before the oral challenge with the allergen under suspicion. In the eleven positive reactors, the symptoms on challenge were chiefly gastrointestinal although these children were suffering from chronic asthma. This study shows the close relationship between the gastrointestinal and respiratory tract in allergy, and raises again the question of what it is that determines the organ in which symptoms manifest themselves.

THE MODE OF INHERITANCE

Gerrard et al.[13] have shown that most allergies tend to involve the same target organ in parents and children. In other words, if one or both of the parents had asthma, the children were more likely to have asthma than any other allergy. The same held true for hay fever, recurrent rhinitis, recurrent bronchitis, and eczema.

Various modes of inheritance have been suggested for atopic disease: a single dominant gene with partial penetrance, a single recessive gene with partial penetrance, and a multifactorial mode of inheritance.[1,30,33] Since environmental as well as genetic factors contribute to the appearance of atopic disease, not all susceptible individuals will be included in frequency estimates based on population surveys.

The data of Kjellman[21] summarized in Table 1-II confirm that atopic disease is a common condition with a deviation in the sex ratio of the affected. The morbidity in the siblings of the proband increases from 12.5 percent when no parent is affected, to 19.8 percent when one is affected, and to 42.9 percent when both parents are affected. A similar increase, by the number of affected parents, was observed in the frequency of two or more affected siblings per family. These observations correspond to characteristics of conditions caused by polygenic inheritance.[5] Van Arsdel and Motulsky observed similar results in families of students with asthma and allergic rhinitis.[35]

TABLE 1-II

Atopic disease in a group of unselected school children and their family members.*

		No. examined	*Atopic diseases in* 1 sibling or more		2 siblings or more	
			No.	*%*	*No.*	*%*
General population	Total	1325	200	15.1	13	1.0
	Male	678	114	16.8		
	Female	647	86	13.3		
Parents affected						
None		990	124	12.5	2	0.2
One		293	58	19.8	5	1.7
Both		42	18	42.9	6	14.3

*Compiled from data of M. Kjellman, with permission.

SERUM IMMUNOGLOBULIN E AND FOOD ALLERGY

Following the discovery of immunoglobulin E (IgE) as the most important of the reaginic antibodies,[19] it was established that this immunoglobulin was often raised in serum of patients with atopic disease.[21] This association is not invariable, and high IgE levels may occur in the absence of atopy (such as in parasitic disease) while many atopic individuals have low levels of total IgE. High levels of IgE are one factor, but not the only one, associated with the development of allergy, and a tendency to high levels of IgE may be inherited. Marsh et al.[25] observed that IgE levels in allergic families have a bimodal distribution with a cut-off point of 95 units/ml distinguishing between allergic individuals with high IgE levels and nonallergic phenotypes with low levels. Gerrard et al.,[13] setting their cut-off point at 150 units/ml, studied three mating types: those with neither, one, or both of the parents having raised levels of IgE. The authors concluded that the low levels of IgE were determined by two dominant genes, the absence of one or the other permitting high levels to occur. Recently, Gerrard et al.[15] applied path and complex segregation analyses to IgE levels in 173 families. They had evidence of polygenic inheritance with a heriditability of 0.425 and of a major regulatory locus (RE) for serum IgE levels. Homozygosity for the recessive allele of *RE*, namely *re/re*, causes high levels of IgE.

Studies on mono– and dizygotic twins confirm the heritability of IgE levels. IgE levels in monozygotic twins were usually very similar, while levels for dizygotic twins are intermediate between the distribution obtained for identical twins and between pairs of individuals chosen at random from the population.[29]

IgE levels in food allergy have been studied by Heiner and Rose,[18] who observed that seven out of sixteen patients had raised serum levels of IgE. As these authors do not record the age and the clinical state of their patients, we cannot compare their results with a group of children investigated by us with food (mostly milk) allergy. The diagnosis in our cases was established according to the criteria of Goldman et al.,[16] which require that three separate challenges with the allergen under suspicion produce identical clinical responses.

In our infants, gastrointestinal symptoms predominated; thus the group was not representative of the spectrum of atopic disease that is encountered in food allergy.

The following groups of children were investigated: group 1, comprising sixty-six normal infants and children without symptoms of gastrointestinal or other allergy. Their ages ranged from one month to thirteen years. Group 2 included twenty-one infants with cow's milk allergy aged one to thirteen months. IgE was measured at the time of presentation, while on the allergen-containing diet. Children on hypoallergenic diets not less than one month following the diagnosis represented group 3. These were thirty-six children aged from four months to two years and four months. The hypoallergenic diet given to this group almost always consisted of a "casein" hydrolysate formula. Children who no longer showed any clinical signs of milk allergy were included in group 4. There were thirty-two children in this group, but two "outliers" with very high IgE levels were excluded. Their ages ranged from five months to eight years. In group 5 there were five children aged two years and two months to four years and three months with allergies to foods other than milk.

Assuming a linear relationship between IgE and age, a linear regression of IgE on age was fitted for each group (Fig. 1-1). Comparing group 2 with group 1, it is obvious that children with cow's milk allergy have very high levels of IgE. The high inter-

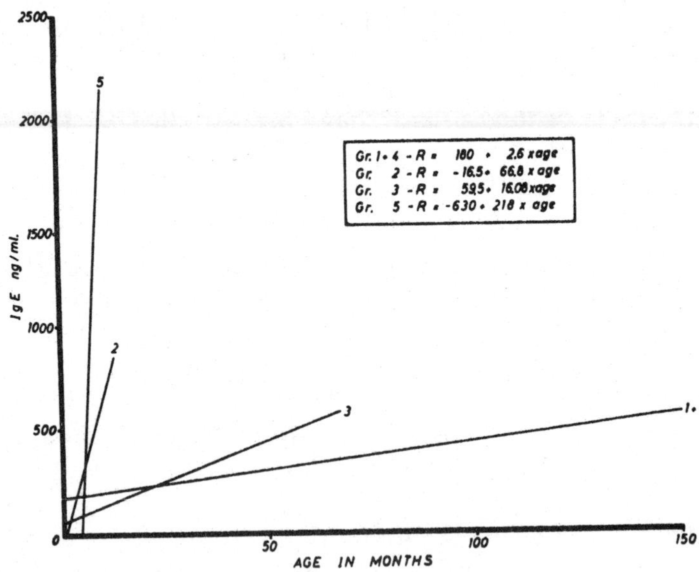

Figure 1-1. R=Regression. Group 1—Normal. Group 2—receiving allergen. Group 3—on hypoallergenic diet for at least one month. Group 4—cured. Group 5—receiving allergen other than milk. As there was no statistical difference between Group 1 and 4, a common regression curve was constructed.

cept for group 1 (180 ng/ml) gives a misleading impression, as most children at one month had IgE levels of 25 ng/ml or less. It is possible, therefore, that the linear relationship assumed for the lower age range is not valid. The levels of IgE tend to be lower when the children are placed on hypoallergenic diets (group 3) and return to normal when symptoms of food allergy disappear. As we found no statistical difference between group 1 (normal) and group 4 (cured), a common regression curve was fitted for both groups. It is likely, therefore, that in most of our cases high IgE levels are an expression of exposure to allergen and are not due to innate inherited high IgE levels. The two children in the "cured" group who had high IgE levels (1680 and 2640 ng/ml respectively) may have inherited a high IgE gene or they may have been exposed to an unidentified and unsuspected allergen.

The levels of IgE found in the group of children allergic to food proteins other than cow's milk did not differ substantially from those of children with cow's milk protein intolerance. These children, too, following recovery from their food allergy, had normal levels of IgE.

It may therefore be concluded that high IgE levels in food allergy reflect a state of sensitivity to a food protein: levels return to normal upon recovery. There is no evidence that children with food allergy belong to a hereditary "high IgE" group that predisposes them to food allergy.

So far the study of the heredity of reagin-mediated allergic disease in man has centered on IgE values and on the association between human histocompatibility antigens (HLA) and allergy.[10, 29] However, the inherited characteristic may not reside in the amount of IgE being produced but in any of the other steps or cells involved in the anaphylactic response, such as the number of mast cells, the ease with which histamine is being liberated, tissue histamine content, ability of the basophil to be sensitized, and the variation in the reactivity of target organs. Most of these aspects have not been fully investigated. In a recent publication, May claimed that spontaneous release of histamine from mast cells is a feature pathognomonic of food allergy;[26] others have found that this is a feature of mast cells from patients with any atopic condition (W. E. Parish, personal communication).

INHERITANCE OF THE IMMUNE RESPONSE

When simple synthetic polypeptide antigens are used in small doses to immunize mice, certain inbred strains will respond to a given polypeptide while others are unable to produce antibody against it. This observation has given rise to the concept of immune response (Ir) genes.[2] These genes are thought to be responsible for determining whether antibodies (including reagins) will be produced against specific antigens. The Ir genes are independent of the genes that control the overall level of reagin production.

Two major findings in immunology have contributed to the understanding of allergy and atopic diseases. The identification that immunoglobulin E is the main antibody class involved in atopic hypersensitivity and the discovery in experimental animals, particularly rats, mice, and guinea pigs, of genes controlling the immune response (Ir genes) to specific antigens.[2] Furthermore, it was shown that the Ir genes are linked to the major histocompatibility complex (MHC). At present, it appears that in experimental animals at least two distinct types of genetic control of IgE responsiveness exist: first, genes controlling the overall ability to produce IgE, and second, antigen-specific control as a result of Ir genes.

In man, the vast majority of studies aimed toward the detection of Ir genes specific for natural allergens were based on immediate skin reactions due to specific IgE. In two studies, it was distinctly shown that skin hypersensitivity to antigen Ra5, a small, highly purified allergen molecule from ragweed pollen, is associated with HLA-B7 and HLA-B7 cross-reacting group. In family studies, Levine et al.[22] were the first to claim a linkage between hypersensitivity to ragweed antigen E and HLA haplotypes. Other family studies have described HLA-linked genetic control of specific response to natural antigens such as alternaria, hormodendrum, and mumps virus. The response to grass, tree pollen, and house dust seems to be linked to the human MHC. These results may indicate that in man, as in experimental animals, Ir genes linked to HLA do exist.[24,17]

In view of the foregoing observations we investigated HLA

antigen frequencies in children under our care with allergy to cow's milk protein. The diagnosis was based in each case on the criteria mentioned above. The children were placed on a milk-free diet and rechallenged with milk at intervals of two months. When symptoms of milk protein allergy subsided, the children were discharged from the clinic. For the purpose of this study, all our known cases of cow's milk allergy were invited to attend the clinic, and the aim of this research was explained to them.

Forty-six unrelated children suffering from milk allergy and family members of eight of these children were studied. The majority of the patients were born in Israel. Twenty-six of them were the offspring of Ashkenazi Jews, originating from Central and Eastern Europe, and twenty were born to non-Ashkenazi parents of Mediterranean and Middle Eastern origin. The controls were 912 individuals unrelated to the patients. They included blood donors, hospital personnel, and volunteers whose parents, and in most cases grandparents, were born in the same country. Four hundred and fifty-three were Ashkenazi Jews, whereas 459 were non-Ashkenazi Jews.

Lymphocytes were separated from defibrinated blood samples by Ficoll-Hypaque flotation density equilibrium centrifugation.[4] The fluorochromasia cytotoxicity test was employed for HLA typing of fresh and frozen (−180°C) lymphocytes.[3] Each individual was typed at least twice for the following specificities: HLA-A1, 2, 3, 9, 10, 11, 25, 26, 28, 29, W19, W23, W24, W30, W31, W32, W33, and HLA-B5, 7, 8, 12, 13, 14, 15, 17, 18, 27, 37, 40, W16, W21, W22, W35. Generally, four alloantisera were used to test each specificity. Typing sera were obtained from the National Institutes of Health (NIH) serum bank, from colleagues, and some were obtained locally.

Of forty-six patients, twenty-four were males and twenty-two were females. Their ages ranged from three months to eight years. The twenty-six Ashkenazi patients originated from Poland (9), Russia (6), Germany (3), Rumania (3), and mixed origin (5); twenty non-Ashkenazi patients were from Morocco (11), Iraq (4), Iran (3), and Yemen (2) (Table 1-III). The HLA antigen frequencies of forty-six patients with milk allergy and of the control group are summarized in Table 1-IV. Our data were examined for possible associations between HLA antigens and milk allergy. In general we looked for positive associations; the *p*-values quoted in Table 1-IV are for a one-sided test of the null hypothesis that the incidence ratio (relative risk) is unity. Since there were too few patients to make specific ethnic comparisons, the data were pooled, using the Mantel-Haenzel method.[23] Three separate analyses were made: of the whole patient sample, of patients of Ashkenazi origin, and of those of non-Ashkenazi origin. In the total sample (Table I-IV), no significant association between any of the twenty-five HLA antigens tested and milk allergy was observed. However, when the patient population was subgrouped by origin and analysed separately, some indications for associations were noted.

Among twenty-six Ashkenazi milk allergy patients, the frequency of HLA-A29 was 0.27 as compared to 0.09 among the controls, with a one-sided *p*-value of 0.0062. However, since the present analysis is exploratory in nature, and twenty-five antigens were tested for, the *p*-value should be corrected. A conservative method is to multiply the calculated *p*-value by the number of antigens tested. After such a correction, the *p*-value for A29 was 0.1548. When the non-Ashkenazi subgroup was subjected to a separate analysis, none of the twenty-five HLA antigens tested showed any association with the disease. Twenty patients were in the non-Ashkenazi subgroup; eleven of these originated from Morocco. HLA antigen frequencies in these eleven patients

TABLE 1-III

Origin of milk allergy patients, studied for HLA antigens.

Population	*Origin*	*Patients*	*Controls*
Ashkenazi	Poland	9	127
	Russia	6	123
	Rumania	3	1·30
	Germany	3	73
	Mixed Origin	5	
Non-Ashkenazi	Morocco	11	141
	Iraq	4	121
	Yemen	2	197
	Iran	3	
TOTAL		46	912

TABLE 1-IV

HLA Antigen Frequencies in Food Allergy Patients and Controls

Phenotype Frequency

HLA	Patients N=46	Controls N=912	*P*-value
A1	.261	.300	.7475
A2	.348	.308	.2773
A3	.174	.164	.5276
A9*	.370	.321	.1080
A10*	.304	.186	.0995
A11	.087	.087	.5118
A25	.043	—	—
A26	.196	—	—
A28	.087	.100	.4216
A29	.196	.079	.0240
AW19*	.087	.252	.9838
AW23	.087	—	—
AW24	.261	—	—
AW30**	.000	—	—
AW31	.000	—	—
AW32	.000	—	—
AW33	.022	—	—
B5	.174	.188	.4890
B7	.065	.093	.7570
B8	.043	.064	.6514
B12	.239	.203	.1827
B13	.065	.085	.7337
B14	.152	.165	.5250
B15	.022	.051	.7518
B17	.109	.114	.5368
B18	.130	.083	.1106
B27	.022	.046	.7024
B37	.000	.019	.6620
B40	.087	.067	.3827
BW16	.283	.187	.1060
BW21	.109	.128	.4162
BW22	.065	.045	.4229
BW35	.348	.286	.3465

*The splits of HLA-A9 (AW23, AW24), A10 (A25, A26) and AW19 (AW30, AW31, AW32, AW33) were examined only in the patient group.

**When the antigen was absent in the patient group, the probability of zero occurence of this antigen under the null hypothesis of no difference between patients and controls was calculated.

showed that three carried HLA-A11, as compared to three out of 138 individuals in the Moroccan control group. The one-sided p-value for A11 in this group of patients was 0.0005. When the p-value for A11 was adjusted for the twenty-five HLA antigens studied, it was 0.0012. Thus, in this small sample of Jewish Moroccan patients we observed a significant association between A11 and milk allergy.

HLA antigens were determined in eight families, which included seventeen affected and nine healthy children (Table 1-V). To test for linkage between HLA and genetic factors causing milk allergy, we compared the haplotypes of the younger siblings to the oldest affected child in the family. Among nine affected siblings, three shared both haplotypes, whereas also among nine unaffected siblings, three had the same haplotypes as the oldest affected sibling. This segregation ratio of $\frac{1}{3}$ of identical haplotypes is similar to the expected $\frac{1}{4}$ in siblings. Thus, no linkage between the HLA complex and factors causing milk allergy was observed.

This study was designed to investigate a possible association between HLA antigens and milk allergy in the Israeli population and within its various communities. The data show that in the Israeli population as a whole, none of the twenty-five HLA-A and B locus antigens were significantly associated with the disease. In the subgroups of the patient population by origin, HLA-A29 showed a positive association within Ashkenazi milk allergy patients at a p-level of 15 percent, only a very mild indicative evidence. Among eleven non-Ashkenazi patients of Moroccan origin, HLA-A11 showed a significant association with the disease ($p = 0.001$). Still, since the patient sample included only eleven individuals of Moroccan origin, this observation needs confirmation.

An increased frequency of HLA-B5 in six of twenty-one patients with milk allergy observed by Dausset and Hors[7] was not confirmed in the present study. Recently, Mougenot et al.[28] noted that the distribution of twenty-eight HLA antigens in thirty-nine Caucasian children, from Europe and North Africa, with intolerance to cow's milk proteins was not different from that in normal subjects, a result similar to ours.

In summary, allergy to milk protein and probably also to other

TABLE 1-V

HLA GENOTYPES IN EIGHT FAMILIES WITH MILK ALLERGY

Family		Parents	HLA Haplotypes		Affected Children	HLA Haplotypes	Unaffected Children	HLA Haplotypes
1	F	A29,B12 / A28,B14	a/b	1	A29,B12 / A1,B17	a/c		
	M	A1,B17 / A2,B40	c/d	2	A29,B12 / A2,B40	a/d		
2	F	A26,BW21 / A2, B40	a/b	1	A26,BW21 / A28,BW22	a/c		
	M	A28,BW22 / AW19,B40	c/d	2	A2,B40 / A28,BW22	b/c		
3	F	AW24,B5 / AW33,B17	a/b	1	A24,B5 / A1,B12	a/c		
	M	A1,B12 / AW19,B17	c/d	2	AW24,B5 / A1,B12	a/c		
				3	AW33,B17 / A1,B12	b/c		
4	F	AW23,BW35 / A28, B14	a/b	1	AW23,BW35 / A2,B17	b/d		
	M	A2,B17 / A26,BW16	c/d	2	A28,B14 / A26,BW16	a/c		

TABLE 1-V — (cont'd)

Family		*Parents*	*HLA Haplotypes*		*Affected Children*	*HLA Haplotypes*		*Unaffected Children*	*Haplotypes HLA*
5	F	A3,BW35 / AW31,B13	a/b	1	A3,BW35 / A11,BW21	a/c	3	A3,B13 / AW31,B13	a x b/d*
	M	A11,BW21 / AW31,B13	c/d	2	A3,BW35 / A11,BW21	a/c	4	A3,BW35 / A11,BW21	a/c
							5	A3,BW35 / A11,BW21	a/c
6	F	AW24,BW16 / A1,B17	a/b	1	AW24,BW16 / AW23,BW21	a/c	3	AW24,BW16 / AW23,BW21	a/c
	M	AW23,BW21 / A2,BW35	c/d	2	A1,BW17 / AW23,BW21	b/c	4	AW24,BW16 / A2,BW35	a/d
							5	A1,BW16 / A2,BW35	b x a/d*
7	F	A29,B5 / AW24,BW16	a/b	1	A29,B5 / AW19,BW35	a/c	4	AW24,BW16 / AW19,BW35	b/c
	M	AW19,BW35 / A2,B5	c/d	2	A29,B5 / AW19,BW35	a/c			
				3	A29,B5 / A2,B5				
8	F	A1,BW16 / AW33,B14	a/b	1	A1,BW16 / A11,B5	a/c	2	AW33,B14 / A11,B5	b/c
	M	A11,B5 / A28,B12	c/d				3	AW33,B14 / A11,B5	b/c

*Child with HLA recombinant; F = Father; M = Mother

food proteins is a familial condition. The evidence presented here suggests that it is associated with a higher frequency of "atopic" diseases such as asthma, chronic sinusitis, hay fever, chronic rhinitis, and eczema in first degree relatives. No association could be observed with celiac disease (gluten-sensitive enteropathy). Data from the literature indicate a polygenic inheritance of allergy. Levels of the major reaginic immunoglobulin, IgE, have also been shown to be influenced by hereditary and environmental factors.

In children with allergy to milk or other food proteins, IgE levels were raised when compared to children without such allergy. These high IgE levels were probably secondary to the ingestion of the allergenic protein; after a short period on a hypoallergenic diet, IgE levels dropped. After spontaneous clinical recovery, normal IgE levels were obtained.

HLA studies on a group of forty-six children with milk allergy have shown that the human major histocompatibility complex is not linked and probably not associated with milk allergy.

REFERENCES

1. Adkinson, J.: The behavior of bronchial asthma as an inherited character. *Genetics, 5*:363, 1920.
2. Benacerraf, B. and McDevitt, H.O.: Histocompatibility linked immune response genes. *Science, 175*:273, 1972.
3. Bodmer, W., Tripp, M. and Bodmer, J.: Application of a fluorochromatic cytotoxicity assay to human leukocyte typing. *Histocompatibility Testing,* Copenhagen, Muunksgaard, 1967, pp. 341-349.
4. Boyum, A.: Separation of leukocytes from blood and bone marrow. *Scand J Clin Lab Invest (Suppl), 97*:7, 1968.
5. Carter, C.O.: Genetics of common disorders. *Br Med Bull, 25*:52, 1969.
6. Coe, B. and Mausman, H.C.: Similar multiple milk protein intolerance in non-fraternal twins. *Ann Allergy, 24*:307, 1966.
7. Dausset, J. and Hors, J.: Some contributions of the HLA complex to the genetics of human diseases. *Transplant Rev, 22*:44, 1975.
8. Davies, W.: Cow's milk allergy in infancy. *Arch Dis Child, 33*:265, 1958.
9. Despres, P., Plainfosse, B., Papiernik, M., and Seringe, P.: Les intolérances digestives aux proteines du lait de vache chez l'enfant. *Ann Pédiatrie, 18*:464, 1971.
10. de Weck, A.L., Blumenthal, M., Junis, E., and Jeannet, M.: HLA and Allergy. In Dausset, D. and Svejgaard, A. (Eds.) *HLA and Disease:* Copenhagen, Muunksgaard, 1977, pp. 196-203.

11. Finkelstein, H.: Kuhmilch als Ursache Akuter Ernahrungstoe rungen Bei Sauglingen. *Monatsschr Kinderheilk, 4*:65, 1905. Quoted by Dees, S.C., Allergy to cow's milk. *Pediatr Clin North Am, 6*:882, 1959.
12. Gerrard, J.W., Heiner, D.C. Ives, E.J., and Hardy, L.W.: Milk allergy: Recognition, natural history and management. *Clin Pediatr, 2*:634, 1963.
13. Gerrard, J.W., Horne, S., Vickers, P., MacKenzie, J.W.A., Goluboff, N., Garson, J.Z., and Maningas, C.S.: Serum IgE levels in parents and children. *J Pediatr, 85*:660, 1974.
14. Gerrard, J.W., Lubos, M.C., Hardy, L.W., Holmlund, B.A., and Webster, D.: Milk allergy: Clinical picture and familial incidence. *Can Med Assoc J, 97*:780, 1967.
15. Gerrard, J.W., Rao, D.C., and Morton, N.E.: A genetic study of immunoglobulin E. *Am J Hum Genet, 30*:46, 1978.
16. Goldman, A.S., Sellars, W.A., Halpern, S.R., Anderson, D.W., Furlow, T.W., and Johnson, C.H.: Milk allergy: Skin testing of allergic and normal children with purified milk proteins. *Pediatrics, 32*:572, 1963.
17. Goodfriend, L., Santilli, J., Jr., Schacter, B., Bias, W.B., and Marsh, D.G.: HLA B-7 cross reacting group and human IgE mediated sensitivity to ragweed allergen Ra.5. HLA and Allergy. In de Weck, A. (Ed.) *Monogr Allergy, 11*:80, 1977.
18. Heiner, D.C. and Rose, B.: Elevated levels of IgE in conditions other than classical allergy. *J Allergy, 45*:31, 1970.
19. Ishizaka, K., Ishizaka, T. and Hornbrook, M.M.: Physiocochemical properties in reaginic antibody. *J Immunol, 97*:840, 1966.
20. Johansson, S.G.O., Bennich, H.H., and Berg, T.: The clinical significance of IgE. In Schwartz, R. (Ed): *Progress in Clinical Immunology*, vol. 1, New York, Grune and Stratton, 1972 p. 157.
21. Kjellman, M.: Immunoglobulin E and atopic allergy in childhood. Linkoping University Medical Dissertations, No. 36, 1976.
22. Levine, B.B., Stember, R.H., and Fontino, M.: Ragweed hay fever: Genetic control and linkage to HL-A haplotypes. *Science, 178*:1201, 1972.
23. Mantel, N. and Haenszel, W.: Statistical aspects of the analysis of data from retrospective studies of disease. *J Natl Canc Inst, 22*:719, 1959.
24. Marsh, D.G., Bias, W.B., Hsu, S.H., Goodfriend, L.: Association of the HLA 7 cross reacting group with a specific reaginic antibody response in allergic man. *Science, 179*:691, 1973.
25. Marsh, D.G., Bias, W.B., and Ishizaka, K.: Genetic control of basal serum immunoglobulin E level and its effect on specific reaginic sensitivity. *Proc Natl Acad Sci USA, 71*:3588, 1974.
26. May, C.D.: High spontaneous release of histamine in vitro from leuko-

cytes of persons hypersensitive to food. *J Allergy Clin Immunol, 58:* 432, 1976.

27. ———: Objective clinical and laboratory studies of immediate hypersensitivity reactions to foods in asthmatic children. *J Allergy Clin Immunol, 58:*500, 1976.
28. Mougenot, J.F., Hors, J., Schmid, M., Cathelineaul, L., Navarro, J., and Polonovski, C.: Les antigènes HLA et l'intolérance digestive aux proteines du lait de vache chez l'enfant. *Gastroenterol Clin Biol, 1:* 507, 1977.
29. Orgel, H.A.: Genetic and developmental aspects of IgE. *Pediatr Clin North Am, 22:*17, 1975.
30. Ratner, B. and Silberman, D.E.: Allergy—its distribution and the hereditary concept. *Ann Allergy, 9:*20, 1952.
31. Rosenblum, A.H. and Matheson, A.: Gastrointestinal food allergy in infants. *Pediatrics, 29:*153, 1962.
32. Talbot, F.B.: Idiosyncrasy to cow's milk; its relation to anaphylaxis. *Bost Med Surg J, 175:*409, 1916.
33. Tips, R.L.: A study of the inheritance of atopic hypersensitivity in man. *Am J Hum Genet, 6:*328, 1954.
34. Tufts, L.: Foods and their relation to allergy. *Clinics, 5:*414, 1946.
35. Van Arsdel, P.P. and Motulsky, A.G.: Frequency and hereditability of asthma and allergic rhinitis in college students. *Acta Genet, 9:*101, 1959.
36. Withers, O.R. and Hale, R.: Food allergy: a review of the literature. *Ann Allergy, 14:*384, 1956.

Chapter 2

ATOPIC ECZEMA

VIDA H. GORDON

INTRODUCTION

A DISCUSSION of the relationship of atopic eczema to food allergy must necessarily include an understanding of the nature of atopic eczema, its pathophysiology, its immune mechanisms, the natural history, clinical appearance, and diagnostic criteria, as well as its management.

Atopic eczema is one of the most commonly diagnosed dermatoses seen by family physicians, dermatologists, and allergists. Its importance is emphasized by the severity and, frequently, the long-term morbidity. This disease entity was first described by Besnier and Brocq in 1885 and was known in Europe as prurigo Besnier. In 1934 Boca first used the name *atopic dermatitis* because of his observation of the association between flexural eczema, dermatitis, allergic rhinitis, and bronchial asthma in a single patient. About 70 percent of patients with atopic eczema have a family history of atopy.[10,33,42]

Some confusion that has developed regarding this disorder is related to the diversity of the nomenclature. American non-dermatologic physicians often call it "eczema, allergic dermatitis, or allergic eczema." Another source of confusion regarding the natural history is the divergence of opinion between allergists and dermatologists regarding the pathogenesis of this disease. Dermatologists usually see the patient for the first time as an older child or adult, whereas pediatricians and allergists are more apt to see an infant or young child on a first consultation.

NATURAL HISTORY

The pediatrician, and many times the allergist, has firsthand knowledge of the family history, revealing the allergies in the parents and siblings of the eczematous patient.[19] Atopic eczema affects a significant number of infants and young children, probably 3.8 percent[45,22] or higher (6.4 percent)[41] if both parents have hay fever or asthma. In interpreting incidence statistics, one needs to divide atopic eczema into three groups: infantile eczema, childhood eczema after three years, and the adult form. Seventy-five percent[33,49] of all eczema patients we see have infantile eczema starting at about the second or third month of life.

According to Stewart,[45] 1 percent of all young school children and at least 0.5 percent of teenagers and young adults have atopic eczema. The majority of the latter patients clear by thirty years of age, but a few have atopic eczema that persists throughout life. There is evidence that infantile atopic eczema is decreasing in the United States. Hill[18] pointed out that in a five-year period from 1930 to 1935 an average of 435 children a year reported with eczema to the outpatient department of Boston Children's Hospital, in contrast to fifty-two admitted during 1959. In the experience of the author, both in the public allergy clinic and in private practice, this same trend persists. The author and others[1,7,8,9,10] attribute this to the increasing use of processed milk and the return of breast-feeding by the young adult mothers today.

PATHOPHYSIOLOGY

Atopic eczema is characteristically an exudative papule, which may or may not go on to true vesiculation. Excessive oozing is not common, and it may be a dry eruption until the *tremendous itching* causes scratching and extensive trauma to the skin,[10] resulting in lichenification.

Histologically, in the more acute lesion, there are pyknotic nuclei retained in the thickened keratin layer of the skin. The granular layer is less prominent or absent. The epidermis is more hyperplastic, and the corium has more signs of edema and less perivascular infiltration. The cellular exudate is composed mostly of lymphocytes with an occasional plasma cell and neutrophil.

Eosinophiles are not conspicuous.

The chronic lichenified eczematous patches show hyperkeratosis and hyperplasia of subjacent squamous eipthelium (acanthosis). The rete ridges extend into the corium to a fairly uniform depth. The infiltrate, which is mainly lymphocytic, is extensive around the vessels.[37]

The skin of 80 percent of patients with atopic eczema reacts differently from that of a normal individual when stroked with a blunt instrument. The usual red line appears within fifteen seconds but is replaced in five to fifteen seconds by a slightly larger line of paleness. This persists for two to five minutes and may be surrounded by a red flare. Whealing does not occur, and this phenomenon is referred to as *white dermatographism.*

Response to acetylcholine (an intradermal injection of 0.1 cc of 1:1000 dilution) is different in patients with atopic dermatitis. They get an area of *blanching* rather than erythema. It lasts for fifteen to thirty minutes and is restricted to the involved skin. This physiological characteristic is presumed to be due to edema rather than vasoconstriction.

Blanching rather than the normal erythematous response follows application of nicotinic acid esters to the skin of atopic eczema patients. *Histamine* injected intradermally causes blanching instead of flaring. Blanching instead of flaring also occurs after the intradermal injection of *serotonin.* Blanching instead of erythema occurs after the intradermal injection of *bradykinen.*[5]

The *itch threshold* in the skin of patients with atopic eczema is markedly reduced. There is disagreement whether this is a primary abnormality or a secondary one produced by repeated trauma to the skin in an effort to relieve the increased itching. The extreme itching may be triggered by numerous different stimuli, such as dry skin, sweating, friction, overheating (wool clothing) or overcooling (severe cold of winter), anxiety-producing situations, and sometimes by food or inhalant allergens.

IMMUNOLOGIC CONSIDERATIONS

Many dermatologists even today persist in using the term *atopy* to describe a condition that they say is nonallergic and without atopic immunologic mechanisms. In the light of recent advances in immunological techniques, eczema should be more precisely defined as with or without an atopic component. This can be accomplished by various immunologic investigations. The atopic state may be identified by demonstrating the presence of IgE antibody to specific allergen by the RAST or measuring the serum IgE levels using PRIST.*[2] The levels of serum IgE in atopic eczema are usually the very highest. The serum of the patient Ishizaka first used to identify IgE had a level of 16,000 units. This patient had severe generalized atopic dermatitis, hay fever, and asthma.[21] Johansson and Juhlin found that the increased IgE level was restored to normal when the patient was free from atopic eczema for at least two years.[23]

Hamburger,[15,35] however, has shown that serum IgE levels are genetically determined, and less than 20 to 40 percent of the marked variant of serum IgE levels is due to environment and other influences. From animal studies[15] it appears that two genetic loci control total serum IgE levels, and segregation of *human* populations into distinct groups with regard to IgE levels suggests a similar mechanism in man.[15]

Several workers have demonstrated that food allergens can produce humoral antibodies with increased IgE levels. The indirect basophil degranulation test of Shelly[44] was used by the author in 1966–67 to detect food-specific atopic antibodies[12] (see Table 2-I). Although these studies were done on sera from patients prior to knowledge of their clinical symptoms, it was later found that they all fitted into the class of patients with immediate hypersensitivity. The direct skin test and the indirect basophil degranulation test may pick up the humoral antibodies causing the immediate food reactions. They do not pick up the delayed food reactions that occur in a large proportion of the food-sensitive individuals. The results shown in Table 2-I correlated well with the clinical symptoms of the patients whose sera was tested.

The same tests, using the same antigens, were performed on the sera of a control group of twelve patients who had no known allergic symptoms and ranged in age from twenty-four to forty-two years, with three females and nine males.[12] They had no history of serum hepatitis. All direct skin tests for all antigens were nega-

*PRIST—test for measurement of IgE.

TABLE 2-I

Food allergy study group with results of direct skin tests and in-direct basophil tests of their sera using food antigens suspected of causing symptoms.

Subject	*Age*	*Sex*	*Food*	*Clinical Manifestations*	*Direct Skin Test*	*Baso Test**
W.M.	23	M	Egg	Infantile Eczema, Asthma	3+	80
			Tuna	Nummular Eczema (adult)	1+	66
P.N.	36	M	Shrimp	Nausea	4+	70
			Catfish	Asthma	1+	40
G.B.	18	M	Shrimp	Rhinitis. Chronic Sinusitis, Asthma	3+	63
T.P.	30	M	Tuna	Rhinitis	4+	76
			Catfish	Asthma	2+	50
			Chocolate	Urticaria	2+	63
B.S.	30	M	Peanut	Urticaria, Abd. pain, Rhinitis, Vertigo	4+	76
M.G.	37	F	Milk	Urticaria, Abd. cramps	2+	66
			Chocolate	Diarrhea	1+	60
R.H.	19 mo.	F	Milk	Diarrhea	2+	63
C.L.	1	M	Milk	Runny nose, Asthma	4+	70
R.S.	5 mo.	M	Milk	Asthma	4+	70
E.M.	3 mo.	M	Milk	Rash, Diarrhea, Vomiting	3+	80
J.E.	34	F	Shrimp	Nausea in 2 min after ingestion	4+	73
			Tuna	Vomiting, Nausea	1+	56
			Catfish	Nausea	0	30
N.M.	39	F	Milk	Diarrhea, Abd. distension (esp. in pollen season)	2+	50

*Percentage Basophils Degranulated. 30% of 30 cells counted = Positive Reactor tive. The average percentage of basophils degranulated with any antigen was 3 percent. The test done with catfish antigen was 10 percent, and this was the only one that high.

The serum IgE levels are the highest in atopic eczema combined with co-existing allergic respiratory disease.[36] However, that IgE is a tissue-fixing antibody complicates the problem, since serum levels do not necessarily indicate total body levels. Skin IgE levels in patients with atopic eczema may be elevated independent of serum levels.[22] Ogawa et al.[35] found no difference in intradermal tests in patients with atopic dermatitis and two control groups; the first had psoriasis, the second were nonatopic volunteers. The minimal amounts of anti-IgE required to elicit a standard wheal and flare reaction were used. They found no correlation between the results of intradermal testing and the severity of the dermatitis. In patients with atopic dermatitis there was strong correlation between the level of serum IgE and the severity of dermatitis, whether or not positive history for asthma or hay fever was obtained.

Increased frequency of IgA deficiency has been reported in atopic eczema. Kaufman and Hobbs[27] demonstrated this in a population of 641 atopic patients. IgA deficiency at three months was reported by Taylor et al.[40] and was associated with development of atopy (eczema plus positive prick tests) within the first year in offspring of atopic parents. Kaufman and Hobbs[27] found that the IgA deficiency was transient and in later life may be high. Presumably, once the IgA system matures it is exposed to overstimulus by antigen as a result of ready entry of antigen through mucosa rendered permeable by reaginic reaction. The transient nature of the immunodeficiency has therapeutic implications. If potentially atopic infants were identified early and protected from excessive antigen stimulation during the susceptible early months, much atopic disease might be prevented. Reduction of contact with the allergens most likely to induce atopy could be helpful, such as house dust-mite, pets, feathers, allergenic fabrics, and cow's milk.

Foods most commonly causing daily atopic symptoms, including eczema, are often those ingested frequently but causing the reactions hours to days afterwards. In this instance the detailed history, physical examination, and skin tests for the suspected foods, but especially good food elimination followed by food challenge, are essential for pinpointing the cause of delayed onset food reaction.[9,10,48,51]

The Rebuck skin window technique was used by Galant et al.[6] for testing certain foods. They observed inflammatory exudation and particularly allergen-induced eosinophilia.[6] They found an excellent correlation between positive skin windows, skin tests, and immediate onset food reactions, while those patients with delayed onset symptoms were negative. They also found a 70 percent correlation between positive skin tests and positive leukocyte histamine release tests, if the patients had immediate reactions to food antigens. They found far less correlation between delayed reactions to foods and the battery of immunological tests used on the nineteen patients tested. Three of these patients had eczema. However, they concluded that *in vitro* tests for IgE responses to food allergens may prove to be helpful adjuncts to the clinical evaluation of food sensitivity. These authors cautioned that the major active components of foods in testing for food allergy must be used and that whole food extracts might not be adequate.

Johnstone tested the sera of eighty infants and children known to be clinically sensitive to egg, milk, wheat, chocolate, and peanut. The sera of a large group of normal children were used for controls. Using the bisdiazotized hemagglutinating technique,[25] Johnstone found no significant difference in the titer of antigen-specific hemagglutinating antibody between the food sensitive group and the controls. A small but equal percentage of both groups gave a positive titer.

Abnormalities in the adenylate cyclase-cyclic AMP system have been investigated in studies of skin from individuals with atopic dermatitis. One of the best examples of these abnormalities is the white dermatographism and the delayed blanch phenomenon, which has generally been thought to be due to vigorous vasoconstriction. There is an exaggerated sensitivity of the sweat glands to acetylcholine. Propranolol, a beta-antagonist, enhances stimulation in the sweat glands of normal but not atopic persons.[16,17,40]

There are several evidences of *cell-mediated immune changes in atopic eczema.*[29] McCready and Buckley[29] found that IgE concentrations were significantly lower in patients with milder forms of eczema, but concentrations in these groups were significantly different from normal. They found decreased T-lymphocytes and an inverse correlation between rosette-forming cells (RFC) and IgE levels. There is a dependence of IgE production on T cells, and the question of an RFC serum inhibitor was raised. There is a depression of lymphocyte function in patients with severe atopic eczema. Lymphocyte transformation to PHA is depressed, along with chemotaxis of both the polymorphonuclear and monocyte series.[14,10] There appears to be a compensatory increase in B cells as evidenced by an increased number of EAC rosettes when a rosette assay test for B-lymphocytes is performed.

There appears to be cutaneous anergy in atopic eczema patients. Some patients fail to respond to a battery of naturally occurring antigens, such as tuberculin and candidin, yet have normal *in vitro* lymphocyte responses to nonspecific mitogens.[14] It is known that skin test results disappear long before mitogen response. The explanation of why this is so is not clear. It may be because the skin test is a much less sensitive assay.

CLINICAL AND DIAGNOSTIC MANIFESTATIONS

The clinical signs of this disease vary with the age of the patient. It can occur from two to three months of age to over 80 years. There are a number of manifestations and associated signs that appear in all phases of atopic dermatitis. The most outstanding of these is the *intense pruritus.* Patients respond to the itch with scratching and rubbing resulting in marked excoriation of the skin. Repetition of this sequence of events over a long period of time results in lichenification with resulting increase in the visibility of the normal geometric skin markings. These findings are characteristically present in the antecubital and popliteal fossae.

Dennie's line is a prominent fold on the lower eyelid originating near the inner canthus of the eyelid and extending to one-half to two-thirds of the lower eyelid. Dennie believed that this fold was indicative of a predisposition to allergy, especially eczema, hay fever, and asthma. Dennie never published his observations, but his student Morgan did so.[32] These signs are referred to in the literature as Dennie's or Morgan's lines.

Nutrition is not much interfered with, unless an unwise physician eliminates essential foods from the baby's diet on suspicion alone, leaving him on a most deficient diet in hopes of curing the rash. It is possible to eliminate too many foods suspected of causing the allergy and so "eliminate" the baby.

The presenting signs and symptoms vary with the age of the patient.

PHASE I. Early infantile eczema is characterized by weeping vesicular and crusting lesions mainly on the face, scalp, neck, and extensor surfaces of the extremities. The *itching is terrific.* This phase may improve gradually and disappear between two and three years of life.

PHASE II. The *childhood phase* may follow that of infancy at around four or five years, or at this age atopic eczema may appear for the first time. At this stage there is a predilection for the rash to be located on the flexural surfaces of the extremities as well as the face, although there is apt to be less face and more involvement of the skin of the trunk. There are itching, excoriated papules in the popliteal and antecubital fossae and ankles. The constant scratching produces the lichenification previously described (see Fig. 2-1).

PHASE III. The *adult phase* may be a persistence of the childhood phase, or there may be a few years of no difficulty after ten years of age, late adolescence, or early adult life. The eruption in this period is dry and may be scaly. Large areas may be highly pruritic with prominent lichenification in the flexural regions, forehead, sides of neck, wrists, and feet.

Most patients with atopic eczema have seasonal exacerbations (especially in winter) and remissions (in summer). If they flare up in the summer, they probably have sweat retention syndrome. In a severe atopic eczema it is uncommon for patients to have long symptom-free periods.

Buffed nails may be observed on these patients. They are produced by chronic scratching and rubbing.

Allergic shiners and the *allergic nasal crease* may be obvious in those patients who have atopic nasal allergy in addition to their skin rash. About 76 percent of children[41] with atopic eczema have white dermatographism.

In summary, for diagnosis of atopic eczema the criteria as shown in Table 2-II should exist.[14]

COMPLICATIONS

1. *Bacterial infection* is the *most common* complication of atopic eczema. Much of this is due to the scratching that takes place on a skin that often carries strains of *Staphylococcus aureus* and beta-hemolytic streptococci.
2. *Viral infections* occur because of increased susceptibility to vaccinia, herpes simplex, molluscum contagiosum, and coxsackievirus A16.[34] This is due as much to the suppression of cellular immunity as it is to the damaged skin. Disseminated herpes simplex (Kaposi's varicelliform eruption) is a serious infection with widespread skin lesion, high fever, and encephalitis.

Children with atopic eczema should never be vaccinated against smallpox. Since vaccinations for smallpox are now no longer routine, the danger of getting eczema vaccinatum or Kaposi's varicelliform eruption from contact with a recently vaccinated sibling is very slight.

3. *Fungal infection,* though not common, can occur. *Candida albicans* is the most common and may reach the child's skin because of a vaginal yeast infection in the mother who bathes the infant.
4. *Ocular complications* of atopic eczema include the following:
   a. Anterior subcapsular cataracts (these may occur in the older child and about 10 percent of adult patients with severe atopic eczema).
   b. Thickening of the cornea or keractoconus.
5. *Nummular eczema* is a variant of atopic eczema. The word *nummular* means *coin-line.* These are sharply defined, circular patches of rather dark color, the size of a dime on extensor surfaces of the extremities and face. They are accompanied by far less itching than usual atopic eczema; they are very resistant to treatment. There is a question whether this kind of eczema has an "atopic" basis.

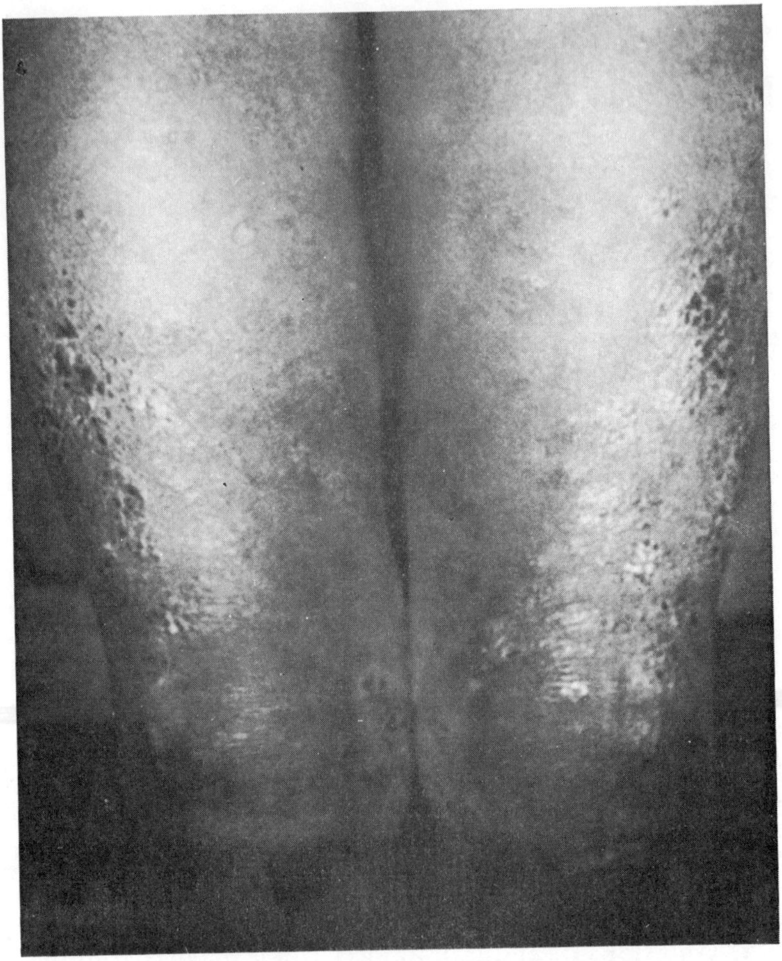

Figure 2-1a. Black female, age 9 years, with chronic atopic eczema, *before* treatment.

DIFFERENTIAL DIAGNOSIS

A careful history is the most important single factor in identifying the child whose rash is on an atopic basis. Other types of common eczematoid dermatoses can resemble atopic eczema. Table 2-III summarizes the clinical differences between the three most common types of dermatitis seen in childhood: atopic, con-

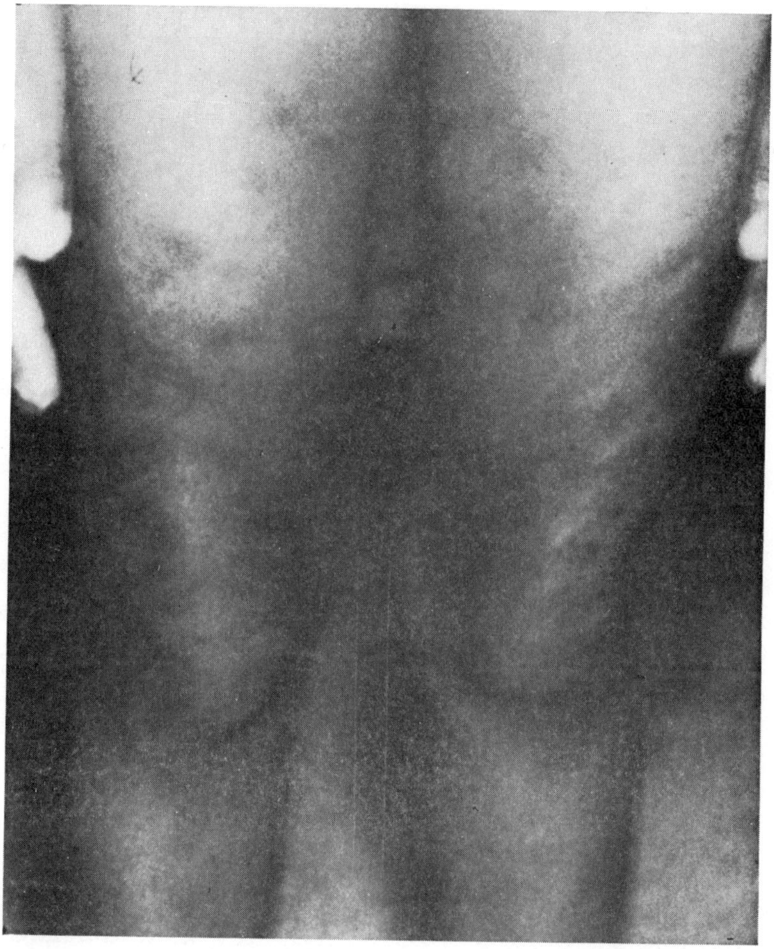

Figure 2-1b. Black female, age 9 years, with chronic atopic eczema, *after* treatment.

tact, and seborrheic.

Seborrheic dermatitis in infancy lacks the pruritus of atopic infantile eczema.[5,10] The onset is usually within the first two months of life with involvement of the scalp, forehead, and postauricular areas. The hallmark lesions of this disease entity are the dry, greasy, reddish orange scales over the above areas of

TABLE 2-II
CRITERIA FOR DIAGNOSIS OF ATOPIC ECZEMA

Major Manifestations	Minor Manifestations
1. Terrific itching	*Specific Signs* 1. Personal or family history of atopic disease
2. Chronic or relapsing dermatitis	2. Immediate skin test reactivity 3. White dermatographism
3. Typical morphology and distribution	*Nonspecific Signs* Four or more of the following: 1. Dennie-Morgan fold
a. Facial and extensor involvement — infancy	2. Facial pallor/infraorbital shadows (allergic shiners) 3. Elevated serum IgE
b. Flexural distribution and lichenification — older children, adolescents, and adults	4. Keratoconus 5. Keratosis pilaris 6. Ant. subcapsular cataracts 7. Repeated cutaneous infections 8. Nonspecific hand dermatitis 9. Pityriasis alba 10. Icthyosis/hyperlinear palms

the body where sebaceous glands are plentiful. These are often referred to as "potato chip" scales. Sometimes seborrheic dermatitis may precede the development of atopic dermatitis, or both can be present at the same time but not be etiologically related.

Contact dermatitis is a papulovesicular or erythematous eruption with no hereditary factor and is due to Type IV hypersensitivity of the epidermis to one or more substances, which may be of almost any composition. Prick or scratch tests are commonly negative, but patch tests may be positive. It is more common in adults.

Additional disease entities included in the differential diagnosis of atopic eczema are as follows:

1. Wiskott-Aldrich syndrome, an X-linked immune-deficiency disease characterized by eczema, thrombocytopenia, and recurrent otitis media. Patients have low or absent IgM and thrombocytopenia.

2. Letterer-Siwe (histiocytosis X), a disease characterized by eczema, petechiae, hepato splenomegaly, generalized lymphadeno-

TABLE 2-III
DIFFERENTIAL DIAGNOSIS OF THREE COMMON DERMATOSES

	Atopic	*Contact*	*Seborrheic*
Usual Age	Infancy or Childhood	Adult	Adult, Occas. Infant
Family History of Allergy	Frequently positive	Negative	Negative
Personal History of Allergy	Frequently positive	Negative	Negative
Type of Excitant	Inhalant, ingestant, usually protein & water soluble	Nonprotein fat soluble	Negative
Eosinophilia	Often positive	Negative	Negative
Scrtach tests	Often positive	Usually neg.	Negative
Characteristics	Dry papular, lichenified, excoriated vesicles only if acute & scratched. Severe pruritus	Papulovesicular erythema, edema	Sharply circumscribed reddish orange, greasy "potato chip" scale. Mild pruritus
Localization	Anticubital & Popliteal spaces. Eyelids, dorsum of hands, sides of neck, face, mouth	Exposed areas usually face, neck, & hands	Scalp, forehead, sides of nose, ears, sternum, hairy areas
Complications	50% have asthma & hayfever in later life	None	None
Serum IgE Levels	Marked elevation (Mean = 493ng/ml)	Normal (Mean = 122ng/ml)	Normal
RAST	Positive for specific allergens	Negative	Negative

pathy, and bone tumors.

3. Patients with phenylketonuria have a high incidence of eczema. The phenylpyruvic acid present in their urine is diagnostic of the condition.

4. Bruton's agammaglobulinemia is an X-linked immunedeficiency disease in which patients may develop eczema indistinguishable from atopic dermatitis.

5. The best examples of contact dermatitis are the diaper rash or ammonical dermatitis, dermatitis venenata, and shoe dye dermatitis. These are diagnosed by history, distribution of the

rash, and the fact that the vesicles are more intraepidermal.[42]

6. Leiner's disease is a generalized seborrheic dermatitis that may resemble atopic eczema. There is familial deficiency of opsonin activity related to dysfunction of C_5 and biotin deficiency.

7. Toxic epidermal necrolysis (Ritter's disease) occurs in the first two weeks of life when atopic eczema is infrequent. It starts as a generalized erythema and then develops large bullae and generalized exfoliation. Nickolsky's sign is always present. Merely touching the skin makes it come off.[11]

8. Scabies in infancy can resemble atopic dermatitis in that both have widespread pruritic eczematoid dermatitis. Infantile atopic eczema usually begins on the cheeks, whereas scabies occurs as large papules on palms, soles, and upper back. The proof of diagnosis is in the finding of mites or ova in the scrapings of vesicles.

9. Hyperimmunoglobulinemia E with susceptibility to infection with depressed immunologic functions such as depressed cell-mediated immunity *in vivo* and depressed polymorphonuclear and monocyte chemotaxis[4] may also have signs of eczema.

MANAGEMENT

Although much is known about atopic eczema, the exact cause is not known. Management therefore, both prophylactic and therapeutic, has to be based on facts that are known and treatment of the symptoms as they arise for the sake of comfort of the patient and the parents, if the patient is a child. This requires a great deal of time on the part of the physician treating the patient and/or the patient's parents. It is important to stress to them that treatment of this condition is not based on a single cause and that how it is managed may vary with the age of the patient and the chronicity of the disease. It is important to convey the idea that atopic eczema is influenced at various times by a variety of factors such as climate, psychic state, contactants, heat, infection, food, and even inhalant allergy.[9,10,47,48]

A *detailed history* and *physical examination* are of paramount importance. Environmental and general medical history as well as personal history should be included. Many factors that trigger the patient's eczema can be identified and pointed out to the patient or parents.

Prophylactic measures in management may be very helpful, especially if a physician has previously treated another sibling in the same family for the same condition. *Environmental control is very important.* It is generally accepted that atopic dermatitis may at times be caused by direct contact of allergens with the skin (transepidermal penetration) as well as by allergens that reach the skin by the bloodstream after inhalation.[47] Avoidance of dust exposure in the nursery, which often is overloaded with dust-catching paraphernalia, pays off in the susceptible family that has had other siblings with eczema. Avoidance of dust is far superior to hyposensitization.

Breast-feeding the infants should always be encouraged in families with a strong allergic history. For many years we have known from clinical experience that if it is necessary to supplement breast-feeding of an infant in a family that had another child with eczema, a nonmilk formula such as a meat base or a soybean formula should be used. The author has had firsthand evidence of this; one family in particular is recalled. The first and second babies had cow's milk formula supplements and developed severe eczema when cow's milk was started; the third and fourth babies were supplemented only with soybean formula. One of the latter two babies was inadvertently given cow's milk and promptly developed severe eczema.

As already stated, there is evidence now that the fetus can develop IgE or allergic antibody as early in its intrauterine existence as eleven weeks.[15] There is evidence that cow's milk antigen ingested by the mother is excreted in her breast milk. The babies who already have IgE antibody specific for cow's milk protein thereby develop eczema. Several workers have reported sensitization of babies, totally breast-fed, to cow's milk protein and egg, having obtained exposure to these proteins solely through the breast milk.[8,15,28] The author remembers well a mother whose breast-fed baby had severe eczema, and toward the end of the interview she asked, "Doctor, does you suppose turnip greens could cause this rash? I just loves them." We removed turnip greens from the mother's diet and the eczema cleared promptly. We know, too, that breast milk provides effective protection against certain common enteric pathogens, *E. coli* for example, as well as relative freedom from allergic disease. The latter is especially true if the mother does not eat excesses of any one food and learns early in her pregnancy to rotate her intake of known potent allergens such as milk, egg, wheat, and chocolate.[10]

Therapeutic measures facilitate keeping atopic eczema under control, though not curing it. Most of all, these patients and/or parents should not be told they will outgrow the eczema. They should be reassured that much can be done to keep it under control. Since there is no single cause, there must be multiple approaches to treatment that require cooperation of the patient and much time and understanding from the doctor.

Topical therapy encompasses both specific anti-inflammatory agents such as corticosteroids and tars, as well as proprietary preparations such as soaps, bath oils, shampoos, and lubricants.

The topical therapy prescribed depends largely on the stage of the eczema, whether acute, subacute, or chronic. It is not sufficient to give the mother a prescription for an ointment or lotion. She needs detailed instruction as to how to apply it and how to prevent scratching.

There is no use in treating at all without covering the skin, since scratching alone can produce much of the picture one sees in neglected cases of eczema. Double thickness cotton restraints for the arms with ties reinforced by tongue blades (inserted into pockets like corset stays) prevent flexion at the elbow and minimize scratching. Soft, washed cotton may be laid directly over the skin, and the arms and legs covered with stockinette. Along with the restraints, drugs can be used for sedation or tranquilization. The ones preferred by the author are diphenhydramine hydrochloride (Benadryl®) and chloral hydrate (Noctec®). Hydroxyzine hydrochloride (Atarax®) is also useful in controlling the pruritus.

In the exudative stage, probably the best treatment is the application of 0.5 percent solution of aluminum acetate in a 1:20 dilution or Burrow's solution. It has been possible to have the mothers carry this out successfully by laying over the cheeks a 3-by-3-inch sterile gauze dressing or soft cotton and holding these in place with a stockinette mask. The dressings are kept wet by adding solution to the mask through the openings, being careful to avoid the eyes. If the rash is badly secondarily infected, potassium permanganate in dilutions 1:5000 or 1:10,000 can be used (or 1 tablet 5 gr in 2 quarts of sterile water). Boric acid is not used because of its potential toxicity.

Other forms of treatment of this stage are collodial baths, soaking for fifteen minutes and patting, not rubbing, the child dry with a solution of 1 to 2 cups of cornstarch in a tub of tepid water. Tar baths also are helpful. Liquor carbonis detergens (N.F.) and saponified alcoholic extract of coal tar (2 cups to a tub of water) soaking four times daily. Tar is not used if much infection is present. If there is some cradle cap along with the eczema, Alvinine® (Westwood) or Sebulex® shampoo is helpful in removing it. Synalar® lotion (a steroid) is more easily applied to hair-bearing areas than creams or ointments.

In the subacute and chronic stages, ointments are best. Topical corticosteroids in a variety of vehicles have potent anti-inflammatory and antipruritic effects. Creams are more widely used because of their tendency to vanish when rubbed into the skin, so that less is wasted. They look better and have a water base. The following steroid ointments are preferred by the author because they contain no parabens (a strong sensitizer) as a preservative: Valisone® cream—0.1 percent (betamethasone valerate) (Schering); Diprosone® cream— 0.05 percent (betamethasone dipropionate) (Schering); hydrocortisone cream—1 percent (E. Fougera Co., Hicksville, N.Y.).

In the chronic, dry, lichenified stage of atopic eczema, which is most frequently seen in the older child and adult, tar ointments can be very effective and inexpensive. In spite of the newer coal tar preparations, white and flesh colored, I still prefer and get better results with the old black crude coal tar in a 3 percent concentration. Two percent ichthyol in Lassar's paste is good in the milder cases. Although steroids have largely replaced the tars, the tar ointment does have definite antipruritic value.

For the infected eczemas a 3 percent concentration of Vioform® in aquafor base put out by Ciba Co. is effective. Bacitracin® and Neo-polycin® ointments are also used. All of these preparations require that the skin be covered.

The latest ointment to be tried for topical treatment of atopic eczema is a 10 percent sodium cromoglycate in soft white paraffin. Haider[13] used this in a double-blind randomized trial to treat forty-two children with eczema of three months to thirteen and one-half years duration. Sixteen out of twenty-one patients in the study group improved and only 2 out of 21 in the placebo group.

Dietary measures on the first visit are very important. A baby is put on an elimination diet, which takes away immediately most of the foods that the history suggests are apt to make him worse. The diet is individualized. If it was learned the rash started when cow's milk was first added to the diet, then milk would be withdrawn and a soybean milk or meat base formula substituted. Whatever diet is prescribed is used for a week to ten days, at the end of which the patient is reexamined. Foods are more important allergens in infancy. The elimination diet usually employed, depending on the age of the patient, consists of Prosobee®, Neo-Mull-Soy® or Isomil®, lamb, rice, or barley cereal, pears or pineapple, carrots, string beans, and Tri-Vi-Sol® 0.6 cc daily or its equivalent in tablets.

Inhalants, especially house dust and ragweed, may become important in the toddler or older child. Immunotherapy is seldom needed. Figure 2-2 shows results in forty of the author's own patients with atopic eczema treated as outlined here. The skin was essentially clear in ten to fifteen days, and only eighteen out of forty had any direct allergy skin tests performed. If, as occurred in these eighteen patients, the clinical signs and test results correlate, we sometimes use immunotherapy. Meticulous care must be taken to adjust the use of the specific extract so as not to exceed the limit of tolerance of the patient, otherwise the eczema is apt to exacerbate. It is not unusual for the patient to require a starting dilution of 1:1,000,000 of a mixed extract. Another fringe benefit of immunotherapy is the decreased likelihood of later development of respiratory allergic disease. One patient, age seven years, with atopic eczema all over her body and with allergic rhinitis, was skin test–positive to house dust and ragweed. Immunotherapy in the above manner with house dust and ragweed extract cleared the skin in six months. She had previously had all kinds of topical therapy.

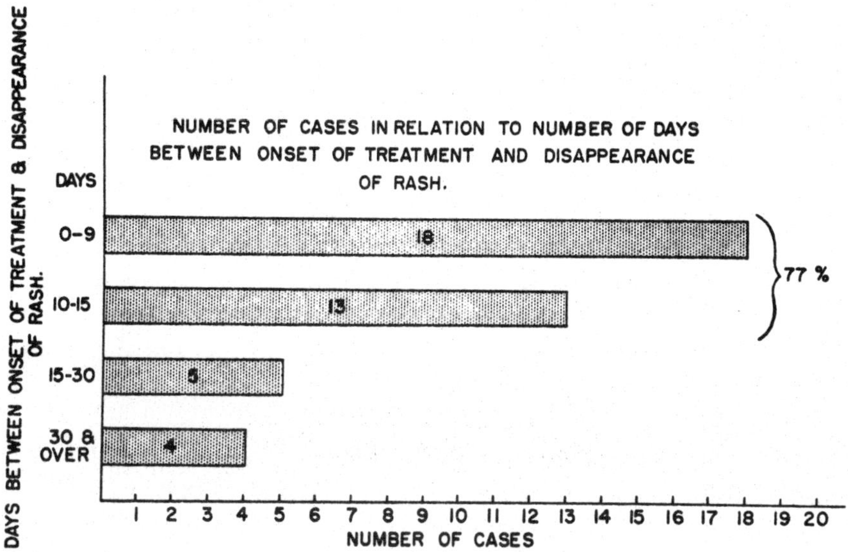

Figure 2-2. Time relationship between onset of treatment and disappearance of rash.

In summary, management of atopic eczema involves the following:

1. Environmental control.
   Avoid a. wool clothing or covered furniture.
   b. dust, feathers, animal danders.
2. Avoidance of soaps, detergents, and too frequent bathing—Use Cetaphil® lotion (Texas Pharm.) for cleansing. Avoid tub soaks unless bath oils such as Alpha Keri®, Domol®, or Lubath® are added.

   Preferred shampoos are Sebulex and Alvinine.
3. Elimination of suspected food allergens and diet manipulation.
   a. Avoid cow's milk before six months.
   b. Encourage breast-feeding of infants, especially in families with strong history of atopic allergies.
   c. Have nursing mothers avoid excesses of any one food and avoid known potent food allergens while nursing.
4. Infection: Use antibiotic ointment.
   a. Use early, if infection is localized.

b. Prevent scratching by covers and elbow restraints.
c. If infection is extensive, use systemic antibiotics for short periods.

5. Adjustment of topical therapy to stage of eczema.
    a. *Acute:* Wet dressings, antipruritic cooling restringents, bactericidal.
    b. *Subacute:* Steroid creams, Valisone 0.1 percent, Diprosone 0.05 percent, hydrocortisone cream 1 percent.
    c. *Chronic, lichenified:* Tar preparations with or without steroids, Cort-Dome®, 0.5 percent, 2 percent ichthyol in Lassar's paste, Alpha-Keri bath oil. Steroids or 10 percent sodium cromoglycate ointment.
    d. Cover extremities—elbow splints.
6. Sedation: Often not much required when other steps are followed. Preferred sedatives: Chloral hydrate (Noctec), diphenhydramine HCL (Benadryl) and hydroxyzine HCL (Atarax).

Food plays a more significant role in infant atopic eczema, but much less in that of the older child and the adult. A physician today must be forever vigilant concerning all ingredients in current food products.

Systemic steroids are rarely indicated in the treatment of atopic eczema.

REFERENCES

1. Barness, L.A., Mauer, A.M., Anderson, A.S. et al. (Committees on Nutrition A.A.P. and Canadian Pediatric Society): Breast feeding, *Pediatrics, 62*:591, 1978.
2. Bellanti, J.A.: *Immunology II,* Philadelphia: Saunders, 1978, p. 511.
3. Blaylock, W.K.: Atopic dermatitis: Diagnosis and pathobiology. *J Allergy Clin Immunol, 57*:62, 1976.
4. Buckley, R.H.: Hyperimmunoglobulinemia E, Undue susceptibility to infection and depressed immunologic function. Symposium on Pediatric Immunology, Los Angeles, CA, February 7, 1978.
5. Ellis, Elliot, F.: Atopic eczema. Seminar: A day in pediatric allergy-immunology, Schumpert Medical Center, Shreveport, LA, September 29, 1977, p. 38.
6. Gallant, S.P., Bullock, J., and Frick, O.L.: An immunological approach to the diagnosis of food sensitivity. *Clin Allergy, 3*:363, 1973.
7. Gerrard, J.W.: Breast feeding: Second thoughts. *Pediatrics, 54*:757, 1974.

8. ----: Allergy in breast fed babies to ingredients in breast milk, *Ann Allergy, 42*:69, 1979.
9. Glaser, J. and Johnstone, D.: Prophylaxis of allergic disease in children. *N Engl J Med, 274*:715, 1966.
10. Gordon, V.H.: Prophylaxis in allergy disease and management of eczematoid dermatoses of infancy and childhood. *Miss Doctor, 28*:115, 1950.
11. ----: Some interesting but rare disorders seen in pediatric practice with recovery. *J Arkansas Med Soc, 54*:358, 1958.
12. ----: Evidence that food can act as an allergen as well as an antigen. Presented at Am. College of Allergists Annual Meeting, El Paso, Texas, March 21, 1967.
13. Haider, S. A.: Treatment of atopic eczema in children, clinical trial of 1070 sodium cromoglycate ointment. *Br Med J, 1*:1570, 1977.
14. Hanifin, J.M. and Lobitz, W.C.: Newer concepts of atopic dermatitis. *Arch Dermatol, 113(5)*: 663, 1977.
15. Hamburger, R.N.: Allergy and the immune system. *Am Sci, 64*:157, 1976.
16. Hemels, H.G.W.M.: The effect of propranolol on the acetylcholine induced sweat gland response in atopic and non-atopic subjects. *Br J Dermatol, 83*:312, 1970.
17. Hemels, H.G.W.M., Thiele, F.A.J., and Bauer, F.W.: Effects of propranolol on the acetylcholine induced response of the human sweat gland. *Br J Dermatol, 86*:206, 1972.
18. Hill, L.W.: Certain aspects of allergy in children, *N Engl J Med, 265*: 1298, 1961.
19. Hovmark, A.: An in-vitro study of depressed cell-mediated immunity and/of T and B lymphocytes in atopic dermatitis. *Acta Derm Venerol, 57*:237, 1977.
20. Huntley, C.C.: Atopic dermatitis and contact dermatitis in children. *Am Fam Physician, 16(2)*:111, 1977.
21. Ishizaka, T., Ishizaka, K., Johansson, S.G.O., and Bennich H: Histamine release from human leucocytes by anti-gamma E antibodies. *J Immunol, 102*:884, 1969.
22. Jansen, C. T., Haapalahti, J., and Hopsu-Havu, V.K.: Immunoglobulin E in the human atopic skin. *Arch Dermatol Forsch, 246*:299, 1973.
23. Johansson, S.G.O. and Juhlin, L.: Immunoglobulin E in "healed" atopic dermatitis and after treatment with corticosteroids and azathioprine. *Br J Dermatol, 82*:10, 1970.
24. Johnstone, D.E.: The natural history of allergic disease in children. *Ann Allergy, 38(6)*:387, 1977.
25. ----: Study of the significance of food antigen precepitins in sera of food-sensitive and normal children. *Ann Allergy, 21*:207, 1962.
26. Knowles, J.A.: Excretion of drugs in milk—a review. *J Pediatr, 66*: 1068, 1965.

27. Kaufman, H.S. and Hobbs, J.R.: Immunoglobulin deficiencies in an atopic population. *Lancet, 2*:1061, 1970.
28. Kuroume, T., Oguri, M., Matsumura, T., Iwasaki, I., Kanbe, Y., Yamada, T., Kawabe, S., and Negiski, K.: Milk sensitivity and soy bean sensitivity in the production of eczematous manifestation in breast fed babies with particular reference to intrauterine sensitization. *Ann Allergy, 37*:41, 1976.
29. McCready, S.J. and Buckley, R.H.: Depression of cell-mediated immunity in atopic eczema, *J Allergy Clin Immunol, 56*:393, 1975.
30. Mears, R.H.: Skin reactions in atopic eczema. *Br J Dermatol, 67*:60, 1955.
31. Miller, D.L., Hirvonen, T., and Gitlin, D.: Synthesis of IgE by the human conceptus. *J Allergy Clin Immunol, 52*:182, 1973.
32. Morgan, D.B.: A suggestive sign of allergy. *Arch Dermatol, Syph, 57*: 1050, 1948.
33. Musgrove, K. and Morgan, J.K.: Infantile eczema: A long term follow up study. *Br J Dermatol, 95*:365, 1976.
34. Nahmias, A.J., Froeschle, J.E., Feronino, P.M. and McCord, G.: Generalized eruption in child with eczema due to Coxsackievirus A16. *Arch Dermatol, 97*:147, 1968.
35. Ogawa, M., Berger, P.A., McIntyre, O.R., Clendenning, W.E., and Ishizaka, K.: IgE in Atopic Dermatitis. *Arch Dermatol, 103*:575, 1971.
36. Orgel, H.A., Kemp, J.P., Meltzger, E. O., and Hamburger, R.N.: Atopy and IgE in a pediatric practice. *Ann Allergy, 39*:161, 1977.
37. Prose, P.H.: Pathologic changes in eczema, *J Pediatr, 66(2)*:178, 1965.
38. Pearlman, D.S.: Management of atopic dermatitis: An allergist's point of view. *Cutis, 13*:1029, 1974.
39. Rajka, G.: Prurigo Besnier (atopic dermatitis) with special reference to the role of allergic factors. II The evaluation of results of skin reactions. *Acta Derm Venereol, 41*:1, 1961.
40. Reed, C.E., Busse, W.W., and Lee, T.P.: Adrenergic mechanisms and the adenyl cyclase system in atopic dermatitis. *J Invest Dermatol, 67*: 333, 1976.
41. Rasmusen, J.E. and Provost, T.T.: Atopic dermatitis. In Middleton, E., Reed, C.E., and Ellis, E.F. (Eds.): *Allergy, Principles and Practice.* St. Louis: Mosby, 1978, p. 1039.
42. Sparks, D.: Atopic dermatitis. In Patterson, R. (Ed.): *Allergic Diseases, Diagnosis, and Treatment.* Philadelphia: Lippincott, 1972, p. 381.
43. Speer, F.: Multiple food allergy, *Ann Allergy, 34*:71, 1975.
44. Shelly, W.B.: Indirect basophil degranulation test for allergy to penicillin and other drugs. *JAMA, 184*:171, 1963.
45. Stewart, W.D.: Atopic Dermatitis: Method of Wm. D. Stewart. In

Conn, H.F. (Ed.): *Current Therapy*. Philadelphia: Saunders, 1977, p. 618.

46. Taylor, B., Norman, A.P., Orgel, H.A., Turner, M.W., Stokes, C.R., and Soothill, J.F.; Transient IgA-deficiency and pathogenesis of infantile atopy. *Lancet, 2:*111, 1973.
47. Tuft, L.: Importance of inhalant allergens in atopic dermatitis. *J Invest Dermatol, 12:*211, 1949.
48. Waisman, M.: Atopic dermatitis: Clinical aspects and treatment, *Postgrad Med, 52:*180, 1972.
49. Walker, R.B. and Warin, R.P.: Incidence of eczema in early childhood. *Br J Dermatol, 68:*182, 1956.
50. Wicker, K., Reisman, R.E., and Arbesman, C.E.: Allergic reaction to penicillin present in milk. *JAMA, 208:*143, 1969.
51. Withers, O.R. and Hale, R.: Food Allergy. A review of the literature. *Ann Allergy, 15:*334, 1956.

Chapter 3

DISORDERS OF THE GASTROINTESTINAL TRACT AND AUTONOMIC NERVOUS SYSTEM IN ALLERGIC PATIENTS.

HSI-YEN LIU

THERE HAS BEEN growing recognition of the role of ingested proteins, particularly bovine milk proteins, in the pathogenesis of clinical disorder. The subject has been well reviewed.[2,9,13,16,26,28,31,33,87] Investigations in recent years have provided increasing data on the gastrointestinal and parenteral manifestations of the disorder,[7,10,14,19,21,22,26,30,35,41,42,45,52-55,58,66,82,90] the intestinal histopathology with or without food antigen challenges,[12,34,37,43,65,72,73,76,84] various immunologic effects in susceptible patients,[7,11,17,24,35,42,48,59,69,70] and newer methods of diagnosis[9,14,29,30,34,38,73,87] and treatment.[6,14,15,19,20,22,30,42,47,81] For elucidation during the years of controversy and confusion, the studies of Gerrard and his colleagues have been invaluable. These investigators have examined multiple facets of cow's milk–induced disease, shedding light on the prevalence,[26] genetic profile[25,26] and varied expressions of the disorder,[10,18,19,21-23,25-27] as well as on the patients' clinical characteristics, including disaccharidase activities,[56] serum immunoglobulin patterns,[24] response to specific pharmacologic control,[81] long-term prognosis[25] and propensity to react to antigens in therapeutic feeds,[21,26] even human breast milk.[22]

This chapter summarizes this author's own findings in allergic patients with intermittent episodes of disturbed gastrointestinal function during exposure to a variety of allergens including bovine milk proteins.

In the ten-year period 1964 through 1973, 508 patients were seen in the Section of Pediatric Gastroenterology of the University of Michigan Medical School. These patients were referred because they had persistent gastrointestinal symptoms that had not responded to conventional diagnostic or therapeutic management. Most had clinical evidence of malabsorption, malnutrition, and growth failure, many had marked weight loss, a few were in shock due to massive fluid and electrolyte deficit.

During the course of our studies we became aware that most of these patients had evidence both of allergy and of a functional disturbance of the autonomic nervous system.

The data presented here were obtained from the first 101 patients selected randomly from our series of 508 provided that they also had one of the following: allergic rhinitis, eczema, asthma, urticaria, and/or angioedema. For the most part they came from Michigan and the surrounding states, and a few were from southern Ontario. Ninety-seven were Caucasian, two were part Mexican, one was part Arabian, and one was black. Most were infants and children; nine were adults. The majority had been brought up on formulae; even the few brought up on breast milk had been early introduced to cow's milk.

METHOD OF CLINICAL DATA COLLECTION

History

To catalog and record the manifestations found in patients on admission, a questionnaire was developed. This was used by the students and staff members. The patients or parents of pediatric patients were also asked to record and report all exacerbations and remissions, as well as environmental changes that accompanied them. Answers were not obtained to all questions. The frequency of occcurrence of a clinical finding is therefore expressed as a percentage of the same finding among all patients in whom the data were complete.

Physical and Laboratory Findings

Whenever permitted by the patient's condition, admission physical and laboratory findings were documented while the patients were fed an unrestricted bovine milk protein–containing diet. Frequently, bovine milk feedings had to be postponed until infections, gastrointestinal disturbances, and acute fluid and electrolyte deficits had been corrected. These delayed milk-related findings were regarded as "admission" clinical parameters since they represented data obtained before diagnosis and before a trial therapy. All the physical signs were re-evaluated after institution of an environmental antigen restriction program, which included dietary exclusion of bovine milk proteins.

Data from Clinical Investigations

In addition to history, physical, and routine laboratory findings in all the patients, data from a few individual clinical research studies are also presented in this discussion. Each investigation was carried out according to a specific protocol on a separate group of subjects. The results of the studies, therefore, apply specifically to the subjects involved.

RESULTS

Occurrence

We do not know how frequently gastrointestinal symptoms form the presenting complaint in allergic patients, or how frequently allergy is found in gastrointestinal patients, but our data indicate that many patients with gastrointestinal problems have evidence of concomitant allergy.

Age

The 101 patients studied were three weeks to fifty-one years of age when first seen. Nine (8.9%) were adults aged twenty-six to fifty-one years, and ninety-two (91.1%) were infants and children three weeks to fourteen years old. Of the ninety-two pediatric patients, seventy-one (77.2%) were three years or younger, more than half (52.2%) were one year or younger, about one-third (30.4%) were four months or younger, and fully a quarter (26.1%) were in their first three months of life. No patient fell in the age groups from five to eight years and fourteen to twenty-six years. Since all patients were referred, virtually none of the admission ages represent the age of onset of initial illness. The preponderance of infants, as well as the presence of some older children and adults, confirms the findings of Gerrard et al. regarding the early onset and occasional persistence of cow's milk–inducible gastrointestinal, respiratory, and dermatologic disease.[25]

Sex

Males were preponderant, comprising sixty-three of the 101 patients (62%), while females made up 38 percent of the group. If the nine adults (2 males and 7 females) are excluded from the series, the male preponderance becomes even more noticeable. Among the ninety-two patients fourteen years and younger, sixty-one were males (66%) and thirty-one were females (34%). This ratio resembles that observed by others in patients with "food allergies."[13,33] Among all the forty-five adults referred to our service, females predominated (62%), with a reversal of the 2 to 1 male to female ratio seen in the younger population.

History of Collateral Allergies

All patients had collateral allergies; these included asthma, allergic rhinitis, eczema, urticaria and/or angioedema. One hundred of the 101 patients (99%) had, at some time, asthma, allergic rhinitis and/or eczema, singly or in combination.

Our experience has confirmed the well-known notion that neither the establishment nor the exclusion of a diagnosis of allergy could be made during the initial evaluations of the younger infants. We had to wait until the children were older and had had several attacks of asthma, wheezy bronchitis, or allergic rhinitis before a diagnosis of atopy could be made. Many of our patients and/or their young parents developed their first signs of allergic disease months to years after the probands were first evaluated for gastrointestinal symptoms. Such patients actually proved baffling at first, when their clinical responses to bovine milk protein ingestion were indistinguishable from those of allergic infants. In families with strongly positive histories of allergy, the patients' collateral allergies appeared to surface at earlier ages.

Family History of Allergy

Eighty-nine patients in this series had recorded family histories. Information could not be obtained on the remaining twelve, either because the subjects were adopted or because there was no contact with the family, and the data were not available. In this analysis, manifestations considered "allergic" included asthma, hay fever, eczema, contact dermatitis, food– and drug-associated urticaria, angioedema, and food-inducible allergic symptoms and signs. All eighty-nine patients with complete family histories gave positive histories of allergy. Sixty-seven (75%) reported allergic manifestations in their mothers; fifty-seven (64%) in their fathers; forty-three (48%) in both parents; fifty-seven (64%) in both maternal and paternal families, including parents; and forty-three (48%) in siblings. Sixty-two of the eighty-nine patients (70%) had family members with "food allergies."

Considering the occurrence of only asthma, hay fever, and/or eczema, eighty of the eighty-nine allergic patients (90%) gave positive family histories; twenty-one out of eighty-nine (24%) in mothers; nineteen out of eighty-nine (21%) in fathers; twenty-three out of eighty-nine (26%) in both parents; forty-three out of eighty-nine (48%) bilaterally, including the parents; and twenty-eight out of eighty-nine (32%) in siblings.

Existing statistics show the incidence of positive family history of allergy to be 48% among "allergic patients,"[5] and 58 percent among college students with asthma or hay fever.[79] However, patients reported by Gerrard et al.,[25] Gryboski,[33] Harrison,[35] and those in the present series exhibit considerably higher incidence (67-100%) of familial allergy. Since the last four studies deal with much younger patients, data suggest an association between a strong allergic family history and the early development of bovine milk–inducible gastrointestinal disease.

Etiology of Inducible Gastrointestinal and Systemic Functional Disorders

The etiology of intermittent gastrointestinal and associated systemic functional disorders is not yet clearly defined. Our own observations suggest that for any given patient the agents that induce symptoms are varied and multiple, and may change with time. In these allergic individuals, the vulnerability of their gastrointestinal tracts appears closely related to their state of hypersensitivity.

During our early studies[50-55] we found that the subjects who developed malabsorption after bovine milk protein ingestion were all allergic, with strong family histories of allergy. When challenged with milk proteins they also developed a wide spectrum of reactions that appeared to be due to functional changes in the autonomic nervous system. The changes included smooth muscle contraction, exocrine gland secretion, and increased vascular permeability.[55] The same changes, as well as the gastrointestinal disturbances, were reversible and repeatedly inducible by the exclusion and repeated reintroduction of bovine milk protein feedings. Before long, it became clear that other foods also often induced gastrointestinal relapses.

In following the early patients, we further noted during one ragweed season that about two-thirds of our first forty patients, who had achieved remission on a milk-free diet, developed gastrointestinal exacerbation along with an allergic rhinitis. These were to become annually recurrent seasonal symptom complexes, usually with diminishing severity of the gastrointestinal component with advancing age. We thus learned that gastrointestinal disorders in some patients could be induced not only by the ingestion of cow's milk proteins and other foods, but also by the inhalation of certain airborne allergens. We noted in addition that in such patients these same disorders often accompanied bacterial[51] and viral infections, less commonly immunization with live viruses, immunotherapy (hyposensitization), and even diagnostic allergy skin tests. The following three case histories give relevant examples.

Case 1. M.P., on admission, was a two-month-old girl who had severe bovine milk protein–inducible vomiting; massive, bloody, mucus-laden acid diarrhea up to twenty times daily; and malabsorption and marasmus. Her father had hay fever, and her mother asthma. She eventually recovered on a soy formula. Her recovery was interrupted by three distinct intercurrent infections. The first was an abscess of her cutdown site, which grew a pure culture of *Staphylococcus epidermidis*. The second was a urinary tract infection with greater than 300,000 colonies of *E. coli*/ml of urine. The third was mumps. Between the bacterial and viral infections she had one to two alkaline (pH 7.5) formed stools and steady weight gain daily during her recuperation from the earlier gastrointestinal disorder. However, accompanying each of her parenteral infections, with no change in her formula, she developed abdominal distention; voluminous, mucus-laden, acid (pH 5.5) diarrhea; and weight loss. In time she also developed allergic rhinitis and asthma. Although a well-developed, well-nourished teenager today, she continues to have milk protein–inducible diarrhea, now associated with abdominal cramps, pruritic eruptions, and periorbital angioedema.

CASE 2. P.M. was a nine-month-old boy who was admitted with vomiting; glucose–, mucus–, and blood-containing, acid diarrhea; marked growth failure; eczema; allergic rhinitis; and asthma. Both parents and his sister had hay fever; his father also had severe asthma. Repeated bovine milk protein challenges induced glucose malabsorption; the baby responded well[55] to a milk protein–free, lamb–corn oil–dextrose formula.[50] At twelve months of age, when he was symptom-free, gaining weight at the rate of 26 gm per day, having one normal, formed, alkaline (pH 7.0), glucose-free stool daily, and exhibiting normal glucose absorption, he was given an injection of live rubeola vaccine. Within six days he developed a fever of 101°F, a morbilliform rash, dry cough, increased expiratory wheezing, normal white blood cell count and differential, and negative stool and respiratory tract bacterial cultures. These were accompanied by the appearance of colic, abdominal distention, flatulence, acid (pH 4.5), glucose-containing diarrhea, and a maximal post-loading venous rise of 20 mg% glucose following a 2 gm/kg oral load of 10% dextrose in water. Without change in his formula, a glucose malabsorption with cessation of weight gain persisted for six weeks before spontaneously abating.

CASE 3. P.G. was a twenty-five-month-old girl from Ontario, referred by the late Doctor John M. Sheldon, with recurrent bouts of vomiting, abdominal distention, colicky abdominal pains, flatulence, 10–12 acid (pH 5.0), mucus-laden, watery stools daily, particularly during her symptomatic episodes of seasonal allergic rhinitis. Both of her parents had hay fever; her father also had angioedema, and her mother eczema and asthma. Doctor Sheldon reported that following a battery of allergy skin tests, many of which had produced strong whealing, she developed abdominal pain followed quickly by voluminous, mucus-containing diarrhea stools. She would develop similar spells of abdominal pain and diarrhea for two to four days following each of her weekly desensitization injections.

The above examples suggest that in highly allergic individuals certain antigens other than foods may trigger gastrointestinal as well as systemic allergic reactions.

Gastrointestinal Symptoms and Signs

Table 3-I lists the gastrointestinal symptoms and signs in the order of descending frequency in the present series of patients.

It can be seen that in more than half, the characteristic gastrointestinal manifestations included abdominal distention, abdominal pain, flatulence, vomiting and diarrhea, with growth failure in the young and rapid weight loss in the older patients. Diarrhea was the most prevalent and troublesome symptom, contributing to the most serious acute morbidity. The incidence of vascular shock with massive fluid and electrolyte loss was high, but could not be calculated because some of the patients had received parenteral therapy prior to their referral.

Besides acute fluid and electrolyte deficit, the most disturbing associated finding was growth retardation among the pediatric patients. Body weight in and below the third percentile was found in 52 percent of the patients, and in and below the twenty-fifth percentile in nearly three-quarters of the total group. Linear growth also was retarded, although less so than body weight. More than one-third of the patients (37%) had height on or below the third percentile, and 61 percent had height on or below the twenty-fifth percentile. Had the nine adults been excluded from these calculations, the incidence of growth failure would have been higher.

Of the physical findings encountered in this group, one of the most interesting was that of disturbed *rhythm* of intestinal peristalsis. Sixty-one of the ninety-two patients surveyed (66%)

TABLE 3-I

Gastrointestinal Symptoms and Signs in 101 Patients Presenting with Gastrointestinal Problems.

	No. with Findings	*No. Surveyed*	%
Diarrhea	96	101	95
Foul stools	91	96	94.8
Abdominal pains	84	97	94.6
Flatulence	90	96	93.8
Mucus in stools	90	98	91.8
Vomiting	90	100	90
Abdominal distention	84	97	86.6
More than 4 stools/day (5–30)	81	100	81
Floating stools	62	78	79.5
Acid stools (pH 6.0)	59	75	78.7
Weight 25th percentile	72	98	73.4
Undigested food in stools	65	90	72.2
Blood in stools	67	96	69.8
Green stools	55	80	68.7
Nonstop bowel sounds	61	92	66.3
Height 25th percentile	52	85	61.2
Weight 3rd percentile	51	98	52
Bowel sounds 0/1–47 min. non-stop	45	92	48.9
Glucose (TesTape+) in stools	19	50	38
Height 3rd percentile	31	85	36.5
Pathogenic *E. coli* in stools	14	41	34.1
Infrequent stools (0/3 days-weeks)	6	100	6
Obstipation, infrequent stools	4	100	4
Ova and parasites in stools	0	101	0

had unremittingly audible bowel sounds during the height of their symptomatology. The continuous peristaltic sounds were not always loud, although they were loudest following controlled bovine milk protein challenge. Occasionally the borborygmi were grossly audible without a stethoscope. At times there were high-pitched "rushes," but without the crescendo in amplitude heard in intestinal obstruction. Even when the bowel sounds were normal in volume, their prolonged periods of nonstop audibility reflected unphysiologically increased gut motility. This hyperperistalsis was investigated in seven atopic subjects and found to be inducible by bovine milk protein feedings. It correlated with rapid transit of gut contents through the proximal small bowel, increased stool frequency, diarrhea, fluid, electrolyte and weight loss and transient intestinal malabsorption (Fig. 3-1).[53] In contrast, forty-five of ninety-two (49%) patients surveyed for the finding showed absence of audible bowel sounds for one to forty-seven minutes, alternating with periods of continuous bowel sounds. Patients with predominantly decreased audible peristalsis tended to show infrequent stools, abdominal distention, anorexia, vomiting, and radiological signs of prolonged gastric, colon, and, at times, ileal retention following bovine milk protein ingestion (Fig. 3-2).[54]

The existence in the same individuals of both hyper– and

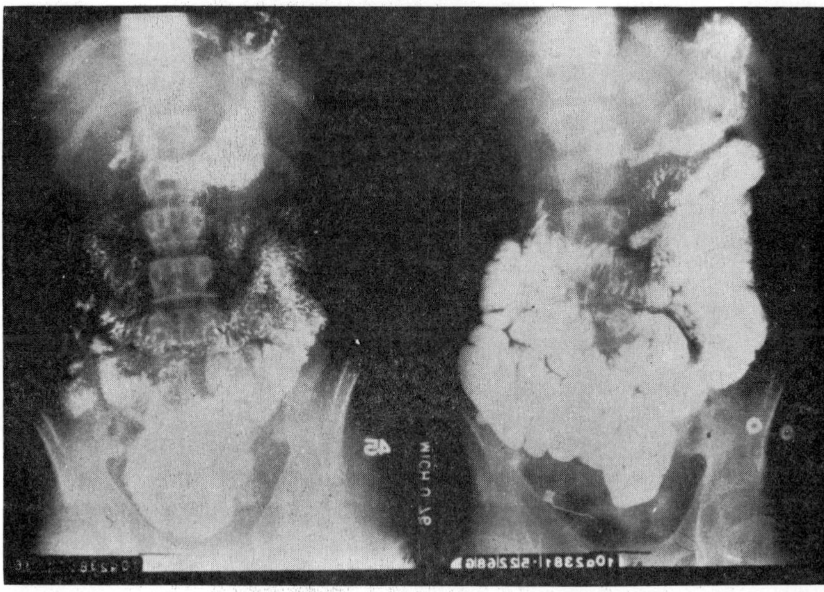

Figure 3-1. Proximal small bowel transit pattern in a 14-year-old boy. (Left) while ingesting a bovine milk–containing diet and 8 hours after a feeding of 240 ml of whole cow's milk, and (right) while ingesting a milk-free lamb–corn oil–dextrose (LCD) formula and 8 hours after a similar feeding of LCD. These radiographs were taken 45 minutes following the intragastric installation of 40% $BaSO_4$ U.S.A. in distilled water, 13.8 ml/kg body weight. After ingesting bovine milk (left) there was a more rapid transit of $BaSO_4$ through the proximal small bowel, with a relative lack of lingering of the contrast medium in the duodenum and jejunum in contrast to the leisurely transit of the barium meal through the same segment of gut after the feeding of LCD (right).

hypoperistalsis has long been noted in patients with gluten-sensitive malabsorption.[3,38,39,57,61] In the current series of patients, 6 percent had chronic, recurrent episodes of obstipation lasting three days to more than two weeks, and 4 percent had obstipation alternating with abnormally increased stool frequency.

Despite the correlation of the audible hyperperistalsis with rapid transit of gut content through the proximal small bowel, and of hypoperistalsis with segmental stasis of luminal content found in short-term milk protein challenge experiments, the overall frequency of disturbed audible persistalsis did not correlate with that of abnormal stool frequency. This discrepancy may be due to a number of factors. In the experimental situations, clinical parameters were monitored and measured over short-term, well-defined time periods, and under strictly controlled conditions, using each patient as his own control. Thus, the comparisons of data obtained were reproducible and more interpretable. On the other hand, this survey recorded only the admission history and physical findings among patients in diverse clinical states. The auscultatory findings at the time of admission may not have represented the long-term intestinal transit patterns of each patient. Besides, stool frequency, which reflects net gut transit, depends as much on the duration of gastrointestinal sphincter contraction as on intestinal peristalsis, introducing an important variable that defies auscultatory assessment. In spite of these difficulties with the interpretation of bowel sounds, much has been learned by following this clinical parameter in patients. In states of optimal intestinal absorption, the patients typically exhibited quiet, intermittent bowel sounds six to twelve times per minute, whereas clinical expressions of gastrointestinal dysfunction were usually accompanied by auscultatory signs of disturbed peristaltic rhythm.

Positive stool glucose by TesTape® was found in more than one-third (38%) of the fifty patients surveyed. This finding correlated best with marked hyperperistalsis, glucose malabsorption, and the passing of voluminous, very acid (pH 4.5–5.5), explosive, watery stools. Of the nineteen patients with this finding, one was a baby aged three weeks, thirteen were under one year of age (6 weeks to 11 months), and the remaining five between

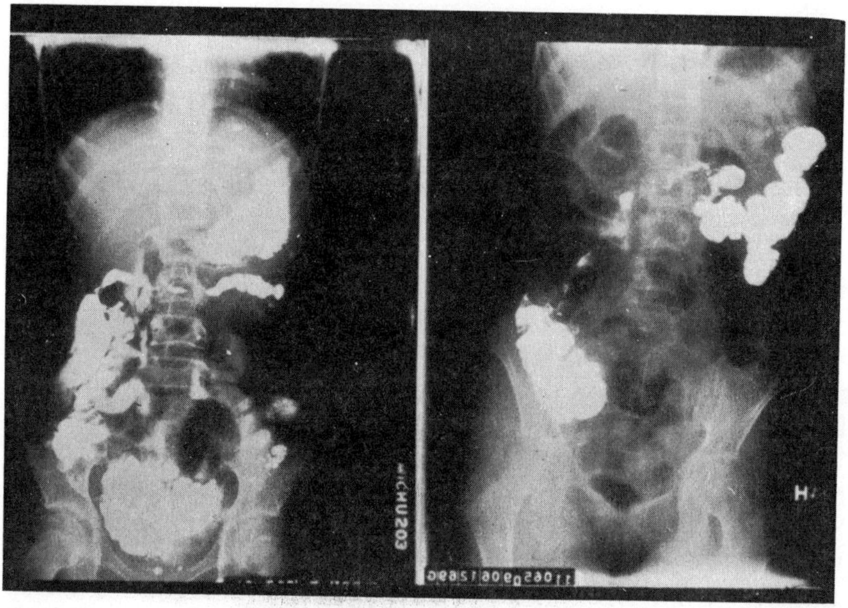

Figure 3-2. A pair of 24-hour abdominal films in a 13-year-old girl after the ingestion of bovine milk (left) and, again, LCD (right). The patient was fed 240 ml of whole cow's milk during the challenge study (left) and the same volume of LCD during the control study (right) before an 8-hour fast each time. The contrast medium transit was investigated with the same technique on both occasions. Note the much slower transit of $BaSO_4$ through the entire gastrointestinal tract after the feeding of bovine milk, with retention of the contrast medium in the gastric, ileal, and colonic segments (left).

thirteen months and fifty-one years of age. The single adult patient developed this sign in association with dramatically rapid gastrointestinal transit. This patient had been recuperating from milk protein–inducible malabsorption and had remained asymptomatic while ingesting 120 gm of glucose each day on a lamb-base, bovine protein–free formula. Ten hours following a challenge with 120 ml of whole cow's milk she was given 50 gm of glucose by mouth. In fourteen minutes she developed abdominal cramps, loud borborygmi and massive, glucose-laden (4+ TesTape), acid diarrhea. In some patients, gut transit can be sufficiently hastened as to preclude both complete absorption and bacterial breakdown of ingested glucose.

No ova or parasites were detected in the stools in any of the patients in this group. Stool cultures in forty-one patients were typed for pathogenic *E. coli,* and fourteen (34%) were positive. The presence or absence of detectable pathogenic *E. coli* in the stools did not correlate with any special symptoms. No other bacterial pathogens were found. The rota virus was not looked for.

Among the 101 patients three had radiologic, sigmoidoscopic, and histologic evidence of ulcerative colitis. One was a four-and-one-half-year-old boy with ragweed hay fever, angioedema, contact dermatitis, and a peripheral eosinophilia of 8 percent. His father had multiple allergies. His mother had abandoned the family early so that the maternal family history was unknown. The second was a twelve-and-one-half-year-old girl with asthma, hay fever, contact dermatitis, food-inducible angioedema, and a peripheral eosinophilia of 11 percent. She had bilateral family histories of asthma. Her gastrointestinal and systemic symptoms and signs could be induced by the ingestion of wheat gluten as well as of bovine milk proteins. The third was a fourteen-year-old boy with hay fever, angioedema, and urticaria due to foods, drugs, and pollens. He had a peripheral eosinophilia of 6 to 13 percent, and a bilateral family history of allergy. The first boy had total remission on an antigen-restriction diet and program. The second patient had symptomatic remission for eight years on the same therapeutic regimen, experiencing brief abdominal cramps and diarrhea with sneezing and serous rhinorrhea only on exposure to the interior of a fabric shop. After remaining well for eight years, gluten and milk proteins were added to her diet; within a day she developed facial edema; nasal pruritis; abdominal distention; cramps; bloody, mucus-laden diarrhea; and weight loss. Further studies are being conducted. The fourteen-year-old boy had a dramatic remission of abdominal discomfort and intestinal malabsorption on an antigen-restriction program and milk protein–free diet. However, his blood– and mucus-containing stools never abated, and after a six-month trial of the medical program he had a colectomy. He has since remained well.

One patient in this series was a three-year-old boy who had a diagnosis of gluten-sensitive enteropathy with flat jejunal mucosa.

He also had hay fever and asthma. Both parents had hay fever and his father also had asthma. He never achieved remission on a conscientious gluten-free diet but continued to have frequent, loose stools, encopresis, enuresis, and growth failure until bovine milk proteins were also excluded from his diet. His symptoms cleared within one week and growth rate accelerated thereafter. His loose stools tend to recur during bouts of respiratory allergy.

The finding of ulcerative colitis in the three children whose gastrointestinal manifestations were partly or wholly relieved on a milk– and gluten-free diet recalls similar experiences of Truelove with milk-provoked ulcerative colitis[78] and Gryboski with milk-induced colitis of infancy.[33] Whether or not these represent varied expressions of the same pathologic state remains to be elucidated.

The prompt cessation of enuresis in the three-year-old boy after milk exclusion closely resembles observations of Gerrard et al.[10,27]

In summary, it would seem that the gastrointestinal symptoms and signs exhibited by patients in this series had an allergic component, for they could be induced by feeding bovine milk proteins as well as by exposure to a variety of antigens; they also tended to accompany systemic allergic reactions.

Parenteral Symptoms and Signs

Table 3-II lists the respiratory and dermatologic manifestations encountered in the patients at the height of their clinical disease. A few random observations on the urinary patterns in these patients are also included.

Most of the respiratory and dermatologic symptoms reflect the presence of collateral allergies. They tended to accompany the gastrointestinal manifestations on admission and during exacerbations.

The history of "easy bruising," with or without signs of ecchymoses, was encountered in 71 percent of the eighty-seven patients surveyed for this finding. Although the data have not been analyzed, similar findings were frequent among the mothers of these patients. This phenomenon was not associated with

TABLE 3-II

Parenteral symptoms and signs in 101 patients presenting with gastrointestinal problems.

	No. with Finding	*No. Surveyed*	%
Respiratory			
Rhinorrhea	97	99	97.9
Sneezing	85	95	89.5
Cough	88	100	88.0
Wheezing	73	98	74.5
Itchy nose	55	84	65.5
Bronchila mucus	25	92	27.2
Pneumonia	25	94	26.6
Dermatologic			
Angioedema	82	99	82.8
Allergic dermatitis	82	100	82.0
Easy bruising	62	87	71.3
Urticaria	38	92	41.3
Eczema	36	92	39.1
Urinary			
Urinary frequency	85	96	88.5
Polyuria	62	86	72.1
Intermittent urinary stream	38	73	52.1

clotting defects and bore no relation to the occasional thrombocytopenia found in 7 percent of the patients.

Eighty-five of ninety-six patients (89%) surveyed had urinary frequency without associated lower urinary tract obstruction or infections. Thirty-eight of seventy-three patients (52%) had had intermittent urinary stream, which was often difficult to initiate. While the former appears to reflect frequent involuntary contractions of the bladder smooth muscle,[10] the latter suggests intermittent involuntary contractions of the trigone and sphincter. During twenty-four-hour urine collections after bovine milk protein feedings, patients often had transient straining dysuria requiring four to six intermittent abortive voidings to empty a full bladder. This dysuria seemed not to be associated with pain.

Unrelated to the lower urinary tract motor changes, sixty-two of eighty-six (72%) young pediatric patients were described by their mothers as having large urine volumes that "soaked through the diapers." This was confirmed in many of these infants and children, especially during infections, allergic reactions, and milk protein challenges. In the face of increased gut water loss through diarrhea and/or vomiting, fully half the patients tended to excrete large volumes of dilute, alkaline urine (see Laboratory Findings). Without diuretics or concurrent large fluid input, twenty-four-hour urine volumes have measured as high as 475 ml in a one-month-old premature infant weighing 2359 gm, 960 ml in a six-month-old, and 3800 ml in a fourteen-year-old. This type of polyuria appeared to be episodic, transient, and vasopressin independent. Such apparent failure of prompt renal tubular compensation for gastrointestinal water loss tended to accelerate hemoconcentration during acute exacerbations of diarrhea and vomiting. Careful measurement of serum and urinary osmolality under controlled water deprivation in such patients should yield invaluable information.

Autonomic Nervous System Functional Changes

By the time the first 200 patients with inducible gastrointestinal symptoms had been seen on our service, it had become evident that (1) bovine milk protein–inducible gastrointestinal disorders tended to occur in highly allergic individuals, (2) antigens other than bovine milk proteins were also capable of inducing similar gastrointestinal disorders, (3) the induced gastrointestinal dysfunction usually was accompanied by autonomic functional changes. The latter included signs attributable to the pharmacologic actions of histaminergic or cholinergic, and alpha- as well as beta-adrenergic mediators. In this respect our observations differ from the concepts of Kuntz[46] and, more recently, Yu et al.,[91] who considered allergy a state of parasympathetic preeminence, and of Szentivanyi[77] who saw in asthma, at least, an unopposed alpha-adrenergic dominance. A survey of the episodic, antigen-related autonomic functional changes was begun in an effort to better understand the relationship between these and the periodic gastrointestinal disturbances.

Table 3-III lists the histaminergic or cholinergic, as well as alpha- and beta-adrenergic symptoms and signs reported and/or observed in our atopic patients during exposure to potentially

TABLE 3-III

Symptoms and Physical Signs of Autonomic Nervous System Functional Changes.

	No. with Findings	*No. Surveyed*	%
Histaminergic and/or Cholinergic			
Exocrine gland secretion			
General sweating	77	94	81.9
Mucus secretion — Respiratory: Nasal	97	99	97.9
Bronchial	25	92	27.2
Gastrointestinal	90	98	91.8
Smooth Muscle Contraction			
Bronchial (wheezing)	73	98	74.5
Gastrointestinal (hyperperistalsis)	61	92	66.3
Bladder (urinary frequency)	85	96	88.5
Vascular Permeability			
Urticaria	38	92	41.3
Angioedema	82	99	82.8
Bruises	62	87	71.3
Alpha- and Beta-Andrenergic			
Increased pulse rate: above normal for age	55	89	61.8
above 140/min (140–212)	52	89	58.4
Widened pulse pressure — diastolic of 0	32	61	52.5
Plantar or palmar sweating	45	92	48.9
Myriasis — pupillary diameter ≥ 6 mm			
Cold extremities	78	88	88.6
Mottled skin	83	91	91.2
Acrocyanosis — dusky lips & nail beds	51	89	57.3
Plantar or palmar sweating	68	87	78.2
Mylriasis — pupillary diameter ≥ 6 mm	38	69	55.1
Functional bladder sphincter contraction (with intermittent urinary stream)	38	73	52.1
Hyperkinesis	68	94	72.3

antigenic stimulation, including bovine milk protein feedings. Symptoms were those reported by parents, older patients, referring physicians, attending nursing and medical staff members, and medical students. Physical signs were those observed and recorded by three examiners. The patients had no concurrent cholinergic or adrenergic drug administration, hypoglycemia, fever, hypothermia, pain, physical exertion, vestibular stimulation, or visible emotional stress. Auscultation for apical pulse rates, brachial arterial blood pressure, and bowel sounds was conducted with the patient supine, at rest, asleep whenever possible, afebrile, and free of visible agitation. Pupil size was estimated while the patient sat on the examining table in a brightly lit examining room staring straight ahead, but not into a light.

Clinical parameters are grouped for convenience under mediator classes according to the latters' best-known pharmacologic actions to which the various clinical signs may be attributed. Such a grouping is not intended to illustrate the complex interaction of all the mediators involved in allergic reactions.[17,63] Findings preceded by question marks are those considered possible, based on effects of mediators under which they are listed. A wide range of autonomic functional disturbances was documented during bovine milk protein challenge. These changes tended to be transient, reversible, repeatedly inducible, and to commonly accompany induced gestrointestinal dysfunction. They appear to reflect a liability of the autonomic nervous system in highly allergic individuals, and are probably mediated by chemical mediators in response to a variety of antigenic stimuli.

Routine Laboratory Findings

Characteristic routine laboratory findings are listed in Table 3-IV. At the height of their gastrointestinal disease, roughly half the patients had the following: anemia due to chronic blood loss with reticulocytosis, large volumes of dilute, alkaline (freshly voided) urine, high hematocrit, hypoproteinemia, hyperchloremic acidosis, and elevated serum IgM. Peripheral eosinophilia of 4 to 51 percent without parasitic infestation or malignancy was found in fifty-two of the eighty-five (61%) patients. About one-third of the patients showed hypokalemia, hyponatremia, hypocarbia, and macrocytosis. Serum IgA was high or low for age in half the patients studied. A fifth of the patients had thrombocytosis.

Special Clinical Investigations

A number of special studies were carried out from time to time to throw light on the nature of the gastrointestinal disturbances. All studies were done when the patients were free of infection, fever, and, unless specified, medications.

1. *Oral Carbohydrate Tolerance Tests.* One hundred and

TABLE 3-IV

Typical Routine Laboratory Findings in 101 Allergic Patients with Gastrointestinal Functional Disorders.

	No. with Findings	*No. Surveyed*	%
LABORATORY FINDINGS			
Urine:			
Low specific gravity: 1.009	43	80	53.8
High pH: ≥ 7.0	40	82	48.8
Serum:			
High chloride ≥ 110 mEq/l	46	81	56.8
≥ 106 mEq/l (107–160)	65	81	80.2
Low proteins: ≤ 5.9 gm/dl	42	79	53.2
≤ 5.5 gm/dl (3.5–5.5)	29	79	36.7
Low pH < 7.35 (6.9–7.34)	29	66	43.9
Low potassium ≤ 3.5 mEq/l (1.9–3.5)	24	80	30.0
Low bicarbonate < 18 mEq/l (10–17.8)	20	68	29.4
Low sodium ≤ 137 mEq/l (98–137)	23	81	28.4
Low calcium ≤ 8.5 mg/dl (3.1–8.5)	14	76	18.4
Hematology:			
Eosinophilia ≥ 4% (4–51)	52	85	61.2
Reticulocytosis > 3.1%	34	68	50.0
Low hemoglobin < 11.0 gm/dl	39	87	44.8
< 10.0 gm/dl (4.2–10.0)	28	87	32.2
MCV: high > 91 μ^3	24	66	36.4
low < 82 μ^3	29	66	43.9
Platelet count: high > 437,000/mm^3	15	69	21.7
low ≤ 150,000/mm^3	5	69	7.25
Hematocrit: high: > 40% in 71 children	(23	122 tests	18.9)

SERUM IMMUNOGLOBULINS:

	High for Age	*Low for Age*
IgA	in 13/51 (25.5%)	in 12/51 (23.5%)
IgG	in 7/50 (14.0%)	in 6/50 (12%)
IgM	in 22/51 (43.1%)	in 2/51 (3.9%)

fifty-three tests were performed on seventy-two patients. The tests, according to the method of Weijers et al.,[89] were performed following six– to eight-hour fasts, with oral loads of 10% glucose, beta lactose, or starch in distilled water, 2 gm/kg of body weight, up to a maximal dose of 50 gm. Venous samples were obtained over a period of two-and-one-half hours before and at thirty-minute intervals after loading; during this time patients were recumbent and asleep without sedation. All blood was collected and maintained on ice, until analyzed in duplicate for glucose immediately after the last venous collection, using a glucose oxidase method. Consecutive tests were performed at intervals of no less than seventy-two hours.

In new patients, all tests were carried out eight hours after the last bovine milk feed. Those with flat oral glucose tolerance curves and/or acid diarrhea following glucose loading were not given further carbohydrate loading tests. All those with normal glucose tolerance curves had subsequent lactose tolerance tests. A few with normal glucose and lactose absorption curves, but histories of other carbohydrate-inducible abdominal distention, flatulence and acid diarrhea, were given starch, sucrose, and additional sugar tolerance tests.

Of the sixty-three patients in this series who had oral glucose tolerance tests, thirty-six (57%) showed flat curves with venous glucose peaks of 0 to 39 mg%. Using the criteria of Weijers et al.,[89] who considered a peak rise of 50 mg% or more to be normal, 65 percent of the current patients had "flat curves" eight hours after milk challenge. In these patients the milk-inducible signs of carbohydrate malabsorption could not be attributed to lactase deficiency.

Twenty of the forty patients who had oral lactose tolerance tests showed maximal post-load plasma glucose peaks of less than 20 mg%. Seven of fourteen starch tolerance tests yielded flat curves with maximal post-load plasma glucose peaks of less than 50 mg%. Five of these seven patients had had normal glucose and lactose absorption, but frequent gastrointestinal manifestations of carbohydrate malabsorption.

In the author's experience, selected oral carbohydrate tolerance tests eight hours following bovine milk challenge have been useful screening tests for milk protein–inducible, transient carbohydrate malabsorption in infants and children.[50,53-55] In some older patients, or after repeated rechallenges, the induced carbohydrate malabsorption may be associated with dramatic gastrointestinal symptoms but without, necessarily, a flattening of the tolerance curves. This discrepancy has been reported before[32,40,53,

[60,67] and must be considered in the interpretation of the oral tolerance test results. The percent differences between the results of well-controlled, paired studies in the same individual patient with and, again, without milk protein challenge yielded more meaningful information regarding the milk protein effect on carbohydrate absorption than did the "normality" or "abnormality" of single test values.

2. *Fat Balance.* Seventy-two-hour fat balance studies were conducted in twenty-seven patients while they were ingesting a bovine milk protein– and, in patient number eight, gluten-containing diet. Daily fat ingestion was more than adequate by Anderson's criteria,[2] ranging from 25 gm in a one-month-old premature baby to 250 gm in a fourteen-year-old. Urine and fecal collections were completely separate so that any fecal wet weights presented here were free of dilution effects from urinary sources. Fecal fat analyses were carried out in triplicate using the method of van de Kamer.[80] Results were expressed as percentage of ingested fat.

Data are complete in only twenty of these patients. Of the twenty, fourteen had steatorrhea ranging from 7.8 percent in a twelve-and-one-half-year-old girl to 100 percent in a nine-year-old boy. Nine of the twenty patients also had "control" fat balances on a therapeutic exclusion diet. Seven of the nine were infants from two and one-half to seventeen months of age; the remaining two were thirteen and fourteen years old. In eight of the nine patients the therapeutic "control" diet consisted exclusively of a milk– and gluten-free, lamb–corn oil–dextrose (LCD) formula (see Treatment). The ninth patient was a thirteen-year-old, wheat-sensitive boy whose "control" balance study was conducted while he was ingesting a gluten-free diet that contained bovine milk proteins. For the "bovine milk protein feeding period," three of the nine patients (#3, 4, and 7) were fed bovine casein hydrolysate (Mead Johnson, Evansville, Ind.) 10 gm twice a day in addition to LCD formula.

Table 3-V lists the fecal fat in these nine patients on milk (or gluten, in patient #8) and, again, on "control" feedings.

Compared to established norms for infants, children, and adults,[2,3,33,75,88] results of the above study revealed remarkably low values of fecal fat excretions in all nine patients while they were

TABLE 3-V
Fecal Fat (% of ingested fat during 72-hour balance) on Different Diets.

Patients	*Age*	*Milk Diet*	*LCD*	*Gluten-free with Milk*	*% Decrease in Fecal Fat on Therapeutic Diets*
1. AF	2.5 mos.	12.0	1.7		85.8
2. MV	3.5 "	22.75	1.2		94.7
3. KH	6 "	9.2	3.17		65.5
4. SL	8 "	1.24	0.49		60.5
5. WS	8 "	10.71	0.68		93.7
6. AH	9 "	11.2	0.77		93.1
7. DF	17 "	1.15	1.34		0
8. GA	13 yrs	14.7*		2.93	80.17
9. TS	14 "	4.85	0.92		81.0

*Value obtained on a gluten-and-milk-containing diet.
LCD = lamb–corn oil–dextrose formula (see Table 3-VIII).
Milk Diet = milk-containing diet.

ingesting diets free from specific food proteins known to precipitate gastrointestinal symptoms and signs. Particularly noteworthy are fecal fat figures below 1 percent of ingested fat in four of the eight patients fed lamb–corn oil–dextrose (LCD), in spite of the young ages (8 months, 8 months, and 9 months) in three of them, and the huge fat intake of 250 gm/day in the fourteen year old. It appears that the hypoallergenic protein, unsaturated fat, and monosaccharide constituents of the LCD formula might have been important in favoring net gut absorption of fat in these allergic patients. Also of note is that in two of the patients (#4 and 9), fecal fat values were significantly (61% and 81% respectively) lower when they were ingesting LCD than when they were ingesting bovine milk, even though the milk-associated fecal fat figures were in the "normal range" for their respective ages. Fecal wet weight in patient #4 was fivefold higher on milk (235.3 gm/day) than off milk (45.3 gm/day) and in patient #9, threefold higher on milk (965.8 gm/day) than off milk (324 gm/day). Thus, bovine milk ingestion had clearly interfered with the efficiency of intestinal absorption in these two patients, even though the diagnosis of steatorrhea could not be made on the basis of absolute fecal fat values. It is conceivable that the established "normal" figures for infants, and even older patients, could have been skewed upwards if some of the "control-normal" subjects had had the same subtle milk protein effects on fat absorption seen in these two patients.

A quantitative comparison of fecal fat in controlled, paired balance studies in the same individual with and, again, without the feeding of a specific food protein should yield more meaningful information about the effect of that protein on intestinal absorption of fat.

In eight of these nine patients, specific dietary exclusion of a suspected offending food protein resulted in 61 percent to 95 percent decreases in fecal fat. One patient (#7) showed no change in fecal fat while ingesting LCD with added bovine casein hydrolysate compared with the period when he ingested LCD alone.

3. *Radiologic Study of Gastrointestinal Transit Patterns Eight Hours Following Bovine Milk Protein Feedings.* As has been mentioned earlier, the patients in this series tended to exhibit auscultatory signs of disturbed intestinal peristaltic rhythm, particularly after oral challenges with bovine milk proteins. Two-thirds showed nonstop bowel sounds, and nearly half also had alternating prolonged periods of absent bowel sounds. The associated symptoms and signs in each group of patients suggested co-existent aberrations in the rhythm of gut transit. The present radiologic study was developed to examine the transit pattern of luminal contents in allergic patients with and without prior bovine milk protein ingestion, each patient serving as his own control.

A 40% suspension of $BaSO_4$, U.S.P. in distilled water, 13.8 ml/kg of body weight, was administered via nasogastric tube to each fasting patient, and its transit followed radiologically at thirty-minute intervals for two and one-half hours in patients with rapid gut transit and for five hours, with an additional twenty-four-hour film, in patients with prolonged stasis of gut content in various segments of the gastrointestinal tract. Bovine milk protein challenges were given as homogenized whole cow's milk, 120 to 240 ml, or 30% bovine casein hydrolysate solution, 20 to 40 ml, eight hours prior to the radiologic study, except in a six-month-old infant who was fed casein hydrolysate one and one-half hours before the $BaSO_4$ administration. Control studies were done after feeding the milk-free control formula, LCD, in comparable volumes and manners as those used in the challenge studies.

Compared to control studies, 7 patients with bovine milk–inducible marked hyperperistalsis and intestinal malabsorption showed significantly hastened transit of ingested $BaSO_4$ through the functionally most active proximal small bowel hours after oral challenge with bovine milk or milk protein solution (Fig. 3-1).[53]

On the other hand, in seven patients exhibiting bovine milk–inducible signs of gut stasis with anorexia, vomiting, abdominal distention, protracted periods of absent bowel sounds, and obstipation, prior milk challenge was followed by radiologic signs of prolonged retention of the contrast medium in the gastric, colonic, and, in one case, ileal segments of the gut (Fig. 3-2).[54]

Among patients presented in this series it was not unusual to see both types of intestinal dysrhythmia in the same individuals at different times, apparently in response to different stimuli. In general, however, the same type of stimuli under the same circumstances tended to elicit the same gastrointestinal responses in any given patient.

Although the small number of patients in this study does not permit generalization, the observed association of slow gastrointestinal transit, radiologic signs of prolonged segmental stasis, and clinical complaints of frequent obstipation does suggest a possible mechanism for milk-associated constipation.

4. *Rectal Mucosal Biopsies Before and After Topical Milk Protein.* Ninety-three gastrointestinal biopsies were performed in sixty-four patients, including thirty-two jejunal mucosal biopsies, eight surgical biopsies, and fifty-three rectal biopsies before and after topical milk application.

Small bowel mucosal biopsies were obtained at the ligament of Treitz with a Quinton-Rubin per oral suction biopsy tube.[4] The position of the biopsy knife was ascertained radiologically in each case. Per oral jejunal mucosal biopsies were performed before the institution of dietary milk exclusion. However, for varying intervals prior to the biopsies, different patients had been fed a variety of diets containing whole milk proteins, casein hydrolysates, soy, gluten, and/or other assorted food proteins. This lack of control precluded any but general descriptions, and permitted no interpretation of the findings. To compensate for this, a controlled study of rectal mucosal biopsies before and after topical milk was devised.

Rectal mucosa was biopsied in twenty-four patients under direct vision before and after the topical application of bovine milk proteins, according to the following procedure. After a "control" biopsy of the anterior rectal mucosa was taken at 12 o'clock, a 10% suspension of nonfat dry milk (STARLAC®, Borden Co. N.Y.) was applied with an applicator for five minutes to an area of posterior rectal mucosa 1 cm in diameter at 6 o'clock. Biopsy of this area was taken exactly one hour after removal of the applicator.

All patients were medicated with secobarbital, U.S.P., 3 mg/kg of body weight, I.M., one hour prior to the biopsy procedure. Tissues were fixed in 10% formalin, imbedded in paraffin, serially dehydrated in alcohol, sectioned, and stained with hematoxylin and eosin.

Small bowel mucosal biopsies during periods of unrestricted milk-containing feedings were "normal" in seven of the thirty-two patients. The remaining twenty-five showed capillary dilatation, varying degrees of villous blunting, crypt elongation, edema, and increased round cell infiltration of the lamina propria, with a preponderance of plasma cells and eosinophils. A few long crypts contained increased numbers of mitotic cells; some specimens contained numerous goblet cells. Most villi showed columnar epithelial cells with intact brush border by light microscopy, others were histologically as well as grossly "flat," with pseudosquamous surface epithelium. Both the tissue and biopsy tubes were commonly covered with mucus. Despite histories of "milk sensitivity" in some of the patients, their jejunal histopathology was difficult to differentiate from that of gluten-induced,[64,68,95] or soy protein–induced enteropathy. The histologic technique used and endocrine status of the patients did not account for the wide variations observed in the specimens.[49]

Of the twenty-four patients who had rectal mucosal biopsies twenty-two were fed a bovine milk protein–containing diet, and two were fed only the milk-free LCD. One of the latter two patients had a "control" biopsy without any topical material. The other had biopsies following topical applications of two nonmilk "control" substances, 10% lactose and gliadin, each on a separate occasion just prior to biopsies of tissue exposed to topical dry milk suspension. The remaining twenty-two milk-fed patients had biopsies before and after topical dry milk applications; one of the twenty-two also had a "control" biopsy after application of 10% lactose.

Histologically, the two patients fed LCD had normal-appearing rectal mucosa whether or not the tissue had been obtained after topical 10% lactose, gliadin, or nothing at all. Biopsies from milk-fed patients often showed minimal to mild edema, even before topical milk. However, in all but two cases, local milk application led to markedly increased mucosal edema (Fig. 3-3).[55]

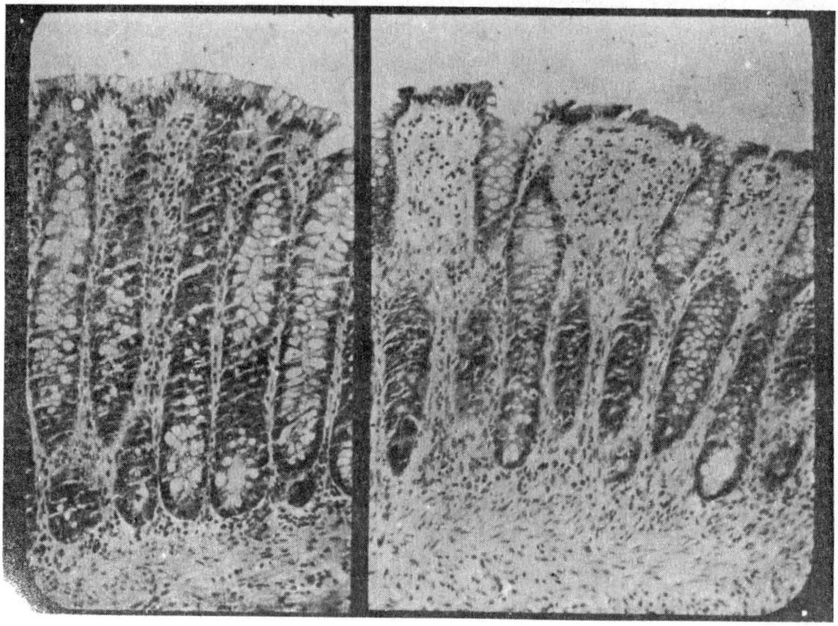

Figure 3-3. Angioedema of the rectal mucosa following topical milk showing (right) capillary dilatation and surface edema one hour following the five-minute application of bovine nonfat dry milk suspension, in contrast to the normal mucosa (left) from an adjacent area biopsied just before topical milk application.

Marked capillary engorgement was commonly but not consistently seen after topical milk. None of the surface vesicles and hemorrhagic vesicles grossly visible following milk application were ever seen in the microscopic specimens.

Grossly, mucosal reactions to the five-minute contact with dry milk suspension were clearly visible. Table 3-VI tabulates the rectoscopic findings recorded individually by three examiners following topical milk application in this study. It can be seen that thirteen of the seventy-five grossly visible mucosal changes were observed before the topical milk application, and all of these were in six patients on bovine milk–containing feedings. Patient #22, who showed the largest number of grossly abnormal mucosal changes *before* topical milk, was a six-month-old boy who had milk-inducible gastrointestinal hemorrhage, a blood-loss type of anemia with hemoglobin down to 6.2 gm/dl, twenty-four acid, watery stools a day, allergic rhinitis, contact dermatitis, and asthma. The most common finding on inspection was that of increased local edema, seen in 91.3% of the patients, accompanied by local hyperemia and/or pallor in nearly two-thirds of them. A local urticaria appeared to develop under the inspecting eyes within five minutes of the first topical application in half of those with mucosal edema. Seven patients had tiny vesicles on the surface of the urticarial lesions, three of these patients had hemorrhagic vesicles, with oozing of blood from the vesicles in one. Topical gliadin application in patient #2, who was not gluten sensitive, produced only pallor of the local mucosal surface. Lactose solution topically produced no visible change in either of the two patients in whom it was tried. All twenty-three patients who had had topical nonfat milk developed grossly detectable mucosal reactions, the least of which was a "mild" local edema.

Systemic autonomic reactions were recorded within one to sixty-three minutes following the mucosal contact with nonfat milk in all of the twenty-three patients. These resembled the manifestations induced during bovine milk protein oral challenge, and included tachycardia, widened pulse pressure with diastolic pressure of 0, mydriasis, peripheral vasoconstriction with icy cold extremities, increased palmar and plantar sweating, loud, nonstop hyperperistalsis, and wheezing. Whether the secobarbital had or

TABLE 3-VI

Gross Appearance of Rectal Mucosa After Topical Nonfat Dry Milk

Pt. #	*Diet*	*Topical*	*Fir.*	*Pet.*	*Pit.*	*Edema*	*Red*	*Pale*	*Muc.*	*Ves.*	*Hem.*	*Bleed.*	*Dusky*
1.	LCD	0	—	—	—	—	—	—	—	—	—	—	—
2.	LCD	10% lactose	—	—	—	—	—	—	—	—	—	—	—
		Gliadin	—	—	—	—	—	+	—	—	—	—	—
		NFM	—	—	—	+	—	—	—	—	—	—	—
3.	Milk	10% lactose	—	—	—	—	—	—	—	—	—	—	—
		NFM	—	—	—	+	+	+	—	—	—	—	—
4.	"	"	—	—	—	+	+	—	—	—	—	—	$+_a$
5.	"	"	—	—	—	+	—	—	—	—	—	—	—
6.	"	"	—	—	—	+	—	+	+	—	—	—	—
7.	"	"	—	+	+	+	+	—	—	—	—	—	—
8.	"	"	—	—	—	+	+	—	—	—	—	—	—
9.	"	"	—	—	—	+	+	—	—	—	—	—	—
10.	"	"	—	—	—	±	—	—	—	—	—	—	—
11.	"	"	—	—	—	+	+	—	+	—	—	—	—
12.	"	"	$+_a$	—	—	+	+	—	+	+	—	$+_a$	—
13.	"	10% bovine cas. hydrol.	—	+	—	+	+	+	—	—	+	+	—
14.	"	NFM	—	+	—	+	+	—	—	—	+	—	—
15.	"	"	—	—	—	+	—	+	—	—	—	—	—
16.	"	"	—	—	—	±	—	+	—	—	—	—	—
17.	"	"	—	—	—	+	—	+	—	+	—	—	—
18.	"	"	—	—	—	+	—	+	—	—	—	—	+
19.	"	"	—	+	—	$+_a$	+	$+_a$	—	—	+	—	—
20.	"	"	—	—	—	+	+	+	+	+	—	—	—
21.	"	"	—	—	—	—	—	$+_a$	+	—	—	—	$+_a$
22.	"	"	$+_a$	$+_a$	—	$+_a$	$+_a$	—	+	—	—	$+_a$	—
23.	"	"	—	—	—	—	+	$+_a$	+	—	—	—	—
24.	"	"	—	—	—	+	—	+	—	+	—	—	—

FRI = friable, PET = petechia, PIT = pits, MUC = increased mucus; VES = vesicles, HEM = hemorrhagic vesicles; BLEED = gross bleeding; LCD = lamb–corn oil–dextrose formula, NFM = nonfat dry milk (Starlac, Borden Co., N.Y.), CAS. HYDROL = bovine casein hydrolysate (Mead, Johnson Co., Evansville, Ind.), a = before as well as after topical milk.

had not modified these autonomic functional changes is not known.

DIAGNOSIS

Although bovine milk protein challenge has turned out to be an effective research tool for the induction of gastrointestinal and autonomic functional disorders in atopic individuals, the positive functional responses do not confer specific diagnosis of either "cow's milk protein allergy" or "gastrointestinal allergy" in such patients. In our experience, symptomatology in these individuals rarely is inducible by bovine milk ingestion alone. As well, the gastrointestinal tract is rarely the only organ disturbed by bovine milk protein challenge. The identifying features of the group seem to be its members' biologic hypersensitivity and their propensity to develop transient systemic, mostly autonomic, functional changes in response to assorted antigenic stimuli. Within the group different individuals, even those from a given family, may become symptomatic on exposure to different combinations of potential antigens, including bovine milk proteins. Furthermore, ingested, inhaled, injected or infectious antigens may produce a variety of parenteral as well as gastrointestinal manifestations. Clinically, the phenomenon appears to be a syndrome of autonomic functional lability among the highly allergic, one that might be considered an *"allergic dysautonomia."*

Thus, diagnostic efforts must be directed towards not only the exclusion of other entities that might share certain clinical expressions of this syndrome, but also the identification of possible allergic tendencies in the patients and their families. The history and physical examination, supplemented by subsequent sessions to confirm the initial findings, usually offer information regarding the inducibility and/or reversibility of the chief complaints as well as the extent and severity of systemic dysfunction. These preliminary data provide guidance regarding the need for hospitalization and the choice of immediate therapy and further diagnostic procedures.

The most common clinical entities considered in the differential diagnosis include intolerance of various constituents of foods, gastrointestinal infections and infestations, infantile diarrhea accompanying parenteral infections, irritable bowel syndrome, inflammatory or granulomatous enteritis, ulcerative colitis, certain immune deficiencies and muscoviscidosis their diagnostic criteria are well known. Clinical and laboratory parameters enumerated in Tables 3-I through 3-IV have been the most useful in identifying and assessing the extent of functional disorders and clinical complications. Additional diagnostic procedures, carried out when indicated, included appropriate microbiologic studies.

The periodicity and inducibility of specific functional aberrations and clinical manifestations were documented with paired evaluations before and after the institution of a trial antigen-restriction diet and program (see Treatment) and, in selected investigations, before and after bovine milk or milk protein challenges, following at least eight days of antigen restriction.

The obvious need in the study of this syndrome for diagnosis, as well as elucidation, of basic pathogenesis is the comprehensive investigation of its underlying immunologic mechanisms. During the decade in which patients in this study were seen, the only accepted criteria for the diagnosis of bovine milk protein–inducible disease state were those of Goldman et al.[29] In recent years Goldman's classical diagnostic precepts have been augmented by the addition of pre- and postchallenge small intestinal mucosal biopsies.[34,43,44,65,72,73,84-86] Particularly interesting have been the demonstrations of increases in IgE plasma cells in the lamina propria,[34,37,43,73] and subepithelial mast cell degranulation[73] following oral challenge with bovine milk. In a recent review,[87] Walker-Smith carefully detailed a thoughtful diagnostic approach that is logical, discriminating, and safe.

In our experience, rectal mucosal biopsies before and after topical milk challenge in allergic patients with gastrointestinal symptoms have shown significant tissue reactions after contact with milk but not with control materials. The nature of the mucosal lesions is compatible with local histaminergic effects that have a systemic counterpart in the simultaneously induced smooth muscle contractions identified as audible wheezing and intestinal hyperperistalsis. With the additional use of immunofluorescent studies in the rectal mucosa,[37] rectal biopsies may become useful diagnostic tools in the future.

TREATMENT

For this group of patients we found it necessary to prescribe a trial diagnostic/therapeutic program that stringently restricted exposure to strongly antigenic environmental stimuli. It was essential to do this quickly, for the clinical manifestations were often serious and life threatening. Also, unless diagnostic challenge could be introduced after the patient had achieved symptom-free baselines, the results of challenges were uninterpretable, or even misleading. In our hands, the conscientious eradication of specific infectious, ingested, and inhaled antigens became an indispensable and effective part of the treatment.

For maximal antigen restriction, all intercurrent infections were identified and, when possible, promptly treated. Prior to the institution of the trial program, the parents were instructed about its nature, rationale, purposes, and limitations. They were given directions on a program of environmental inhalant antigen avoidance, including the removal of household pets and, when economically feasible, installation of air-conditioning and filtering devices if the symptoms and signs in question were disabling or life threatening. A gluten– and milk-free, hypoallergenic, well-balanced, high fluid, high caloric diet was prescribed, supplemented with water-miscible multivitamins and Ca_2HPO_4, ½ gm twice a day. If needed, iron and folate were also added. Infants and severely malnourished children and adults were fed, during the acute phase of the illness, a formula of lamb–corn oil–dextrose (Table 3-VII)[50] with the same supplements described above, except that folate or folate-containing foods were mandatory when intercurrent infections intervened.[51]

TABLE 3-VII

Lamb–Corn Oil–Dextrose Formula (LCD)

CONTENT	
Lamb (strained)	400 gm
Corn oil	40 gm
Dextrose	120 gm
Water to make	1920 gm
CALORIES	
19.6 cal/30 ml of formula	
41% from fat	
39% from carbohydrate	
20% from protein	
SUPPLEMENTATIONS	
Water-miscible multivitamins	0.6 ml bid
Ca_2HPO_4	0.5 gm bid
Folic acid	100.0 μg/day
$FeSO_4$	(as needed)

The designing of "hypoallergenic diets" required individualization. Works of Visakorpi and Immonen,[83] Self et al.,[71] Ament and Rubin,[1] Gerrard et al.,[26] and Freier[14] have shown that milk-sensitive infants often are intolerant of or allergic to other foods, including some commonly used in standard "hypoallergenic diets," such as soy and rice. Gerrard has observed in fifty-four cow's milk–allergic infants the development of clinical reactions to twelve different foods besides milk.[26] His recent report of eighteen breast-fed babies with reactions to food antigens ingested by their lactating mothers has added human breast milk to the list of foods which may be potentially symptom producing.[22] Our own work has demonstrated that carbohydrate malabsorption, radiological signs of disturbed intestinal transit patterns, and gastrointestinal signs and symptoms can be induced in certain allergic infants by the feeding of bovine casein hydrolysate.[53,54] This corroborates the experience of Davidson,[8] cited by Anderson and Burke,[2] and of Freier,[14] who has identified the presence of antigenic oligopeptides in protein hydrolysate formulas. Thus, it must be cautioned that popular "hypoallergenic" infant formulas, using bovine casein hydrolysate as protein source, may or may not be therapeutically effective for bovine milk protein–intolerant patients. Furthermore, experimental data collected in milk-allergic patients while ingesting such a formula may or may not show the full effect of bovine milk protein exclusion.

Patients were monitored and their parents supervised closely during the trial program, and notes were made of infections, factors that produced symptoms, clinical manifestations, and growth patterns.

For the relief of gastrointestinal, nasal, and pruritic dermatological symptoms and signs, diphenhydramine hydrochloride, U.S.P. elixir, often proved effective and safe.

Clinical trials with food additions were postponed until after the patients had attained complete symptomatic relief and normal growth. In most cases these were carried out by the parents under the supervision of family physicians. Specific challenge studies were conducted by the author and colleagues in the Clinical Research Unit.

Methods for the repair of acute fluid, electrolyte, protein, and blood depletion are well known. It needs only to be noted here that facial angioedema tended to mask the severity of hypovolemia in many of these allergic patients during the height of exacerbations, and that the volumes calculated for parenteral fluid therapy must be guided by direct assessment of blood volumes.

PROGNOSIS

On antigen restriction with diphenhydramine hydrochloride therapy, the prognosis for acute symptomatic relief was excellent. Most responsive were manifestations of gastrointestinal and autonomic functional disturbances. Except for patients plagued with recurrent or tenacious infections, conscientious antigen restriction was usually followed within a month by noticeable symptomatic improvement. Table 3-VIII lists the clinical changes observed in patients in this series in response to the program. Data were obtained through history and physical examination on patients during follow-up evaluations, most often one month after institution of the strict antigen restriction. The figures represent the percentage of patients reexamined who showed absence of various symptoms and signs at the time of maximally stringent antigen restriction, but do not, unfortunately, predict long-term course of the disorder.

Besides intercurrent infections, the most common causes for failure to achieve clinical improvement by the time of the one-month checkup were concurrent pollenosis, persistent presence of household pets, and the daily ingestion of foods not suspected but later shown to be symptom producing. These same events were most frequently found to herald recurrent exacerbations, although none were more insidious or more capable of producing severe morbidity than infections. In particular, infections of viral etiology were most apt to be associated with protracted, widespread, and often serious gastrointestinal and autonomic dysfunction.

Mortality rate in this series was 3 percent. Three patients died. All had severe and unusual complications. J.W. was a thirteen-year-old boy with hypogammaglobulinemia, *H. influenzae* sepsis, and copious diarrhea up to 6350 ml/day, and resistant to all available antimicrobial, immunoglobulin, fluid and

TABLE 3-VIII

Clinical response to antigen restriction (symptomatic relief).

	No. Pt. Relieved*	*No. Surveyed*	%
Gastrointestinal Manifestations:			
Vomiting	99	99	100.0
Diarrhea	95	98	96.9
Abdominal pain	86	89	96.6
Undigested food in stools	86	89	96.6
Abdominal distention	90	95	94.7
Blood in stools	83	88	94.3
Mucus in stools	90	97	92.8
Foul stools	87	94	92.6
Flatulence	79	89	88.8
Frequent stools	73	90	80.0
Non stop bowel sounds	38	78	48.7
Autonomic Nervous System Dysfunction:			
Bronchial mucus	87	87	100.0
Urticaria	89	89	100.0
Angioedema	94	95	98.9
Wheezing	93	94	98.9
Acrocyanosis (lips and nail beds)	85	86	98.8
Rhinorrhea	93	95	97.9
Mottled skin	86	88	97.7
Intermittent urinary stream	68	70	97.1
Hyperkinesis	91	94	96.8
Increased generalized sweating	89	92	96.7
Increased palmar and plantar sweating	84	87	96.6
Easy bruising	84	87	96.6
Cold extremities	83	87	95.4
Prolonged absence of bowel sounds	74	78	94.9
Widened pulse pressure (daistolic 0)	50	54	92.6
Mydriasis	63	70	90.0
Urinary frequency	79	90	87.8
Tachycardia	58	67	86.6

Changes in height and weight percentile:

	Increased in *Percentile*	*Decreased* in *Percentile*	*Same Percentile*
Weight	in 76/94 (80.9%)	in 11/94 (11.7%)	in 7/04 (7.4%)
Height	in 52/80 (65.0%)	in 17/80 (21.3%)	in 11/80 (13.8%)

*Pt. = patients.

electrolyte therapy. D.E. was a nine-month-old boy who succumbed to Asian influenza, massive diarrhea, renal tubular failure, associated disseminated intravascular coagulopathy and hypoplastic anemia. Two-month-old S.E. was lost when he developed asthma, ragweed rhinitis, *H. influenzae* pneumonia accompanied by severe vomiting, diarrhea, precipitous hypovolemia, and irreparable acute cerebral ischemia.

The observed mortality of 3 percent in this series was low when it is considered that half the patients had body weights at or below the third percentile on admission.[62] We think, but cannot prove, that prompt and stringent antigen restriction in such patients contributed to their recovery. We hope that future improvements in the control of viral as well as bacterial proliferation in acute infections, especially in immune deficiency states, will further improve the lot of these patients.

SUMMARY

Bovine milk protein–induced gastrointestinal disease is particularly common in patients who have or who later develop evidence of asthma, hay fever, allergic rhinitis, eczema, or food-induced urticaria. Such patients usually come from families with strong histories of atopic disease. The gastrointestinal symptoms in these patients can also often be induced by foods other than bovine milk proteins, as well as by bacterial and viral infections, by exposure to pollens of ragweed (in particular in Michigan), by immunization with live viruses, and even by immunotherapy (hyposensitization). The gastrointestinal disorders are often associated with disturbances of the autonomic nervous system. Treatment entails not only the exclusion of foods, but also of inhalant antigens, as well as the avoidance and prompt treatment of bacterial and viral infections.

REFERENCES

1. Ament, M.E. and Rubin, C.E.: Soy protein—another cause of flat intestinal lesion. *Gastroenterology, 62*:227, 1972.
2. Anderson, C.M. and Burke, V.: *Paediatric Gastroenterology.* Oxford. Blackwell, 1975, pp. 640-641.
3. Bossak, E.T., Wang, C.I., and Adlersberg, D.: Clinical aspects of the malabsorption syndrome (idiopathic sprue). In Adlersberg, D. (Ed.): *The Malabsorption Syndrome.* New York: Grune, 1957, p. 112.

4. Brandborg, L.L., Rubin, C.E., and Quinton, W.E.: A multipurpose instrument for suction biopsy of the esophagus, stomach, small bowel and colon. *Gastroenterology, 37:*1, 1959.
5. Cooke, R.A. and Vander Veer, A., Jr.: Human sensitization. *J Immunol, 1:*201, 1916.
6. Dannaeus, A., Foucard, T., and Johansson, S.G.O.: The effect of orally administered sodium cromoglycate on symptoms of food allergy. *Clin Allergy, 7:*109, 1977.
7. Dannaeus, A., Johansson, S.G.O., Foucard, T., and Ohman, S.: Clinical and immunologic aspects of food allergy in childhood. *Acta Paediatr Scand, 66:*31, 1977.
8. Davidson, M., Burnstine, R.C., Kugler, M.M., and Bauer, C.H.: Malabsorption defect induced by ingestion of beta-lactoglobulin. *J Pediatr 66:*545, 1965.
9. Eastham, E.J. and Walker, W.A.: Effect of cow's milk on the gastrointestinal tract: a persistent dilemma for the pediatrician. *Pediatrics, 60:*477, 1977.
10. Esperanca, M. and Gerrard, J.W.: Nocturnal enuresis: Studies in bladder function in normals and enuretics. *Can Med Assoc J, 101:*269, 1969.
11. Fallstrom, S.P., Ahlstedt, S., and Hanson, L.A.: Specific antibodies in infants with gastrointestinal intolerance to cow's milk protein. *Int Arch Allergy Appl Immunol, 56:*97, 1978.
12. Fontaine, J.L. and Navarro, J.: Small intestinal biopsy in cow's milk protein allergy in infancy. *Arch Dis Child, 50:*357, 1975.
13. Freier, S.: Paediatric gastrointestinal allergy. *Clin Allergy, 3:*577, 1973.
14. ———: Paediatric gastrointestinal allergy. *J Hum Nutr, 30:*187, 1976.
15. Freier, S. and Berger, H.: Disodium cromoglycate in gastrointestinal protein intolerance. *Lancet, 1:*913, 1973.
16. Frick, O.L.: Allergy. In Rudolph, A.M.(Ed.): *Pediatrics,* 16th ed. New York: Appleton-Century-Crofts, 1977, p. 329.
17. Gavani, U.D., Hyde, J.S., and Moore, B.S.: Hypersensitivity to milk and egg white. Skin tests, RAST results and clinical intolerance. *Ann Allergy, 40:*314, 1978.
18. Gerrard, J.W.: Familial recurrent rhinorrhea and bronchitis due to cow's milk. *JAMA, 198:*605, 1966.
19. ———: Gastrointestinal allergy in infants. In Speer, F. and Dockhorn, R.J. (Eds.): *Allergy and Immunology in Childhood.* Springfield: Thomas, 1973, p. 570.
20. ———: Breast-feeding: Second thoughts. *Pediatrics, 54:*757, 1974.
21. ———: Chasing the cause of Crohn's disease. *Br Med J, 1:*1533, 1977.
22. ———: Allergy in breast-fed babies to ingredients in breast milk. *Ann Allergy, 42:*69, 1979.

23. Gerrard, J.W., Heiner, D.C., Ives, E.J., and Hardy, L.W.: Milk allergy: recognition, natural history and management. *Clin Pediatr, 2*:634, 1963.
24. Gerrard, J.W., Ko, C.G., Dalgleish, R., and Tan, L. K-T.: Immunoglobulin levels in white and metis communities in Saskatchewan. *Clin Exp Immunol, 29*:447, 1977.
25. Gerrard, J.W., Lubos, M.C., Hardy, L.W., Holmlund, B.A., and Webster, D.: Milk allergy: Clinical picture and familial incidence. *Can Med Assoc J, 97*:780, 1967.
26. Gerrard, J.W., MacKenzie, J., Goluboff, N., Garson, J., and Maningas, C.S.: Cow's milk allergy: Prevalence and manifestations in an unselected series of newborns. *Acta Paediatr Scand Suppl, 234*:1, 1973.
27. Gerrard, J.W. and Zaleski, A.: Functional bladder capacities in children with enuresis and recurrent urinary infections. In Dickey, L.D. (Ed.), *Clinical Ecology,* Springfield: Thomas, 1976, p. 224-232.
28. Goldman, A.S.: Cow's milk sensitivity: A review. In Hambraeus, L., Hanson, L.A. and McFarlane, H. (Eds.): *XIII Symp Swed Nutr Found,* Stockholm: Almquvist and Wiksell International, 1977, p. 99.
29. Goldman, A.S., Anderson, D.W., Jr., Sellers, W.A., Saperstein, S., Kniker, W.T., and Halpern, S.R.: Milk allergy. I. Oral challenge with milk and isolated milk proteins in allergic children. *Pediatrics, 32*:425, 1963.
30. Goldman, A.S. and Heiner, D.C.: Clinical aspects of food sensitivity. Diagnosis and management of cow's milk sensitivity. *Pediatr Clin North Am, 24*:133, 1977.
31. Goldstein, G.B. and Heiner, D.C.: Clinical and immunological perspectives in food sensitivity. *J Allergy, 46*:270, 1970.
32. Gray, G.M.: Problems with lactose tolerance tests (Letter). *Gastroenterology, 53*:496, 1967.
33. Gryboski, J.D.: *Gastrointestinal Problems in the Infant.* Philadelphia: Saunders, 1975.
34. Harris, M.J., Petts, V., and Penny, R.: Cow's milk allergy as a cause of infantile colic: Immunofluorescent studies in jejunal mucosa. *Aust Paediatr J, 13*:276, 1977.
35. Harrison, M., Kilby, A., Walker-Smith, J.A., France, N.E., and Wood, C.B.S.: Cow's milk protein intolerance: A possible association with gastroenteritis, lactose intolerance and IgA deficiency. *Br Med J, 1*:1501, 1976.
36. Haworth, E.M., Hodson, J.D., Pringle, F.M., and Young, W.F.: The value of radiological investigations of the alimentary tract in children with coeliac syndrome. *Clin Radiol, 19*:65, 1968.
37. Heatley, R.V., Rhodes, J., Calcraft, B.J., Whitehead, R.H., Fifield, R., and Newcombe, R.G.: Immunoglobulin E in rectal mucosa of pa-

tients with proctitis. *Lancet, 2:*1010, 1975.

38. Heiner, D.C.: The use of RAST in the study of allergy in foods. In Evans, R. III (Ed.) : *Advances in Diagnosis of Allergy: RAST.* Proc First NA Conf on RAST. Miami: Medical Book Publisher, 1975, p. 153.
39. Ingelfinger, F.J. and Moss, R.E.: The motility of the small intestine in sprue. *J Clin Invest, 22:*345, 1943.
40. Isselbacher, K.J. and Senior, J.R.: The intestinal absorption of carbohydrate and fat. *Gastroenterology, 46:*287, 1964.
41. Iyngkaran, N., Robinson, M.J., Sumithran, E., Lam, S.K., Puthucheary, S.D., and Yadav, M.: Cow's milk protein-sensitive enteropathy. *Arch Dis Child, 53:*150, 1978.
42. Jakobsson, I. and Lindberg, T.: Cow's milk as a cause of infantile colic in breast-fed infants. *Lancet, 2:*437, 1978.
43. Kilby, A., Walker-Smith, J.A., and Wood, C.B.S.: Small intestinal mucosa in cow's milk allergy. *Lancet, 1:*531, 1975.
44. Kuitunen, P., Rapola, J., Savilahti, E., and Visakorpi, J.K.: Response of the jejunal mucosa to cow's milk in the malabsorption syndrome with cow's milk intolerance. A light and electron-miscroscopic study. *Acta Paediatr Scand, 62:*585, 1973.
45. Kuitunen, P., Visakorpi, J.K., Savilahti, E. and Pelkonen, P.: Malabsorption syndrome with cow's milk intolerance. Clinical findings and course in 54 cases. *Arch Dis Child, 50:*351, 1975.
46. Kuntz, A.: *The Autonomic Nervous System,* 4th ed. Philadelphia: Lea & Febiger, 1953, p. 474-476.
47. Kuzemko, J.A. and Simpson, K.R.: Treatment of allergy to cow's milk. *Lancet, 1:*337, 1975.
48. Law-Chin-Yung, L. and Freed, D.L.J.: Nephrotic syndrome due to milk allergy. *Lancet, 1:*1056, 1977.
49. Liu, H.Y. and Baker, B.L.: The influence of technique and hormones on histochemical demonstration of enzymes in intestinal epithelium. *J Histochem Cytochem, 11:*349, 1963.
50. Liu, H.Y., Tsao, M.U., Moore, B.F. and Giday, Z.: Bovine milk protein induced intestinal malabsorption of lactose and fat in infants. *Gastroenterology, 54:*27, 1968.
51. Liu, H.Y. and Giday, Z.: Effect of a supplemented synthetic liquid formula, LCD, on physical growth in bovine-milk-sensitive infants. *Pediatric Basics,* No. 5, 1972.
52. Liu, H.Y., Giday, Z., and Moore, B.F.: Certain bovine milk protein inducible eye signs in patients with allergic malabsorption. *J Pediatr Ophthalmol, 10:*7, 1973.
53. Liu, H.Y., Whitehouse, W.M., and Giday, Z.: Proximal small bowel transit pattern in patients with malabsorption induced by bovine milk protein ingestion. *Radiology, 115:*415, 1975.

54. Liu, H.Y., Whitehouse, W.M., Horner, J.M., and Giday, Z.: Radiologic and clinical signs of gastrointestinal stasis induced by bovine milk ingestion in allergic patients. *J Pediatr, 86*:977, 1975.

55. Liu, H.Y., Giday, Z., and Moore, B.F.: Possible pathogenetic mechanisms producing bovine milk protein inducible malabsorption: A hypothesis. *Ann Allergy, 39*:1, 1977.

56. Lubos, M.C., Gerrard, J.W., and Buchan, D.J.: Disaccharidase activities in milk sensitive and celiac patients. *J Pediatr, 70*:325, 1967.

57. Marshak, R.H., Wolf, B.S., and Eliasoph, J.: The roentgen findings in the malabsorption syndrome. In Adlersberg, D. (Ed.): *The Malabsorption Syndrome*. New York: Grune, 1957, p. 188.

58. Matsumura, T., Kuroume, T., Oguri, M., Iwasaki, I., Kanbe, Y., Yamada, T., Kawabe, S., and Negishi, K.: Egg sensitivity and eczematous manifestations in breast-fed newborns with particular reference to intrauterine sensitization. *Ann Allergy, 35*:222, 1975.

59. Matthews, T.S., Soothill, J.F.: Complement activation after milk feeding in children with cow's milk allergy. *Lancet, 2*:893, 1970.

60. McGill, D.B. and Newcomer, A.D.: Comparison of venous and capillary blood samples in lactose tolerance testing. *Gastroenterology, 53*:371, 1967.

61. McNicholl, B. and Egan-Mitchell, B.: Infancy coeliac diseases without diarrhea. *Pediatrics, 49*:85, 1972.

62. Metcoff, J.: Regulation of the Body Fluids (Fluid Spaces and Fluid Therapy. In Cooke, R.E. and Levin, S. (Eds.): *The Biologic Basis of Pediatric Practice*. New York: McGraw, 1968, p. 122.

63. Orange, R.P.: Immunopharmacological aspects of bronchial asthma. *Clin Allergy, 3*:521, 1973.

64. Padykula, H.A., Strauss, E.W., Ladman, A.J., and Gardner, F.H.: A morphologic and histochemical analysis of the human jejunal epithelium in non-tropical sprue. *Gastroenterology, 40*:735, 1968.

65. Poley, J.R., Bhatia, M., and Welsh, J.D.: Disaccharidase deficiency in infants with cow's milk protein intolerance. *Digestion, 17*:97, 1978.

66. Powell, G.K.: Enterocolitis in low birth weight infants associated with milk and soy intolerance. *J Pediatr, 88*:840, 1976.

67. Rosenquist, C.J., Heaton, J.W., Jr., Friedland, G.W. et al.: Assessment of a radiographic method for diagnosis of intestinal lactase deficiency: A prospective study. *Invest Radiol, 6*:40, 1971.

68. Rubin, C.E., Brandborg, L.L., Phelps, P.C., and Taylor, J.C., Jr.: Studies of celiac disease. I. The apparent identical and specific nature of the duodenal and proximal jejunal lesion in celiac disease and idiopathic sprue. *Gastroenterology, 38*:28, 1960.

69. Savilahti, E.: Immunochemical study of the malabsorption syndrome with cow's milk intolerance. *Gut, 14*:491, 1973.

70. Scheinmann, P., Gendrel, D., Charles, J., and Paupe, J.: Value of lym-

phoblast transformation test in cow's milk protein intestinal intolerance. *Clin Allergy, 6*:515, 1976.
71. Self, T.W., Herskovic, T., Czapek, E., Caplan, D., Schonberger, T., and Gryboski, J.D.: Gastrointestinal protein allergy. *JAMA, 207*:2393, 1969.
72. Shiner, M., Ballard, J., Brook, C.I.D., and Herman, S.: Intestinal biopsy in the diagnosis of cow's milk protein intolerance without acute symptoms. *Lancet, 2*:1060, 1975.
73. Shiner, M., Ballard, J., and Smith, M.E.: The small-intestinal mucosa in cow's milk allergy. *Lancet, 1*:136, 1975.
74. Shiner, M. and Birbeck, M.S.: The microvilli of the small-intestinal surface epithelium in coeliac disease and in idiopathic steatorrhea. *Gut, 2*:277, 1961.
75. Shmerling, D.H., Forrer, J.C., and Prader, A.: Fecal fat and nitrogen in health, malabsorption and maldigestion. *Pediatrics, 46*:690, 1970.
76. Shmerling, D.H. and Rein, D.: Jejunal biopsy in cow's milk protein intolerance. *Lancet, 2*:272, 1978.
77. Szentivanyi, A.: The beta-adrenergic theory of the atopic abnormality in bronchial asthma. *J Allergy, 42*:203, 1968.
78. Truelove, S.C.: Ulcerative colitis provoked by milk. *Br Med J, 1*:154, 1961.
79. Van Arsdel, W.T. and Motulsky, A.G.: Frequency and hereditability of asthma and allergic rhinitis in college students. *Acta Genet, 9*:101, 1959.
80. van de Kamer, J.H.: Quantitative determination of the saturated and unsaturated higher fatty acids in fecal fat. *Scand J Clin Lab Invest,* 5:30, 1953.
81. Vaz, G.A., Tan, L. K-T., and Gerrard, J.W.: Oral cromoglycate in treatment of adverse reactions to foods. *Lancet, 1*:1066, 1978.
82. Visakorpi, J.K.: Gluten intolerance and its nutritional implications. In Hambraeus, L., Hanson, L.A., and McFarlane, H. (Eds.): *XIII Symp Swed Nutr Found.* Stockholm: Almqvist and Wiksell International, 1977, p. 92.
83. Visakorpi, J.K. and Immonen, P.: Intolerance to cow's milk and wheat gluten in the primary malabsorption syndrome in infancy. *Acta Paediatr Scand, 56*:49, 1967.
84. Vitoria, J.C., Aranjuelo, M.E., and Rodriguez-Soriano, J.: Jejunal biopsy in cow's milk protein intolerance. *Lancet, 1*:722, 1978.
85. Walker-Smith, J.A.: Cow's milk protein intolerance. Transient food intolerance of infancy. *Arch Dis Child, 50*:347, 1975.
86. ———: Jejunal biopsy in cow's milk protein intolerance. *Lancet, 2*:1237, 1977.
87. ———: Gastrointestinal allergy. *The Practitioner, 220*:562, 1978.
88. Weijers, H.A. and van de Kamer, J.H.: Coeliac disease. I. Criticism

of the various methods of investigation. *Acta Paediat, 42*:24, 1953.

89. Weijers, H.A., van de Kamer, J.H., Dicke, W.K., and Ijsseling, J.: Diarrhoea caused by deficiency of sugar splitting enzymes. I. *Acta Paediatr, (Stockholm), 50*:55, 1961.
90. Whitfield, M.E. and Barr, D.G.D.: Cow's milk allergy in the syndrome of thrombocytopenia with absent radius. *Arch Dis Child, 51*:337, 1976.
91. Yu, D.Y.C., Galant, S.P., and Gold, W.M.: The role of the parasympathetic nervous system in human asthma: Inhibition of antigen-induced bronchoconstriction by atropine in asthmatic patients. *J Appl Physiol, 32*:823, 1972.

Chapter 4

FOOD-INDUCED RESPIRATORY DISEASE

John W. Gerrard

In this chapter, cow's milk will be referred to frequently, not because cow's milk is the only food to cause clinical disease, but because it is the food that has been studied most widely. It should, however, be borne in mind that disorders caused by cow's milk can be caused by almost any other food.

It has been recognized for many years that cow's milk can disturb gastrointestinal function, causing colic, vomiting, and diarrhea in infants.[10] The mechanism alone has been in doubt; a lactase deficiency can cause similar symptoms. Lactase deficiencies are rarely primary; more commonly they are induced by gastrointestinal infections,[23] or by the ingestion of cow's milk proteins.[22,29] The latter can induce immunological changes in the gut.[36] When this is the case, the disturbance in function, even though the precise immunological mechanism is not known for certain, is usually referred to as cow's milk allergy.[5]

If cow's milk can cause diarrhea on an allergic basis, and the disorder is as common as we have found,[20] it should also be possible to identify many cases of respiratory allergy also due to cow's milk, and this indeed is the case. In our own series of fifty-nine infants and children with cow's milk allergy,[20] 63 percent had diarrhea and/or vomiting; 60 percent had recurrent rhinorrhea, bronchitis, and/or asthma; and 46 percent had eczema either singly or in combination. In Goldman's[21] series of eighty-nine children, oral milk challenge caused vomiting in 33 percent, diarrhea in 37 percent, colic in 28 percent, rhinorrhea in 35 percent, asthma in 27 percent, and eczema in 35 percent; 77 percent had more than one type of reaction. This is a remarkably even distribution of the major manifestations of cow's milk allergy. Buisseret,[7] in his series of 79 cases, also found a very uniform distribution: 82 percent had eczema, 93 percent had respiratory symptoms (rhinorrhea and/or asthma), and 84 percent had gastrointestinal symptoms (colic, constipation, and diarrhea). The pediatrician is singularly fortunate in seeing the whole range of cow's milk allergy (CMA), and many are very much aware that eczema, diarrhea, vomiting, and recurrent rhinorrhea and wheezy bronchitis can be due to cow's milk, though some still tend to ascribe respiratory manifestations to an infection rather than to an allergy. The above symptoms are, however, often different aspects of the same underlying disorder. The pediatrician, however, when he sees a child with recurrent diarrhea and either eczema or recurrent bronchitis, is more likely than is the subspecialist to ascribe all to a common allergy than the diarrhea to a primary lactase deficiency, the eczema to an allergy, and the bronchitis to a series of viral infections.

This is not to belittle the importance of infections, for viral infections in infants with allergic backgrounds are often followed by, and probably initiate, the development of allergies and a rise in IgE levels.[16] The interplay of infections and even of immunizations and allergy is such, as Liu (Chapter 3) also has shown, that infections can trigger the development of allergies, while allergies can complicate infections.

Although CMA is common, the label often stirs up controversy. There are three principal reasons for this. The first is that the accepted test for an allergic reaction, namely a positive prick test, usually is negative. The second is that symptoms do not differ from those associated with infections such as gastroenteritis, the common cold, and bronchiolitis. The third is that even when cow's milk is a cause of the child's symptoms, simply taking him off cow's milk may not lead to recovery because cow's milk is only one of many allergens—both foods and inhalants—to which the patient is sensitive. Taking the baby off cow's milk and substituting soya may not lead to relief of symptoms because the child often is sensitive to both.[20,33]

For a long time, I was puzzled by the two contrasting characteristics of the common form of cow's milk allergy, namely the ease with which symptoms can be relieved and the predictable regularity with which they return when cow's milk is first avoided and soon afterwards reintroduced, and the complete lack of the usual evidence of allergy, namely the negative prick tests and RAST, and the low or normal IgE level. The reintroduction of breast-feeding, plus the recognition that allergies in breast-fed babies may arise in response to ingredients in the mother's milk, has thrown new light on the problem and has, I think, clarified it.[18]

Allergies in breast-fed babies tend to occur to foods being taken in abundant amounts by the mother, commonly cow's milk; nevertheless, only trace amounts are present in her milk. If the antigen being studied is egg, it is found that there are only 10^{-6} to 10^{-9} parts of egg in the breast milk.[14] These trace amounts in the sensitized baby can precipitate eczema, rhinorrhea, wheezing, vomiting, and diarrhea. In the latter instance, the stools may even contain frank blood. These reactions are commonly associated with positive prick tests and RAST, and if the baby later is inadvertently given a little cow's milk or cheese, he may have a violent, even anaphylactic, reaction. In some instances the baby is sensitized to cow's milk while on the breast but is symptom-free, presumably because of the low antigen load, until given cow's milk, when he has his first violent reaction. Doctor Park's[32] report of the reaction of his own breast-fed child to very small amounts of cow's milk is an excellent illustration of this clinical picture. This type of adverse reaction to cow's milk tends to persist, and even though cow's milk may be avoided scrupulously, the child may react adversely to trace amounts months later.

By contrast, allergies to cow's milk in babies brought up on formulas derived from cow's milk are induced by large amounts of milk. The average baby consumes its own weight as milk in the course of a week, and even though the antigenic load is great, the reaction on the part of the baby is mild, for example recurrent rhinorrhea, bronchiolitis, colic, vomiting, or diarrhea, the latter usually being troublesome but not catastrophic. These reactions are associated with negative prick tests and low or normal IgE levels. The main contrasting features of the two types of food allergy as seen in infants are that the immediate is initiated by trace amounts of antigen and is associated with positive prick tests and often, when studied, positive RAST. The reactions tend to be striking and often severe, for example, angioedema, asthma, and severe diarrhea and vomiting. The delayed type of food allergy is initiated by large amounts of antigen and is associated with negative prick tests and, in our experience, negative RAST. The symptoms produced are less striking and are more characteristic of infections, for example, rhinorrhea, bronchiolitis, and gastroenteritis.[19]

Extrapolating the data on infants to our experience with children and adults, we can infer that there are at least two common types of food allergy. One, which we call immediate, is precipitated by trace amounts of food, is associated with positive prick tests and RAST, and tends to recur whenever the child encounters the food in question even though the food itself has been avoided for months or even years. The second, which we call delayed, is precipitated by large amounts of the incriminated food, is not associated with positive prick tests, and tends to clear if the food is avoided for several months.

RESPIRATORY FOOD ALLERGIES OF THE IMMEDIATE TYPE

These, characteristically, are associated with asthma. They also may be associated with eczema, rhinorrhea, and, in severe cases, with angioedema. They are not necessarily (though they may be) associated with gastrointestinal symptoms such as vomiting and diarrhea. When they occur in the breast-fed baby they are not usually (but they may be) ascribed by the mother to foods that she has recently ingested, but only if the relationship is obvious. One of our mothers, for example, who was successfully breastfeeding her baby, found that when she visited her parents on their farm her baby began to wheeze. She correctly ascribed the wheezing to the large amounts of fresh cow's milk that she herself had started to drink. If reactions occur when unusual foods are introduced, the reaction may be sufficiently obvious and severe that the mother feels certain the food she has ingested has caused the reaction in her baby.

In older children and adults, the relationship between the food and symptoms usually is so obvious that the parent or patient knows the food in question causes wheezing. The clinician is not surprised to find that the appropriate prick test is markedly positive. Wraith[39] has found that when symptoms, usually asthma, have their onset within an hour of ingesting the food, the RAST is virtually always positive. If the onset of symptoms is longer delayed, only 64 percent have positive RAST. Others have found positive RAST to be reliably associated with egg, fish, and peanut sensitivity, and less reliably associated with clinical milk and wheat sensitivity.[1,6,8,9] The latter finding may be more a reflection on the test than on the patient's allergy.

RESPIRATORY FOOD ALLERGIES OF THE DELAYED TYPE IN THE INFANT

The clinical manifestations include nasal stuffiness, recurrent rhinorrhea, recurrent bronchiolitis, recurrent wheezy bronchitis, and recurrent bronchopneumonia with extensive pulmonary infiltrates, sometimes associated with pulmonary hemosiderosis.[24,28] The picture ranges from that of the common cold at one end of the scale to that of a severe, widespread bronchopneumonia at the other. It differs clinically from a simple infection in that it is recurrent. It affects all racial groups in our society, but in Saskatchewan it hits the North American Indians with particular severity.[26,38] The Indians most affected are those in poor socioeconomic surroundings, many of whom come from homes with single rooms heated by wood stoves, and no indoor plumbing—no place for a child in the best of circumstances, least of all in a Saskatchewan winter. The recent substitution of formula for breast-feeding also has contributed to the frequency and severity of the disorder in the Indian child.[15] The substitution of cow's for breast milk is the greatest single change in mankind's feeding habits in the whole of his evolutionary history, and when one considers the important role played by breast-feeding in protection against infection (it provides as much protection against respiratory as against gastrointestinal diseases), it is not surprising that the introduction of formula feeding should have affected more than the baby's nutritional status.

In infancy, respiratory allergies of the delayed type due to cow's milk naturally occur only in formula-fed babies. They should be suspected in any infant (1) brought up on a formula derived from cow's milk whose symptoms date from early infancy or from the time that he was weaned from the breast to a prepared formula, or from a prepared formula to cow's milk; (2) whose symptoms are recurrent; (3) who has multiple system involvement; eczema, colic, vomiting and/or diarrhea, as well as rhinorrhea and bronchitis; (4) if there is a family history of a previously affected sibling; (5) if there is a parent who has recurrent rhinorrhea and bronchitis and who drinks a great deal of milk; (6) if the baby's chest clears between feeds and is aggravated by them; and (7) if the baby has a parent who dislikes or never drinks milk and who is symptom-free.

Respiratory problems caused by cow's milk also can be caused, but less commonly, by other foods, and particularly in infancy by soya,[22,33] for soya is the one food other than cow's milk to which many babies, particularly those sensitive to cow's milk, are commonly exposed in large amounts.

A similar clinical picture can be associated with cystic fibrosis of the pancreas, immunodeficiency disorders, and gastroesophageal reflux. Cystic fibrosis of the pancreas can be identified quickly by measuring sweat chlorides, immunodeficiency disorders by measurement of the serum immunoglobulin levels and, if necessary, an assessment of T cell function, and gastroesophageal reflux by radiological studies. In this context it should be remembered that cystic fibrosis of the pancreas is often complicated by allergies;[2,37] cystic fibrosis and milk allergy, therefore, may be found together. With regard to immunological problems, IgA deficiencies are ten times as common in babies with severe respiratory milk allergies (Heiner's syndrome) [28] as they are in a normal population. An IgA deficiency may therefore predispose to "respiratory milk allergy."

Gastroesophageal reflux may be more commonly associated with recurrent respiratory infections and asthma than is presently realized, for until recently it was not looked for routinely. In Klotz's[27] original series the surgical cure of reflux was followed by cessation of asthma. More recent studies[34,35] suggest that this is not always the case. The role of surgery has still to be determined. It is tempting to speculate that in some instances foods may cause both the respiratory disease and the reflux.

PATHOGENESIS AND PATHOLOGY

In our understanding of any group of disorders, those which focus on the more severe or extreme examples often provide the most clearcut evidence of both pathogenesis and pathology. The original studies of Heiner and his colleagues,[24] which delineated the syndrome often referred to as Heiner's syndrome, and their recent review,[28] together with the studies of Holland,[25] indicate that though precipitins to cow's milk proteins can occur in normal babies, heavy, multiple precipitin lines correlate closely with severe forms of the disease and, in particular, with pulmonary hemosiderosis due to cow's milk. In the severest forms of the disease, levels of IgG and IgA as a whole are elevated, as are specific IgG and IgA antibodies to cow's milk proteins. There is no increase in either IgM or IgE antibody levels or of specific IgM and IgE antibodies to cow's milk proteins. IgD binding to cow's milk proteins is reduced. This indicates that there is a brisk response of IgG and IgA, but not of IgM, IgE, and IgD to cow's milk proteins.

Heiner and his colleagues[28] also found evidence of type 4 hypersensitivity, for lymphocytes from all patients with evidence of cow's milk protein hypersensitivity responded with significantly greater uptakes of tritiated thimidine than did the controls; the latter were age-matched children with nonimmunologic gastrointestinal and respiratory diseases. There was no significant difference in this parameter between the cow's milk–sensitive children with and without pulmonary hemosiderosis. Lung biopsies, carried out by Kniker in two Mexican-American Indians with milk-related pulmonary hemosiderosis, revealed deposits in the lungs of IgG, C3, and cow's milk proteins.

In addition to the laboratory evidence of immunologic involvement there was clinical evidence: when challenged with cow's milk—Kniker's patients and our own experience—the children responded with fever as well as cough, dyspnea, and pulmonary infiltrates. Their reaction to cow's milk paralleled the expected reaction to an infection and was clinically indistinguishable from one.

Anderson[3] has also carried out detailed studies on a black infant with recurrent pneumonia whose symptoms developed while he was on a cow's milk formula and cleared when he avoided it. This child had an elevated IgE and, on cow's milk challenge, an Arthus type of reaction with complement activation, as well as delayed hypersensitivity, a positive LE preparation, and the development of antibody to extractable nuclear antigen (ENA). Anderson[4] and his colleagues have more recently studied a second, similar child who, in addition to making ENA, made DNA. It would seem that the baby can mount one or all of the immune responses to the proteins in cow's milk, and that immune complexes[13] are not unusual in such babies.

The normal child, having recovered from an infection, viral or otherwise, is rarely troubled by the same infection again, and certainly not for a number of years, for the child's immune system, having been alerted and primed by the first infection, rarely allows the organism when encountered a second time to multiply and cause disease. The immune system cannot distinguish between live and dead antigens, hence the use of killed bacteria and viruses in the production of immunity. Once primed, it can prevent the multiplication of bacteria and viruses previously encountered; it is, however, unable to prevent the accumulation of food antigens that cause respiratory and other diseases, for these are thrust upon the child by well-meaning parents and/or physicians who are unaware that the antigens in the formula are provoking an immune response and are indirectly making the child ill. The question to which we should address ourselves is not why so many children have cow's milk allergy, but how so many children, brought up on liberal amounts of cow's milk, manage to avoid it.

Having made sure that the child with a recurrent wheezy bronchitis does not have cystic fibrosis of the pancreas, an immunological disorder, or gastroesophageal reflux, one should not necessarily assume that the baby's symptoms are being produced by cow's milk. We have seen a similar clinical picture due to the following:

PHYSICAL FACTORS. Most babies become excited at the prospect of being fed and will wave their arms and kick their legs. A few actually wheeze, the infant's counterpart I suspect to exertional asthma. Such infants, if exertion is the prime cause of their wheezing, are quiet when asleep and at such times are free from expiratory rhonchi. Their parents should be reassured and the baby followed. Weather changes such as a fall in barometric pressure and rain occasionally cause wheezing. It is generally thought that babies with a wheezy bronchitis benefit by humidity; this is true of some but not of all.

INHALANTS. House dust, cigarette smoke,[11] feathers, and animal danders seem to be the most troublesome inhalants in infancy; pollens and mold spores cause increasing trouble in the older child. I have, however, been surprised by the importance of chemicals, having encountered babies whose respiratory symptoms were precipitated by fumes from oil furnaces, by propane gas, by chemicals used in the construction of trailers, by plastic materials, and by chemicals such as Fleecy® and Downy®, used in the dryer.

With regard to establishing the diagnosis, this is easy if the infant is sensitive only to cow's milk, for within a few days, or at most three weeks in severe instances, of being taken off cow's milk and placed, for example, on a soya formula, his symptoms will clear. If he is then offered cow's milk in liberal amounts his symptoms will quickly return; he may even become obviously ill with fever, dyspnea, cough, and pulmonary infiltrates. If he is not given cow's milk for several months he may remain symptom-free initially, but if he continues to take cow's milk in liberal amounts his respiratory problems will probaby return.

If the baby sensitive to cow's milk is also sensitive to soya, his symptoms will persist on his new formula. When this is the case, it usually is best to place him only on a suitable water, glucose, and electrolyte solution for two to four days. We do not recommend apple or other fruit juices, for we have seen many babies who have become sensitized to these, developing, commonly, a troublesome diarrhea. If symptoms clear, this is presumptive evidence that the forumla was causing his symptoms. If the baby is still being bottle fed, he may then be offered a meat base formula. The formula may be built up in stages, first substituting sucrose for glucose, then adding a meat (chicken, beef, lamb, or ham), followed by a fat (corn oil, safflower oil, or olive oil), a vitamin preparation, e.g. Poly-Vi-Sol,® and finally, calcium. If, with the addition of any food, rhinorrhea or wheezing returns, an attempt should be made to find a suitable substitute.

It not infrequently happens that a new formula is well tolerated for two to three weeks and then begins to precipitate symptoms, the infant reacting to his new formula in the same way that he reacted to his old. When this happens it is sometimes possible by rotating formulas, for example by giving the child a soya formula on day one, a chicken meat base formula on day two, Nutramigen® on day three, and a lamb base formula on day four, to maintain tolerance. An alternative approach is to place the infant on glucose water and to introduce one new food a day. Foods that are tolerated should be given no more frequently than once every four to five days; foods that are not tolerated should be avoided. In infants who appear to react adversely to most foods, I have occasionally used immunotherapy[30] with appropriate food antigens, sometimes, but by no means always, with seemingly beneficial results.

With regard to long-term management, although it is generally believed that infants grow out of their food allergies, this is not in keeping with the experience of some of the veterans in this field. As Deamer[12] has indicated, when a food to which a child once was sensitive is later reintroduced into his diet, symptoms often return but so slowly and insidiously that their relationship to the food remains unsuspected. It is best, therefore, for the child to avoid taking the food regularly on a permanent basis and to be content with a little intermittently in foods, or if the food is cow's milk, to indulge in an occasional ice cream or piece of cheese only, provided no untoward symptoms arise. If the food is taken only infrequently, tolerance may be maintained. Advertising pressures,[31] together with those of well-meaning nutritionists, however, are such that were a similar lobby to be mounted on behalf of the manufacturers of feather pillows, it would generally be believed that no one, even if he were allergic to feathers, could sleep soundly unless he slept on a feather-containing pillow.

RESPIRATORY FOOD ALLERGIES OF THE DELAYED TYPE IN THE CHILD AND ADULT

In the older child and adult with delayed type of respiratory food allergy, symptoms may mainly involve the upper respiratory tract with repeated colds, croup, sinus infections, "sore throats," and fevers. Sore throats are not usually looked upon as a manifestation of allergy, but throats, not tonsillitis, that literally feel raw and sore associated with pain on swallowing can occur as a result of a food, commonly milk, sensitivity. They are due, I suppose, to pharyngeal involvement. Symptoms also may involve mainly the lower respiratory tract with, in the toddler, recurrent bronchiolitis and even bronchopneumonia, and in the adult recurrent bronchitis.[17] The cough is often preceded by rhinorrhea, the patient may complain of chest colds or of "colds settling on his chest," the rhinorrhea being the nasal manifestation of the allergy. Fevers commonly accompany these illnesses and often are associated with a leukocytosis. They resemble infections and differ in this respect from IgE-mediated attacks of asthma. My experience with adults is limited, but in both the child and the adult symptoms produced by foods are more commonly akin to recurrent or chronic bronchitis than to asthma. Cough and sputum, rather than episodes of wheezing, are the main complaints. The adults do not have the increase in airways resistance that is characteristic of the asthmatic.

With regard to investigations, chest x-rays may show some degree of hyperinflation, with thickening of the bronchial walls, with or without patchy infiltration, segmental collapse (collapse of the right upper lobe is particularly common in infants, for they spend much of their time lying on their backs), and of the right middle lobe in the older child (due to the appropriate bronchus being plugged with thick, tenacious mucus). Prick tests are usually, if not invariably, negative where cow's milk is concerned. Intradermal tests as outlined by Miller (Chapter 10) often are positive and may indicate, if a food is causing symptoms, which food should be suspected. Intradermal tests should also be carried out on the older child and the adult against the inhalants that cause problems locally. Treatment should not be based only on the results of prick and intradermal tests. The allergist, like a detective, takes a careful history, does a thorough physical examination, unearths all the available clues, carries out the necessary tests, sifts the evidence, and then decides on his plan of action, being prepared to re-examine the evidence if his first line of attack is fruitless. He should persist in his endeavors until he has found a solution to his patient's problems and has put the latter on the road to recovery.

With regard to the management of food allergy in children and adults, it is sometimes possible, on the basis of the patient's and the family history, to be fairly certain that a given food is causing symptoms. When this is the case the patient should avoid the food, and if his symptoms settle he should, a week later, once more take the food in question. If symptoms return the food should be avoided, and this is all that may be needed. In most instances, however, it is necessary to carry out preliminary prick, followed by intradermal tests. If these indicate that the patient's symptoms are primarily due to inhalants, and if the findings fit in with the clinical history, environmental control with or without immunotherapy and appropriate medications is all that will be required. If the history and intradermal tests indicate that foods may be playing a part in the patient's symptomatology, it will be necessary to confirm this by avoidance and challenge and then to institute dietary management, with or without appropriate immunotherapy.

REFERENCES

1. Aas, K.: The diagnosis of hypersensitivity to ingested foods. Reliability of skin prick testing and the radioallergosorbent test with different materials. *Clin Allergy, 8*:39, 1978.
2. Allen, J.D., Moss, A.D., Wallwork, J.C., and McFarlane, H.: Immediate hypersensitivity in patients with cystic fibrosis. *Clin Allergy, 5*:255, 1975.
3. Anderson, J.A., Weiss, L., Rebuck, J.W., Cabal, L.A., and Sweet, L.C.: Hyperreactivity to cow's milk in an infant with LE and tart cell phenomenon. *J Pediatr, 84*:59, 1974.
4. Anderson, J.A., Yanari, S.S., Niemes, W.J., Heinzerling, R.H., and Hayashi, H.: Antibodies to DNA in patients with hyperreactivity to cow's milk. *J Allergy Clin Immunol, 63*:182, 1979.
5. Bahna, S.L. and Heiner, D.C.: Cow's Milk Allergy: Pathogenesis,

Manifestations, Diagnosis and Management. In Barness, L.A. (Ed.): *Advances in Pediatrics.* Chicago: Year Bk Med, *25*:1, 1978.

6. Björkstén, F., Backman, A., Järvinen, K.A.J., Lehti, H., Savilahti, E., Syränen, P., and Kärkkäinen, T.: Immunoglobulin E specific to wheat and rye flour proteins. *Clin Allergy, 7*:375, 1977.
7. Buisseret, P.D.: Common manifestations of cow's milk allergy in children. Lancet, *1*:304, 1978.
8. Chua, Y.Y., Bremner, K., Lakdawalla, N., Llobet, J.L., Kokubu, H.L., Orange, R., and Collins-Williams, C.: In vivo and in vitro correlates of food allergy. *J Allergy Clin Immunol, 58*:299, 1976.
9. Chua, Y.Y., Bremner, K., Llobet, J.L., Kokubu, H.L., and Collins-Williams, C.: Diagnosis of food allergy by the radioallergosorbent test. *J Allergy Clin Immunol, 58*:477, 1976.
10. Clein, N.W.: Cow's milk allergy in infants. *Ann Allergy, 9*:195, 1951.
11. Colley, J.R.T., Holland, W.W. and Corkhill, R.T.: Influence of passive smoking and parental phlegm on pneumonia and bronchitis in early childhood. *Lancet, 2*:1031, 1974.
12. Deamer, W.C., Gerrard, J.W. and Speer, F.: Cow's milk allergy: A critical review. *J Family Practice, 9*:223, 1979.
13. Delire, M., Cambiaso, C.L., and Masson, P.L.: Circulating immune complexes in infants fed on cow's milk. *Nature, 272*:632, 1978.
14. Donnally, H.H.: The question of the elimination of foreign protein (egg white) in woman's milk. *J Immunol, 19*:15, 1930.
15. Ellestad-Sayet, J., Coodin, F.J., Dilling, L.A., and Haworth, J.C.: Breast-feeding protects against infection in Indian infants. *Can Med Assoc J, 120*:295, 1979.
16. Frick, O.L., German, D.F., and Mills, J.: Development of allergy in children. I. Association with viral infections. *J Allergy Clin Immunol, 63*:228, 1979.
17. Gerrard, J.W.: Familial recurrent rhinorrhea and bronchitis due to cow's milk. *JAMA, 198*:605, 1966.
18. ———: Allergy in breast-fed babies to ingredients in breast milk. *Ann Allergy, 42*:69, 1979.
19. ———: Oral cromoglycate: Its value in the treatment of adverse reactions to foods. *Ann Allergy, 42*:135, 1979.
20. ———: MacKenzie, J.W.A., Goluboff, N., Garson, J.Z., and Maningas, C.S.: Cow's milk allergy: Prevalence and manifestations in an unselected series of newborns. *Acta Paediatr Scand (Suppl), 234,* 1973.
21. Goldman, A.S., Anderson, D.W., Sellers, W.A., Saperstein, S., Kniker, W.T., and Halpern, S.R.: Milk allergy: 1. Oral challenge with milk and isolated milk proteins in allergic children. *Pediatrics, 32*:425, 1963.
22. Harrison, M.: Sugar malabsorption in cow's milk protein intolerance. *Lancet, 1*:360, 1974.

23. Harrison, M., Kilby, A., Walker-Smith, J., France, N.E., and Wood, C.B.S.: Cow's milk protein intolerance: A possible association with gastroenteritis, lactose intolerance and IgA deficiency. *Br Med J, 1:* 1501, 1976.
24. Heiner, D.C., Sears, J.W., and Kniker, W.T.: Multiple precipitins to cow's milk in chronic respiratory disease. *Am J Dis Child, 103:*634, 1962.
25. Holland, N.H., Hong, R., Davis, N.C., and West, C.D.: Significance of precipitating antibodies to milk proteins in the serum of infants and children. *J Pediatr, 61:*181, 1962.
26. Houston, C.S., Weiler, R.L., and Habbick, B.F.: Severity of lung disease in Indian children. *Can Med Assoc J, 120:*1116, 1979.
27. Klotz, S.D. and Moeller, R.K.: Hiatal hernia and intractable bronchial asthma. *Ann Allergy, 29:*325, 1971.
28. Lee, S.K., Kniker, W.T., Cook, C.D., and Heiner, D.C.: Cow's Milk–Induced Pulmonary Disease in Children. In Barness, L.A. (Ed.): *Advances in Pediatrics.* Chicago: Year Bk Med., *25:*39, 1978.
29. Liu, H.Y., Tsao, M.U., Moore, B., and Giday, Z.: Bovine milk protein–induced intestinal malabsorption of lactose and fats in infants. *Gastroenterology, 54:*27, 1967.
30. Miller, J.B.: *Food Allergy: Provocative Testing and Injection Therapy.* Springfield: Thomas, 1972.
31. Oski, F.A. and Bell, J.D.: *Don't Drink Your Milk.* New York: McKay, 1977.
32. Park, A.E.: A case of hypersensitivity to cow's milk. *Am J Dis Child, 19:*46, 1920.
33. Powell, G.K.: Milk– and soy-induced enterocolitis of infancy. *J Pediatr, 93:*553, 1978.
34. Rachelefsky, G., Byrne, W., Strobel, C., Ament, M., Katz, R., Siegel, S., and Euler, A.: Gastroesophageal reflux and recurrent pulmonary disease in children. *J Allergy Clin Immunol, 61:*138, 1978.
35. Shapiro, G.G., Christie, D.L., Pierson, W.E., Bierman, C.W., and Furukawa, C.T.: Gastroesophageal reflux (GER) in asthmatic children. *J Allergy Clin Immunol, 61:*137, 1978.
36. Shiner, M., Ballard, J., Brook, C.D.G., and Herman, S.: Intestinal biopsy in the diagnosis of cow's milk protein intolerance without acute symptoms. *Lancet, 2:*1060, 1975.
37. Turner, M.W., Warner, J.O., Stokes, C.R., and Norman, A.P.: Immunological studies in cystic fibrosis. *Arch Dis Child, 53:*631, 1978.
38. Upadhyay, Y.N. and Gerrard, J.W.: Recurrent pneumonia in Indian children. *Ann Allergy, 27:*218, 1969.
39. Wraith, D.G., Merrett, J., Roth, A., Yman, L., and Merrett, T.G.: Recognition of food-allergic patients and their allergens by the RAST technique and clinical investigation. *Clin Allergy, 9:*25, 1979.

Chapter 5

CARDIOVASCULAR DISEASE TRIGGERED BY FOODS AND CHEMICALS

WILLIAM J. REA AND CHARLES W. SUITS

INTRODUCTION

THE CONCEPT of immunity is generally perceived as serving two main functions, defense and surveillance. At the turn of the century, Von Pirquet[62] coined the term *allergy* to mean an altered reactivity of the host to commonly occurring substances. In this chapter we shall use the term *allergy* to mean an altered or unusual response to any ingested or inhaled chemical.

We have focussed our attention on the abnormal effects of foods and inhaled chemicals on the cardiovascular system. A broad approach that takes into account the effect of all environmental incitants, whether IgE mediated or not, is essential. This chapter will outline the ecological principles and diagnostic techniques necessary for the recognition of environmentally triggered diseases, the suspected pathophysiology, the broad mechanisms involved in the spectrum of inflammatory vascular disease, and the available laboratory tests. We will give examples of the part played by the environment in inducing disease and will conclude with a section on treatment.

PRINCIPLES

When searching for the etiology of vascular inflammation, one must be familiar with several principles so as to identify specific incitants. Selye[52] originally described the stages of alarm, adaptation, and exhaustion to explain how animals coped with their environment. Adolph[1] further expanded these ideas to include individual differences in response to specific stresses. Rinkel[47] then applied this principle to food susceptibility, but changed the terminology to unmasked, masked, and maladapted. He showed that when an individual avoided for four days in succession a food to which he was sensitive, his symptoms would subside or clear. If he then took this food, his symptoms would return, usually in an acute, clearly defineable, and reproducible form. However, if he were to take the food several times a day for several days, adaptation or masking would again occur, and symptoms would not appear to be related to the food in question. Randolph[41] confirmed these observations and later discovered that inhaled and ingested chemicals reacted similarly.

Patients with recurring or cyclic food and chemical sensitivities often experience biphasic responses to the substances to which they are susceptible. When they first take the food they often have an initial feeling of well-being, or even of euphoria. This is then followed by a return of their symptoms, or withdrawal reactions. To avoid the latter, the patient with food and/or chemical susceptibilities tends to repeatedly eat or inhale the substances to stave off the unpleasant reactions. An addictive eating pattern develops in which each reaction builds on the last, never allowing the body to recover. In doing this, the patient masks the substances to which he is sensitive. The masking process eventually gives way to a stage of exhaustion, and a noncyclic, irreversible disease state develops. This bipolarity of response can be very misleading because the individual often feels euphoric when in contact with the harmful substances. He believes the substances are harmless because he does not realize that his severe reactions when he avoids them are due to withdrawal symptoms. For the above reasons, the effect of the environment in triggering vascular inflammatory disease has often been overlooked.

Triggering agents or incitants can be divided into three major categories: (1) natural inhalants, which include pollens, dusts, mold spores, animal danders, etc. (2) foods and their odors, (3) inhaled or ingested chemicals. Many patients with simple sensitivities or few incitants can be adequately investigated in the physician's office. However, to do this it is nearly always necessary for the office to be appropriately constructed. Those with complex sensitivities can be studied adequately only in environmentally controlled units such as those pioneered by Randolph.[40] The program of provocative challenge with foods and inhalants plays an essential role in determining incitants. The Environmental Unit makes it possible to decrease exposure to fumes and particulates, reducing the total load of the body to these factors.

The Environmental Unit that we have developed is specially constructed so as to be as free as possible from fumes and particulate contamination. After studying more than 300 patients in such a unit, it has become apparent that reactions in very sensitive patients can be triggered by picomolar amounts of outgassing chemicals or particles contained in many building materials.[45] It is, therefore, extremely important to pay attention to details of structure. To treat patients with varying sensitivities, rooms of different types have been designed. The first is constructed with specially painted wallboard and is employed for the least sensitive patients. The second is lined with aluminum, used for moderately sensitive patients. The third type is constructed with ceramic tile and wallboard; these are required for the most sensitive patients, who often have metal sensitivities. The best environmental room is probably one that is constructed of a special porcelain-coated steel. This same material is also used to line the walls of the corridors of our Unit. The ceiling is sealed with a special non-synthetic plaster, which also acts as an acoustical barrier. All building materials used in the Environmental Unit are carefully screened and tested.

The creation of a specialized unit, as described above, reduces the total load of environmental incitants exerted on a patient. A hypothesis that has evolved from the study of patients in such an environment is that of "total body load." This is the sum of all external agents to which the body is exposed. Each individual seems to possess a limited capacity to handle this load, and if he is chemically susceptible, the quantity of incitants that his body can handle may be markedly reduced. One might make the analogy of a barrel. The patient is represented by a barrel, with the brim of the barrel being a reaction threshold (Fig. 5-1). Constant pouring of foods, synthetic chemicals, or common allergens

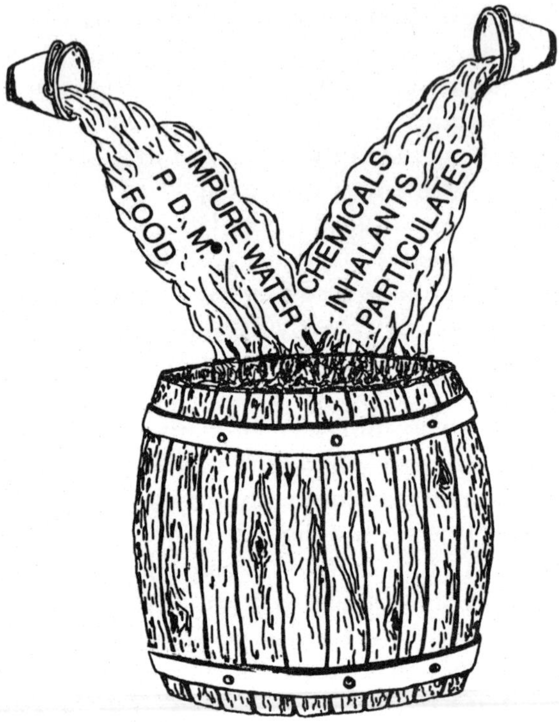

TOTAL BODY LOAD

•pollen, dust, mold

Figure 5-1. Total body load.

to which the patient is susceptible into the barrel causes it eventually to fill to the brim. Continued exposure causes the barrel to overflow and symptoms to be produced.

A major constituent of this total body load is ambient air pollution. Air pollution has long been recognized as potentially dangerous. However, since most research workers are unaware of the concept of the "total body load," they have not taken into account both indoor and outdoor pollution along with foods. Whitby[64] has shown that city air may be 3000 to 4000 times more polluted than sea air. Coupling this fact with increased air pollution on the job, and adding to this the levels of the most contaminated place in our environment, which is the home, one can appreciate the gigantic chemical load that must be handled daily.

It is becoming apparent to us that places of work, including most offices, are often highly "polluted." Attempts to keep them clear often are thwarted because most people are not aware that the total load is not safe, even though the levels of the individual components may be. In one situation in which a patient became ill at work, the total load of the chemicals to which he was exposed was 400 times as great as that in the outside air.[18] Nevertheless, the concentration of each individual chemical was found to be in the federally accepted "safe" normal level. The importance of the total body load cannot be emphasized strongly enough. Apparently, overload will disrupt, and in some patients even destroy, the food handling as well as the chemical handling mechanisms, and it will produce widespread sensitization and illness. An example of this is the patient who cannot tolerate certain foods at home, but who can tolerate them in an area with less air pollution because of the decrease in his overall load. Since the home is where individuals spend most of their time, it is essential to reduce the pollutant load there if the individual is to have a chance to recover. In the susceptible patient, sensitive to chemicals and foods, the home load can usually be reduced by eliminating all gas appliances, including the heating system, foam rubber, synthetic upholstery, and most soft plastics. The patients themselves wear cotton or silk rather than synthetic materials.

AIR

In our Environmental Unit, we constantly monitor the air. Currently, the air quality studies are conducted using 100 ml direct readout gas detector tubes and a particulate fractionator. This system is accurate only to 1 ppm with a standard deviation of 20 percent.[33] It is important to note that some patients react to much lower concentrations. Therefore, future air analyses must be done at the molecular level by gas chromatography, colorimetry, and mass spectrometry. In addition, no one entering the unit wears perfumes of any kind, and of course, no one smokes.

WATER

Chemically contaminated water is another major component of the total environmental load. In a recent analysis in which local city water was compared to various spring waters, city water was shown to contain 1,000 to 30,000 times as many synthetic compounds.[20] Experience has shown that both chlorinated and nonchlorinated waters, including numerous spring, charcoal filtered, and distilled waters, often cause symptoms in chemically sensitive patients. These, if undetected, frequently distort the food and chemical testing. Therefore, spring waters from around the world are used for severely sensitive individuals. Following three days in the controlled environment, double-blind studies are performed to determine the best water for each patient.

DIAGNOSTIC TECHNIQUE

After an acceptable water is found and the patient has cleared his symptoms by fasting for three to seven days in the controlled environment, food testing is started with chemically less contaminated source foods. These are biologically pure foods whose origin is known and include wheat, oats, cane sugar, beet sugar, chicken, duck, turkey, etc. These foods have been grown, stored, and prepared in the relative absence of synthetic chemicals. They are given to the patient one at a time, and no more than three foods are given in any one day. Any adverse reactions are carefully noted. Adverse reactions can be confirmed by double-blind Levine's tube challenge. Gelatin capsules also may be used, but their suitability is limited by the volumes they contain and the frequency with which they can be given. Individuals being tested also may be or may become sensitive to the substances, beef or pork, from which the gelatin is made. Repetition of a positive challenge on three separate occasions is accepted as evidence of food susceptibility.

When sixteen tolerated foods have been identified, this allows a four-day rotation of four different foods a day; the patient is rechallenged with the same foods but this time acquired from a commercial market. These foods are often contaminated by preservatives, additives, plastic packaging, or pesticides. They may also be contaminated in preparation by natural gas stoves or from the Teflon® from a frying pan.

At the conclusion of food testing, double-blind studies are conducted on most potential inhalant chemical incitants, using ambient doses. These include alcohol, phenol, formaldehyde, pesticides, perfumes, chlorine, synthetic fabrics, and work chemicals. Testing is done in a specially constructed stainless steel and glass booth for a maximum of fifteen minutes for each chemical. Natural gas challenge is done by exposing the patient to a gas pilot light.

Objective measurements to substantiate clinical observations have been developed. Through constant monitoring of the homeostatic mechanism, including the immune, mediator, and enzymatic systems, one is better able to assess the efficacy of the less chemically contaminated environment. Laboratory parameters can be observed returning to within normal limits during the period of environmental control (Figs. 5-2 through 5-5). All tests are performed at the time of the patient's entrance into the Environmental Unit and at the beginning and end of testing. In addition to routine blood counts, SMA-22, and clotting studies, the following laboratory tests are performed on each patient: protein electrophoresis by the cellulose acetate method (Helena Labs); quantitative immunoglobulins; complement components C_3 and C_4; alpha$_1$-antitrypsin; C-reactive protein by the radial immunodiffusion method (Behring); total hemolytic serum complement (CH_{100} and CH_{50}) and serum complement components using differential reagents and sensitized sheep erythrocytes (Cordis); C-1-esterase inhibitor by immunoelectrophoresis (Behring); B-lymphocytes; and T-lymphocytes by the sheep red cell rosetting method.

The assays have helped in the diagnosis and identification of environmentally triggered diseases. Kinetic monitoring during challenge testing allows the investigator to observe fluctuations of the immune response and of some mediator systems. The author's previous studies have shown transient changes of several parameters following incitant challenge (Figs. 5-6 through 5-9). There is no set pattern of response, but patients who enter the Environmental Unit often have reduced numbers of T-lymphocytes; these

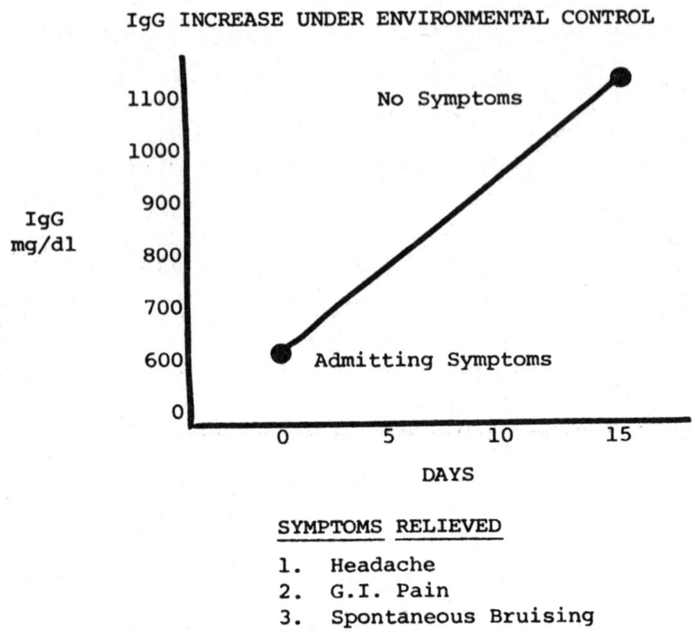

Figure 5.2. IgG rise in Environmental Unit.

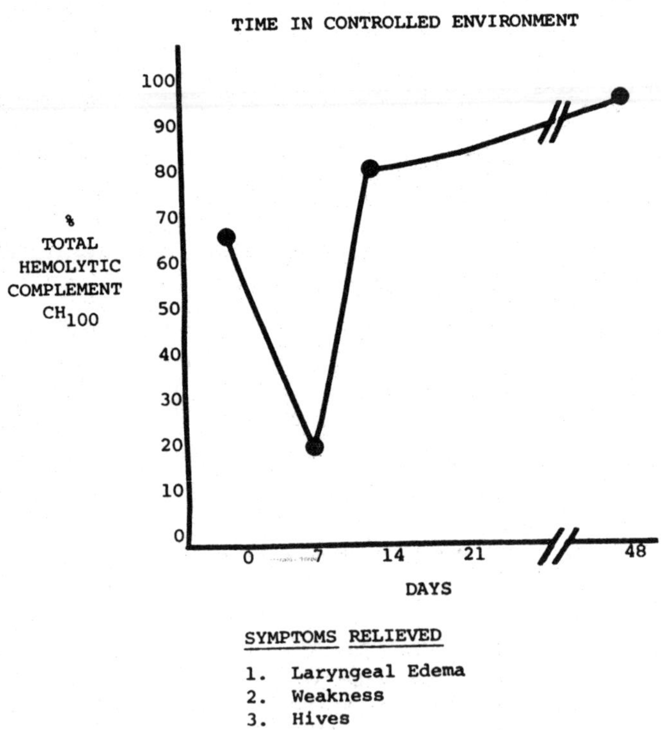

Figure 5-3. Hemolytic complement rise in Environmental Unit.

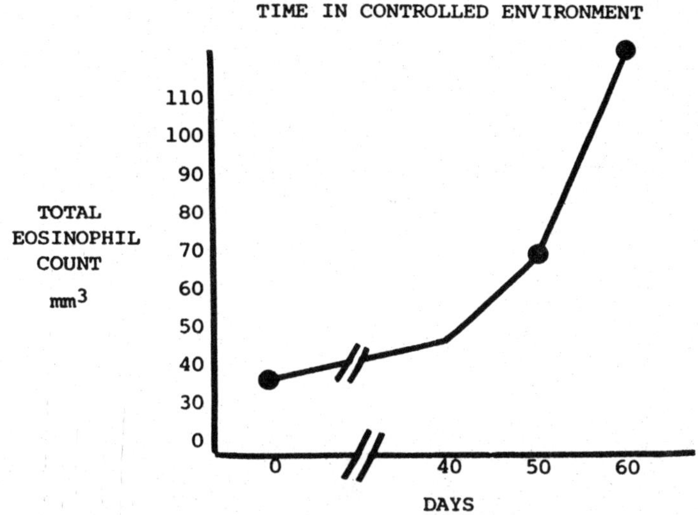

SYMPTOMS RELIEVED

1. Arrhythmia
2. G.I. Upset
3. Confusion

Figure 5-4. Eosinophil count rise in Environmental Unit.

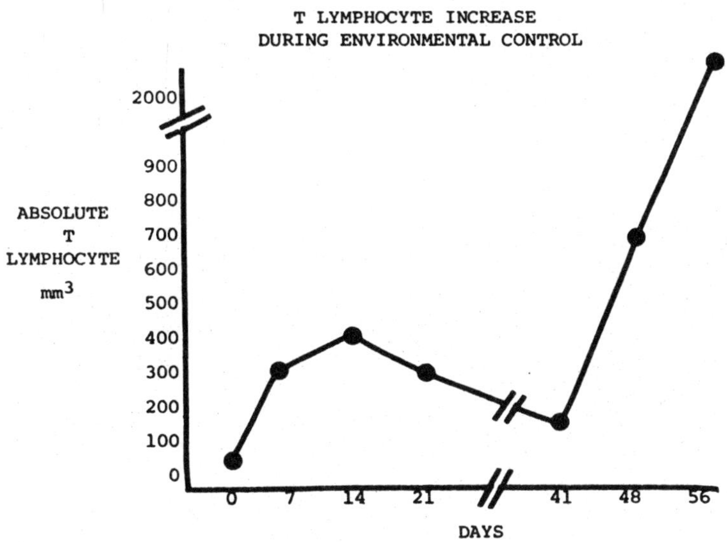

SYMPTOMS RELIEVED

1. Speech Difficulty
2. Fugue-like States
3. Depression

Figure 5-5. T-lymphocyte rise in Environmental Unit.

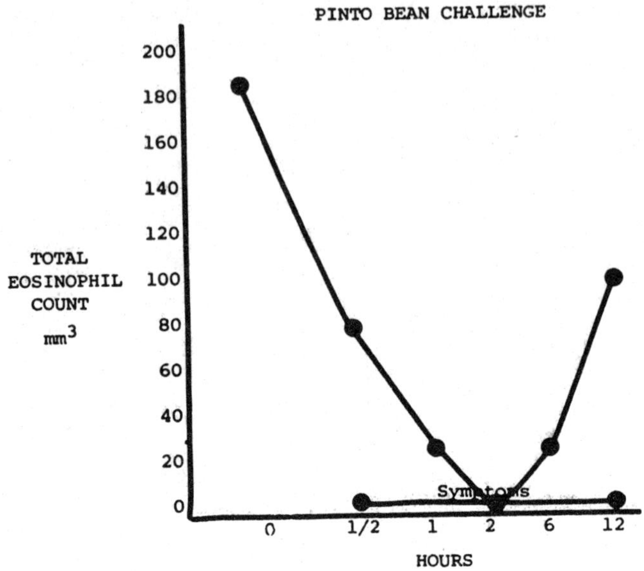

SYMPTOMS REPRODUCED

1. Depression
2. Generalized Edema

Figure 5-6. Eosinophil fall on food challenge.

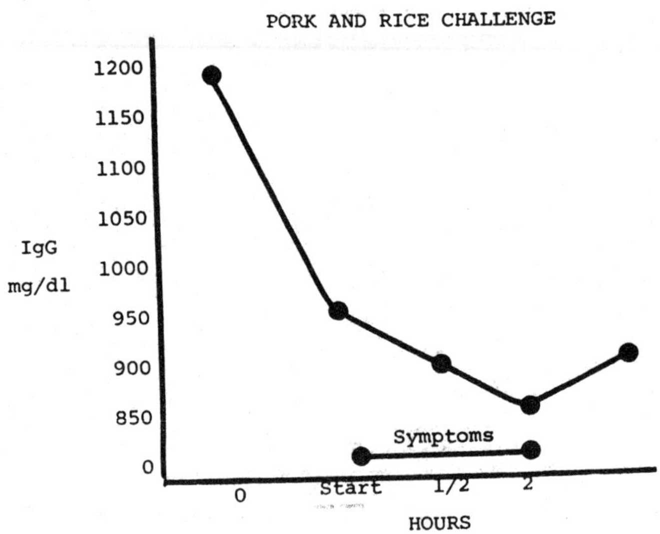

SYMPTOMS REPRODUCED

1. Edema
2. Headache
3. Peripheral Arterial Spasm
4. Peripheral Cyanosis

Figure 5-7. IgG fall on food challenge.

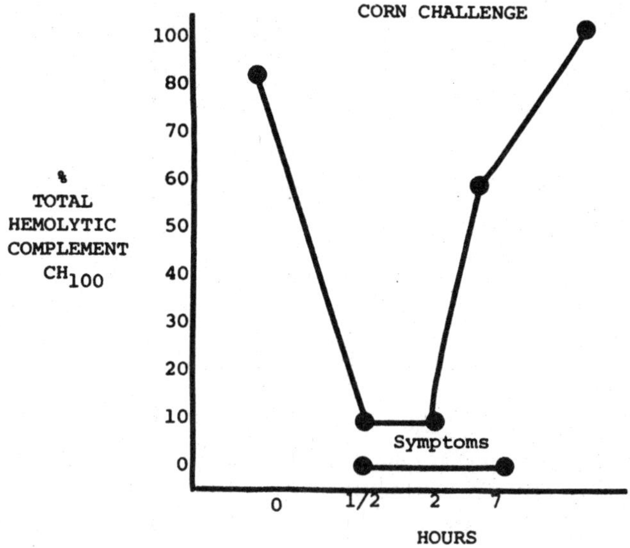

SYMPTOMS REPRODUCED

1. Headache
2. Depression
3. Edema
4. Spontaneous Bruising

Figure 5-8. Hemolytic complement fall during food challenge.

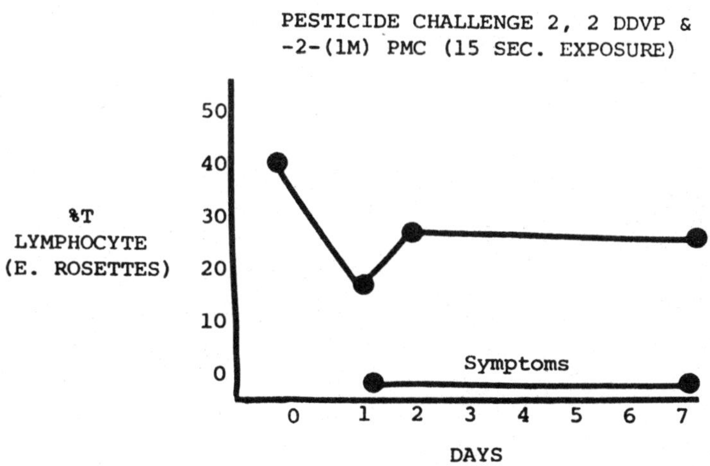

SYMPTOMS REPRODUCED

1. Coronary Spasm
2. Peripheral Vascular Spasm
3. Gastrocolic Spasm
4. Spontaneous Bruising

Figure 5-9. T-lymphocyte fall on inhalant challenge.

return rapidly to normal during the patient's initial fasting period. More than 80 percent of patients experience a drop in their circulating eosinophil level when challenged with an incitant. This is contrary to the eosinophilia commonly found in IgE-mediated reactions. Eosinophilia is observed, however, in most of the asthmatics we have studied, and in them eosinophils rise on incitant challenge. The exact mechanism underlying the decrease in our nonasthmatic patients is unclear, but the drop often parallels concurrent decrease in circulating IgG and/or complement. Complement activation is observed in approximately 40 percent of the patients. Kinins, prostaglandins and other mediators need to be monitored as tests become available. Buisseret[12] et al. have shown changes in prostaglandin levels after challenge with mollusks.

ETIOLOGY

It is clear that the bulk of research has focussed on the study of infectious agents as causative factors in the triggering of abnormal vascular responses. It is well known that streptococci, gonococci, meningococci and hepatitis B virus can cause vasculitis,[34] but chemicals in the form of drugs can also cause abnormal vascular reactivity.[34,38] Sometimes symptoms are mild, for example, local itching, urticaria, and localized edema;[26] sometimes they are more severe.[9,30] Daughters[17] et al. reported studies on a sixty-eight-year-old female who developed an uriticarial and anaphylactoid reaction after topical application of chlorethamine hydrochloride. Intracutaneous testing with chlorethamine produced a wheal and flare reaction. The patient had used this chemical intermittently for the previous five years without any hypersensitivity reactions. Delayed hypersensitivity was reported with neomycin, bacitracin, and penicillin ointments.

The effects of foods and inhaled or ingested chemicals on disease processes are rarely suspected or mentioned in most discussions on environmental influences because of the lack of understanding of the principles mentioned earlier in this chapter.

MECHANISMS OF INFLAMMATION

It will be helpful to examine briefly the mechanisms underlying vascular inflammation. For the purpose of this review, vasculitis will connotate any inflammation that primarily begins in the walls of the blood vessel (Fig. 5-10). Vascular inflammation can result from one or more of the following: (1) direct infection of blood vessels by microbial agents, (2) deposition of antigen-antibody complexes in vessel walls, (3) alteration of a native component of the vessel so that it becomes antigenic and induces humoral or cellular immunity, or (4) deposition of an antigenic foreign substance within the vessel wall resulting in immunologic attack.

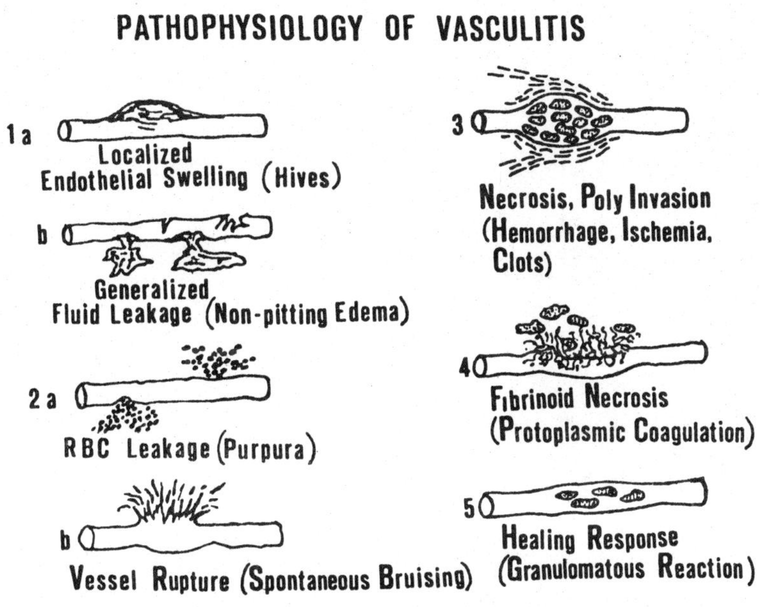

Figure 5-10. Pathophysiology of vasculitis.

Inflammation can result from direct mediator activation, i.e. activation of the alternate complement pathway, or Hageman factor activation generating kallikrein and kinin. Once inflammation is instituted in the vessel wall, various pathologic responses occur.[2] There is frequently an overload phenomenon, which causes the body's normal defense mechanisms to be broken down or altered. This overload may be triggered by infections, foods, or chemicals. Physiologically, this initial step between incitant and defense breakdown leading to inflammation still is not well understood. Nevertheless, once homeostasis has been disrupted, any of the aforementioned mechanisms can be triggered, resulting in vascular inflammation. Often, early stages of triggering are reversible by withdrawal of incitants, but following years of constant overexposure, or an acutely massive incitant overload coupled with individual susceptibility, irreversible vasculitis may occur. The disease then appears to be self-perpetuating.

The symptoms depend on the size, number, and location of the vessels involved, together with the quantity and number of the triggering substances. Pathologically, the degree of vasculitis depends on the extent to which the vascular wall is affected. Zeek[60] has delineated a pathologic classification and stages of vasculitis that encompass the various clinical entities observed (Fig. 5-11).

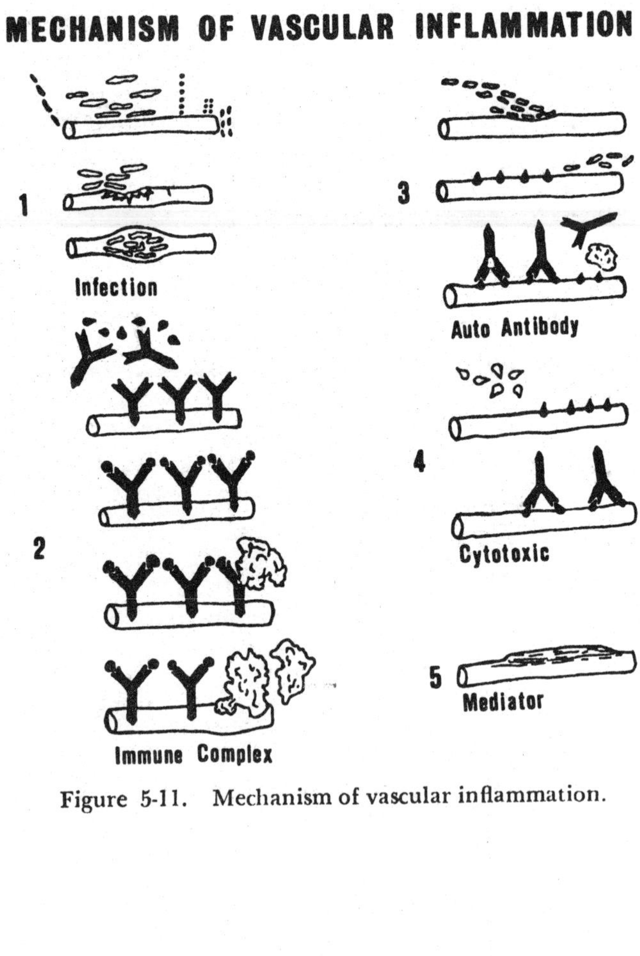

Figure 5-11. Mechanism of vascular inflammation.

Stage 1 vasculitis involves an increase in vascular permeability with consequential endothelial swelling. This can result in localized or generalized edema, the extent depending on the number of vessels involved. Localized edema is usually manifested as urticaria and is well recognized. Generalized edema (some patients will gain or lose 5 kg in weight in twenty-four hours) is often not recognized for what it is, and is less well understood.

Stage 2 presents a greater increase in vascular permeability with the escape of red cells into the perivascular spaces, often associated with perivascular monocellular infiltration. Patients present with purpura, spontaneous bruising, and/or petechiae.

Stage 3 is characterized by ulceration of the vessel wall, with infiltration and swelling of the endothelium. Occlusion may occur following vessel wall necrosis and platelet aggregation. Thrombosis is common with resulting hemorrhagic necrosis and ischemia. Apparently, the more acute leukocytoclastic inflammation occurs here.

Stage 4 is classified as fibrinoid necrosis. This is commonly precipitated by infarction and is characterized by protoplasmic coagulation. Small amounts of fibrin or fibrinoid material are seen microscopically in the necrotic areas.

Stage 5 represents the proliferative, healing response. This is characterized by an increased number of perivascular fibroblasts. Granulomatous reactions as well as plaque formation may occur.

The important feature of this classification is that there is a wide range of vessel wall involvement from localized edema to organ necrosis. Several investigators have elaborated on these classifications. Parish[36] has divided the pathology into the monocytic and leukocytoclastic types. Gilliam[19] later elaborated on Zeek's and Parish's classification of the leukocytoclastic types. The clinical manifestations of leukocytoclastic vasculitis have been more thoroughly investigated than the etiology. It appears that the leukocytoclastic, as defined by Parish, may be the more severe of the two types.

INCITANTS

As already mentioned, an increase in the total body load of any or all of the common environmental substances may disrupt the ability of the body to handle adequately pollens, dusts, mold spores and foods; this allows vascular inflammation to occur. Edema, hemorrhage, spasm, and dilation may follow. The symptoms will depend on the size and location of the blood vessels.

Theorell[60] et al. reported their observations on a thirty-two-year-old female and a forty-year-old male with cutaneous vasculitis. They demonstrated positive allergic responses to foods and airborne allergens in both patients. Laboratory analysis of skin biopsies revealed IgG and C_3 deposition in the vascular wall, apparently resulting in cutaneous vasculitis. We also have studied patients, including ten with Raynaud's disease, whose vascular symptoms were triggered by the inhalation of pollens, dusts, and mold spores.[46] These studies were confirmed using controlled inhalation tests and the intracutaneous injections of individual pollen, dust, and mold extracts. The extent to which these substances affect the vascular tree is unclear, but sensitivity to molds appears to be a major factor in causing inflammatory vascular disease.

An ever increasing portion of the total load of incitants influencing the vascular tree are the synthetic chemicals. Nour-Eldin[35] found the affinity of the vessel wall to phenol to be fifteen times greater than that of any other tissue in the body. That plastics are largely phenol derivatives and are the products that outgas the most makes this observation highly relevant. Both inhalation of chemical odors and ingestion of chemicals in food and water appear to have a major influence on how blood vessels react. Chemical toxins such as benzenes and toluenes are known to cause irreversible immunodeficiencies due to bone marrow suppression, while milder doses apparently cause vascular alterations. Combinations of urethane and toluene produce one of the most highly sensitizing groups of chemicals, the isocyanates. Many chemical substances such as formaldehyde, polyvinyl chloride, and acetone have been shown to trigger the kinin system, which can use the smooth muscle of the vascular tree as its target organ.[6] Perhaps different environmental incitants can trigger other immune mediators. Microaneurysms of digital arteries have been reported in a large number of vinyl chloride workers.[15]

Many of my previous studies, conducted in a rigidly controlled environment relatively free from fumes and particles, also have shown activation of the complement system following ambient dose chemical challenge with resultant abnormal vascular response. These responses have spanned the spectrum of inflammatory vascular disease.

We will now examine some defined clinical entities and then focus our attention on various affected portions of the body. Emphasis will be placed on symptoms that pathologically fall into Stage 1 and 2, since these are much more commonly observed by the general physician and are more easily preventable. Perhaps control of these can prevent advanced irreversible disease.

Historically, patients with early vascular disease often have bizarre symptoms such as fleeting aches and pains, frequently misinterpreted as being psychosomatic. Symptoms often fluctuate for years before becoming fixed. The vascular tree is so vast and dynamic that malfunction of any part can cause both local and segmental dysfunction. Patients may present with complaints localized to one side of the body or to one limb. Frequently, symptoms do not fit comfortably into segmental nervous system distribution, but can be explained in terms of vascular dysfunction to many nerves at one time. Hypothalamic regulation may also be disturbed.[7]

In what follows, we have given examples of diseases triggered by exposure to foods and chemicals. These diseases have involved the central nervous system: migraine, hemiparesis, seizures, and spells of apnea; the vascular system: vasculitis, periarteritis nodosa, and cardiac arrhythmias; and systemic disorders such as rheumatoid arthritis and lupus erythematosus. In all these examples, the vascular system has been directly or indirectly involved. All disease states have responded to environmental control, suggesting that at least in some patients with these disorders the diseases have arisen as a result of "faulty" interaction between the environment and the patient. They all might well be called "maladaptation syndromes."

STAGE 1 AND 2

These stages appear to be reversible; they can be considered to be pre-disease stages. They can occur after a brief massive exposure to an incitant, but more usually occur as a result of repeated multiple exposures to one or more low level incitants.

It has long been recognized that food is a causative agent in certain clinical manifestations of abnormal small vessel reactivity. Hare,[24] in the early 1900s, first observed peripheral vascular phenomena following withdrawal and subsequent rechallenge with certain foods.

Most reports of localized vasculitis describe various manifestations of urticaria. These may be of a "fixed food" or IgE-mediated type in that urticaria is produced whenever the food is eaten no matter how long the food is avoided. Frequently, however, urticaria is triggered by multiple incitants, including cold and heat, and this susceptibility may even be cyclical. A common offending group of agents involved in at least a third of the cases has been salicylates and related compounds.[54] British investigators have suggested that certain molds, especially *Monilia* and *Alternaria,* may also cause urticaria.[48] The complexity of the triggering agents is often overlooked, and the urticaria is sometimes unjustly classified as emotional.

In the course of treating over 300 patients with vasculitis, we have observed a common manifestation of Stage 1 to be a mild, cyclical, frequently generalized edema. This entity is not well recognized and is poorly understood, but Randolph,[42] Rowe,[49] Brown,[11] Rinkel,[47] and Rea[45] have shown that it can be caused by a sensitivity to multiple foods and chemicals. Sandberg's[50] studies on edematous nephrotic and non-nephrotic patients have further confirmed this impression. This mild, generalized edema may precede more advanced stages of vasculitis.

One well-documented manifestation of Stage 2 vasculitis is nonpalpable purpura where simple vascular leakage occurs, allowing extravasation of red blood cells into the subcutaneous tissue or mucous membranes. Purpura is commonly classified as: (1) thrombocytopenic, associated with a significant reduction in the number of platelets, and (2) nonthrombocytopenic, in which platelet levels are normal, and bleeding is the result either of qualitative platelet abnormalities or of vascular disorders. Either form may result from environmental overload. Infectious purpura has been well described in standard texts and will not be discussed here.

Evidence for susceptibility to environmental triggering agents as a cause of purpura is growing. Quick[39] described purpura produced by the ingestion of certain drugs that act as haptens when combined with blood platelets. Siroty[55] described patients with quinine-induced purpura, or the "Gin and Tonic Syndrome." This syndrome was described originally by Belkin[5] when he noted purpuric manifestations in patients after drinking alcoholic beverages. He later was able to link the purpric manifestations to the quinine used in the preparation of the drinks.

Parish[30] described other patients with C-reactive protein in the vascular lesions and rheumatoid factor in the blood. Marquez-Julio[31] et al. described the occurrence of an acidotic state in patients with vascular purpura. These patients also commonly demonstrated hypergammaglobulinemia.

Usually, Stage 2 vasculitis is manifested as cutaneous bruising, petechiae, and edema. For example, a fifty-eight-year-old white female seen by us[46] presented with a nine-year history of recurrent dragging of her right foot. Physical examination revealed extensive noninflammatory purpura, eczema, petechiae, and spontaneous bruising. The patient was admitted to the Environmental Unit. Her symptoms subsided following a five-day fast, at which time challenge food testing was begun. Banana, chicken, honey, avocado, corn, cantaloupe, codfish, and beef each given individually produced headache within five minutes, followed by severe right-sided pain and spontaneous bruising, culminating in widespread noninflammatory purpura. Angiography (Fig. 5-12) revealed spasm of the peripheral arteries. Early on we were able to clear ten patients with cutaneous vasculitis and reproduce their edema and petechiae by challenging them with simple foods and chemicals. Biopsies always showed monocellular infiltrates, usually in the precapillary arterioles, but often also in the venules. We have now studied over 150 patients. Inhalation and intracutaneous injection of pollen, mold, and dust extracts have triggered both local and generalized vasculitis in these patients.

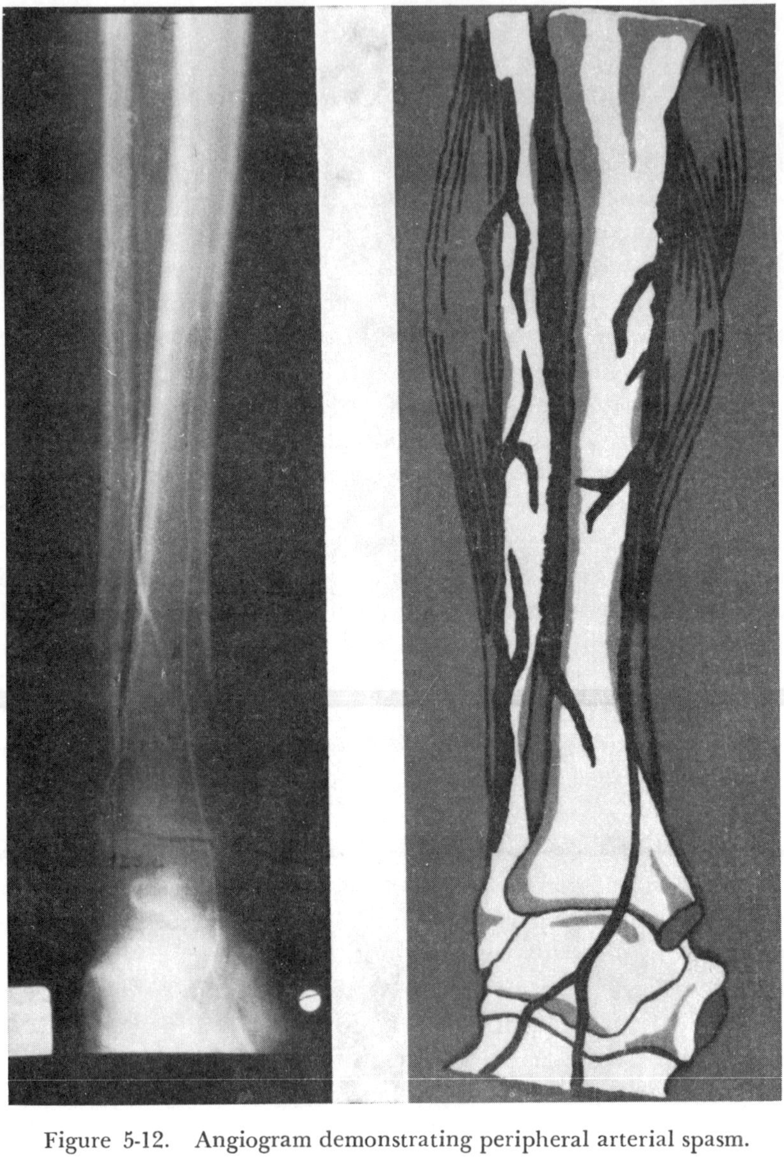

Figure 5-12. Angiogram demonstrating peripheral arterial spasm.

1. Migraine

Vascular headaches probably are caused by abnormal reactivity of one or more of the intra- and extracranial branches of the carotid artery with associated mild edema of adjacent tissues. Although the etiology of most vascular headaches is unknown, some precipitating factors have been identified. Among these are foods[61] and, less commonly, pollens, dusts, molds, weather changes, and sunshine. In 1953, Randolph[41] first demonstrated migraine induced by the fumes of natural gas and paint. Selby and Lance[51] found that fatty foods, chocolate, and oranges were the most common foods to cause migraine in the patients they studied. The subject has been well reviewed by Speer.[56]

In 1963, Blackwell[8] reported that patients given monoamine oxidase inhibitors (MAOI) occasionally developed severe headaches after eating cheese and other foods. Later, Hanington[22] and others linked the attacks of migraine to the high levels of tyramine contained in these foods. In the presence of MAOI, tyramine and other monoamines are absorbed directly into the bloodstream without being broken down. The monoamines then enter the cranial blood vessels and produce headache through their vascular effect. Double-blind studies by Hanington,[23] using tyramine and lactose placebo, reinforced the role of monoamines in the etiology of migraine. In a later study by the same group, 500 patients with dietary migraine were examined. It was found that chocolate, cow's milk and dairy products, citrus fruits, and alcohol were the four foods that most consistently precipitated attacks. All these foods contain high levels of tyramine and phenylethylamine. In a survey of 2,313 spontaneous migraine attacks, Dalton[16] substantiated the role of these foods. During this study, a relationship was noted between food sensitivity and hormonal fluctuations in women taking oral contraceptives. Grant[21] confirmed the observation that women taking oral contraceptives were more likely to experience migraine; she additionally implicated cigarette smoke. Although cranial vessels could not be biopsied, she demonstrated vascular changes in uterine biopsies.

Lord, Duckworth, and Charlesworth,[28] in a study on serum complement levels, have demonstrated significant reductions in

C_4 and C_5 levels during attacks of migraine. The changes in C_4 suggest that complement is activated via the classical pathway. Our studies have shown that both foods and chemical agents can activate the complement system in this type of patient, but as C_4 is often elevated, the alternate pathway may also be involved.

The recent studies of Miller,[32] Rea,[44] Randolph,[42] and Rapp[43] have independently established that any food, as well as food odors and chemicals, can trigger the cerebrovascular response of migraine in susceptible patients, symptoms clearing following avoidance of incitants or appropriate immunotherapy. The following is an example.

CASE 1. A forty-nine-year-old, white female who had been employed as a factory worker in a plant that produces trichloroethylene adhesives was admitted to the Environmental Unit. She had had headaches and sinusitis for two years prior to admission to the unit. She also had had occasional spells of hoarseness, chest pains, edema, spontaneous bruising, and abdominal bloating. Following an eight-day fast with spring water her symptoms cleared, and ingestion food testing was begun. Her symptoms were reproduced by turkey, carrots, pecans, blackberries, lamb, rice, oats, apricots, and asparagus. Challenge with safe foods in chemically contaminated commercial form produced severe headache, fatigue, weakness, mental confusion, eye pain, and chest pain. Symptoms also were reproduced following exposure to phenol, methyl alcohol, cigarette smoke, formaldehyde, and insecticide. Debilitating headache was produced following exposure to trichloroethylene. She is presently well and symptom-free while living in a chemically less contaminated environment. We have, to date, cleared thirty patients with severe vascular headaches, using rigid food and chemical avoidance and food neutralization injection therapy.

2. *Hemiparesis*

Neurovascular involvement, however, causes much more than headaches. General malaise, dizziness, fatigue, occasional paralysis, seizures, and even cerebral apnea have been observed in these patients. Some even have mental symptoms such as hyperactivity, depression, and paranoia. The following is an illustration of severe cerebrovascular spasm resulting in hemiplegia.

CASE 2. A thirty-one-year-old, white female had a history of asthma since childhood. She had been employed as an occupational therapist for eight years prior to current hospitalization. Four years before admission she had had several transient ischemic attacks. This had left her with right-sided weakness, repetitive motor behavior, and an inability to form words properly. Later she developed occasional facial drooping, which became more frequent as time progressed, culminating in transient right-sided paralysis. Following admission to the Environmental Unit and a four-and-one-half-day fast, she lost all her admitting symptoms. Twenty-four out of 40 foods tested in less chemically contaminated form reproduced these symptoms. Challenge test with one meal of commercially available foods reproduced her general weakness and facial paralysis, as well as headache, hoarseness, and nausea. All symptoms were reproduced following test exposure to ambient doses of natural gas, phenol, formaldehyde, insecticide, alcohol, and chlorine. She was discharged without medications on foods to which she had no reactions. She was also instructed to avoid as many synthetic chemicals as possible. She has remained relatively symptom-free for the past nine months.

3. Seizures

Seizures are not usually considered to be triggered by food or chemicals, but it has become increasingly clear to the author that under certain circumstances they can. The following is an example.

CASE 3. A twenty-nine-year-old, white male entered the Environmental Unit with a chief complaint of seizures. He had had fainting spells and seizures for the previous four years. Other symptoms included double vision, tachycardia, dizziness, edema, and spontaneous bruising. He was employed as a bookkeeper and had been a heavy smoker prior to the onset of these attacks. Electroencephalograms were completely normal. He had been placed on Dilantin® and other anticonvulsants prior to referral to us. His seizures were only partially controlled. Following a six-and-one-half-day fast, his symptoms cleared. Subsequent challenge with pork, cane sugar, milk, eggs, brazil nuts, corn, chicken, green peas, and raisins reproduced admitting symptoms. Grand mal seizures were reproduced following a double-blind Levine's tube rechallenge with peanuts, as well as with the intradermal injections of extracts of egg, chicken, corn, and peanut. Exposure to cigarette smoke and phenolated compounds also precipitated his seizures. Laboratory changes accompanied the challenges.

We have encountered four other patients with a history of similar seizures in which triggering agents have been identified. Mackarness[29] has also induced seizures with the sublingual ingestion of foods, and has recorded this in an excellent film.

4. Apneic Spells

Occasionally, environmental triggering can be so severe as to result in death. The frequency of this type of reaction is unknown, but it may be more common than most think. Two patients have been studied, both of whom had a peripheral vasculitis, who developed respiratory arrest with food challenge. The following case is an example.

CASE 4. A fifty-year-old, white female who was employed as a cosmetic salesperson had a thirty-year history of vascular headaches and a twenty-year history of recurrent sinusitis and shortness of breath. Headaches were triggered by exposure to perfumes, hair sprays, cigarette smoke, and pesticides. Treatment with Cafergot® gave no relief. Two years before admission to the Environmental Unit she had noted cramping abdominal pain related to certain foods, ingested chemicals, and inhaled odors. She had experienced rapid weight gain and the development of severe respiratory distress six months before current hospitalization.

On physical examination, edema and mild peripheral cyanosis were noted in fingers and toes. Petechiae and non-nodular bruising were observed on the arms and legs. Biopsy showed lymphocytic infiltrates around a venule. In the Environmental Unit her symptoms cleared following a seven-day fast. She was then challenged with individual foods. A total of eighteen foods were tested, all of which reproduced admitting symptoms. Challenge with cantaloupe during the tests produced apnea, which lasted for five minutes. At the conclusion of food testing, the patient was tested intradermally with extracts of pollens, dust, and mold spores. During the course of skin testing, near apnea was experienced following injections with dilute extracts of marsh elder, mountain cedar, and alternaria. At the time of discharge, she replaced her natural gas heating and appliances with electricity to further lower her chemical load.

The etiology of the apnea in the two patients studied is unknown. Blood gases and pulmonary function studies at the beginning of the spells suggested a central nervous system reaction, perhaps localized to the respiratory center. An alternative hypothesis would involve some disturbance of the autonomic nervous system.

5. Vasculitis Associated with Muscle Pain

Environmentally triggered large vessel vasculitis can be an isolated entity or, more often, it can be accompanied by additional symptoms due to sensitization of the smooth muscle of the respiratory, gastrointestinal, or genitourinary tracts. Frequently, other parts of the vascular system, ranging from the heart to the precapillary arterioles and postcapillary venules, are involved.

Rea[46] has published details of twelve patients with environmentally triggered large vessel vasculitis. The following is an illustrative case report.

CASE 5. A forty-one-year-old, female vocational nurse reported a 20-year history of vague complaints associated with fatigue and mild muscle aches, and a two-year history of near-incapacitating lower extremity arterial spasm, which resulted in absent dorsalis pedis and posterior tibial pulses. She developed incapacitating spasm of the left gastrocnemius and required narcotics and antispasmodics to relieve the unrelenting, painful spasms. Liver toxicity developed from the antispasmodics. She had a history of sensitivity to chemical inhalants such as chlorine, perfumes, pesticides, and cigar smoke, and also to various drugs. The history and clinical course suggested environmentally triggered disease. She was placed in the Environmental Unit. After six days without food or medication, all signs and symptoms cleared. When a safe water was found, she was challenged singly with chemically less contaminated foods. A typical example of the sequence of her reactions was as follows: two bites of squash gave immediate vomiting, then generalized aching and malaise and, within five minutes, aching of legs with spasm and loss of dorsalis pedis and posterior tibial pulses. Within the next five minutes, severe left pedal and gastrocnemius muscle spasm (Fig. 5-13) occurred with excruciating pain that required intravenous sodium bicarbonate and narcotics for relief. Within the next twelve hours, noncontact cutaneous bruising occurred. The muscle and vessel spasm lasted for between 24 and 144 hours. Twelve different foods reproduced these same sequential symptoms.

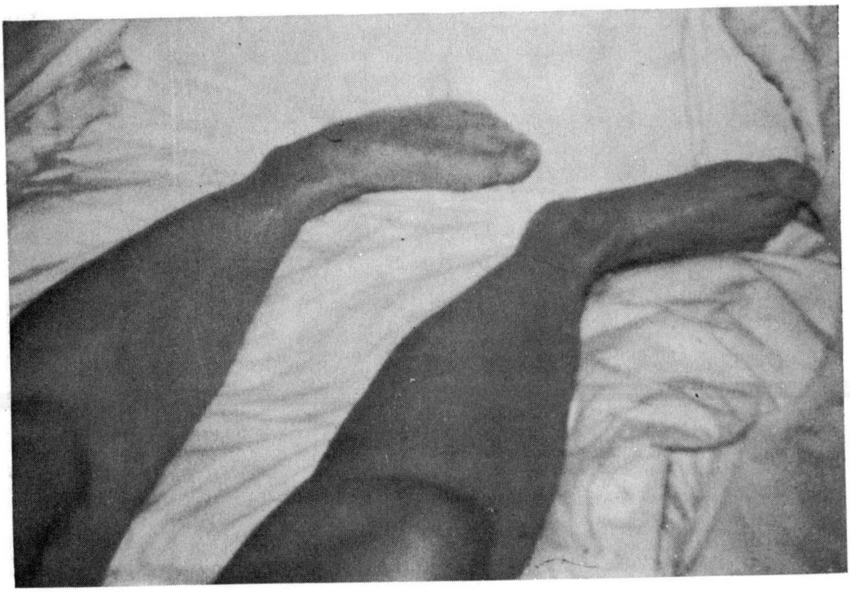

Figure 5-13. Case 5. Spasm of left gastrocnemius and foot.

6. Vasculitis—Recurrent Phlebitis

Another form of Stages 1 and 2 vasculitis starts as recurrent phlebitis and frequently develops into capillary and/or arterial involvement over a period of months to years. Descriptions of these patients are rare in the early literature. Harkavy[25] discussed two patients whose phlebitis was triggered by fish and citrus fruits. The authors have treated a series of patients with environmentally triggered phlebitis and have isolated triggering agents in these patients while in the Environmental Unit (Table 5-1). From long-term follow-up studies on these patients, it has become apparent that phlebitis in some patients is only part of a more generalized and severe vasculitis. The following case follows the progression of the disease from phlebitis to systemic vasculitis.

Case 6. A fifty-four-year-old, female beauty operator was first seen in July, 1975. She presented with pain and swelling in her left leg, and a six-month history of thrombophlebitis. She had been admitted to another hospital with influenza and gastrointestinal symptoms one and a half years prior to current hospitalization. She had for several years experienced recurring ear, nose, and throat infections. Her phlebitis was being treated with anticoagulants, with a measure of relief. She entered the Environmental Unit with active phlebitis. Following a seven-day fast, all her symptoms cleared. Her phlebitis returned following challenge with apples, oranges, and milk, and exposure to natural gas, methyl alcohol, and floor wax. She was discharged eating safe foods and was well, after having cleaned up her home environment, six months after discharge. At this time, she suffered a spider bite and developed pain in her right hip and leg. Shortly thereafter she began to experience dizziness. She was then admitted to her local hospital, where constant chemical exposures apparently caused her condition to deteriorate. She was readmitted to the Environmental Unit with severe hip and leg pain, purpura, and gastrointestinal upset. At this time her T-lymphocyte level was 25 percent of normal. Her symptoms cleared following a five-day fast, and within a week her T-lymphocyte level had returned to within normal limits. She was discharged on a rotary diet of her safe foods. During the following year, repeated inadvertent chemical exposures caused her condition to repeatedly return. In September, 1977, she was readmitted to the Environmental Unit with acute vasculitis. She complained of generalized neck, hip, and leg pain; spontaneous bruising, joint stiffness; petechiae; muscle cramps; and vaginal bleeding.

The basic mechanisms underlying this type of smooth muscle involvement are unclear. However, it appears that continued incitant exposures may lead to progressive vascular disease in sensitive patients. That this patient's symptoms cleared when she

TABLE 5-I

PATIENTS WITH ENVIRONMENTALLY TRIGGERED PHLEBITIS

Age	Anticoagulant	Pulmonary	Episodes of	Caval Interruption	Substances to which sensitive	Signs & Symptoms	Phlebitis Reproduced by
1. 33 W.F.	C	3	20	+	Beef, chicken, cigarette smoke, shrimp, pork, gas heat, ingested chemicals	Diarrhea, pulse increased 30 b/m, nasal stuffiness, bigemeny, multifocal premature ventricular contractions	Pork, shrimp, inhaled chemicals
2. 26 W.F.	C	3	8	+	Wheat, rice, inhaled chemicals	Vomiting, pulse increased 40 b/m, catatonia	None of the foods or chemicals tested
3. 55 W.F.	C	0	2	0	Corn, cane sugar, eggs, inhaled chemicals	Wheezing, rhinorrhea, red nose, nasal stuffiness, tender muscles, cystitis	Corn, eggs, inhaled chemicals
4. 44 W.F.	C	4	5	+	Beef, potatoes, corn, ingested chemicals	Peripheral pulse from 4 to 1+, tachypnea, dyspnea, cyanosis, belching	Beef, corn, ingested chemicals
5. 53 W.F.	H	4	10	+	Pork, pork fumes, ingested chemicals, inhaled chemicals	Edema-generalized, tender muscles, colitis, dizzy	Pork, cane sugar, inhaled chemicals
6. 39 W.F.	C	0	6	0	Legumes, seafood, cane sugar, wheat, chicken, cigarette smoke, ingested chemicals, inhaled chemicals	Syncope, wheezing, muscle tenderness, hives, paroxysmal atrial tachycardia	Cigarette smoke, ingested chemicals, inhaled chemicals, sea food
7. 52 W.F.	C	3	4	+	Beef, chicken, lettuce, ingested chemicals, inhaled chemicals	Bloating, belching, diarrhea, premature ventricular contractions, ventricular tachycardia	Wheat, potatoes
8. 65 W.M.	C	3	1	+	Turkey, chicken, peas, beef, cigarette smoke, inhaled chemicals	Decrease in pulse in left arm only, left neck and arm tenderness, tender over arm veins	None of the foods or chemicals tested
9. 33 W.F.	C & P	0	3	0	Coffee, peanut butter, cane sugar, ingested chemicals	Dyspnea, wheezing, eyes watering, hoarse, pulse increase 50 b/m	Apples, corn, wheat, inhaled chemicals
10. 50 W.F.	C	2	8	+	Corn, wheat, beef, eggs, inhaled chemicals	Cystitis, diarrhea, skin rash, itching, dyspnea, pulse increase	Chicken, beef, inhaled chemicals

C-Coumadin; H-Heparin; P-Persantin; W-White; F-Female; M-Male was in the Environmental Unit but returned when she left it, even after extensive attempts to control her home environment, indicates that even very small amounts of ambient incitants can trigger the syndrome. The most important exposures in her case appeared to be agricultural pesticides and herbicide sprays near her home.

The entity of nontraumatic phlebitis has long been an enigma. It is well known that pulmonary emboli are one of the major causes of death in this country. We have been able to establish the etiology of thirty cases of nontraumatic phlebitis over the past four years. In the initial series, ten patients, with environmental control, lost their intractable phlebitis. In eight of these patients, symptoms returned during challenge testing. Long-term follow-up has yielded only four transient episodes of phlebitis. None of these required anticoagulants, and all cleared within 48 hours of withdrawal of the incitant.

7. *Cardiac Arrhythmias*

Hare,[24] as early as 1905, described vasoactive phenomena including tachycardia in patients after food challenge. Lichtwitz[27] later demonstrated the first causal relationship between food and angina pectoris. In the next decade, numerous case reports showed a direct cause and effect relationship between food ingestion and arrhythmias.[10,25,54,63] Harkavy[25] demonstrated that angina could be triggered by cigarette smoke, and Randolph,[42] using a semi-controlled environment, demonstrated a spectrum of arrhythmias in patients challenged with synthetic chemicals.

Recently, much has been written about the ill effects produced by aerosols and fluorocarbons. This may have been stimulated by Taylor's[59] report of a cardiac death in a sixteen-year-old boy as a result of sniffing an aerosol. The harmful effects of fluorocarbons were reinforced by Speizer,[57] who found that arrhythmias increased with increasing exposure to fluorocarbons.

Certainly, Nour-Eldin's[35] studies showing that the vascular tree has an increased affinity to phenol, coupled with Yevick's[65] demonstration of inflammatory and fibrotic changes in the cardiovascular system of sea animals exposed to oil spills, suggests that pollutants can harm the heart. Stewart[58] has described a case of fatal arrhythmia after repeated exposure to furniture paint remover.

CASE 7. The senior author became suspicious of a more than casual relationship between environmental incitants and arrhythmias when he had the opportunity to resuscitate a sixty-year-old male truck driver with ventricular fibrillation. He remained hypotensive for two days, requiring vasopressors. When he was out of shock, off vasopressors, and recovering satisfactorily, he was fed. He immediately developed bloating accompanied by premature ventricular contractions and a fall in blood pressure. After this had happened on three different occasions, each instance appearing to be life threatening, an ecological history was obtained. This revealed that every time he had had milk or eggs in the past, the above sequence of events had occurred. At the age of seven he had remained in a coma for two weeks, and upon awakening had been placed on an elimination diet consisting solely of potatoes; this resulted in his recovery. Subsequently, whenever he had experienced bloating and irregular heart beats, he had returned to his diet of potatoes to clear his symptoms. In addition, during his childhood, similar reactions had occurred after exposure to gasoline fumes. This reaction caused problems during his trucking career. He frequently had to stop by the roadside to get away from his truck to allow his symptoms to clear. Avoidance of offending foods and chemicals allowed an uneventful recovery.

After this incident, formalized prospective studies were begun. We have since been able to reproduce a spectrum of arrhythmias in many patients. It has long been known that coffee and cigarettes will cause atrial arrhythmias. The following case illustrates how many different incitants can cause these irregularities.

CASE 8. A sixty-five-year-old female presented with an eight-year history of recurrent atrial fibrillation. She also complained of arthritis, blurring of vision, spells of coughing, and generalized muscle pain. During hospitalization in the Environmental Unit, we discovered that her symptoms could be reproduced by exposure to natural gas, phenol, formaldehyde, and insecticides.

We have been able to clear and reproduce a spectrum of

arrhythmias, including ventricular tachycardia, in twenty patients hospitalized in our Environmental Unit. These patients usually had normal large vessels on coronary angiogram. Some patients presented with spasm of various arteries on coronary arteriography. A few patients had plaque formation, and apparently had arteriosclerosis in addition to vasculitis. The following is an example.

CASE 9. This thirty-seven-year-old, white male had a twenty-year history of recurrent fatigue, gastrointestinal distress, sinusitis, tendonitis, joint pains, and headaches. During the two years before referral he began experiencing severe chest pain, bronchitis, and cardiac arrhythmias; a diagnosis of angina pectoris was made. One year prior to referral he was given four coronary jump bypasses in the hope of relieving his symptoms. He was then placed on Inderol,® Valium,® Librox,® and Persantin.® His condition continued to deteriorate. It is important to note that this patient was a mortician, as was his father, who died at the age of forty-six from cardiac disease. His living quarters were directly over his mortuary. His symptoms were precipitated and perpetuated by repeated exposure to formaldehyde.

The patient was admitted to the Environmental Unit, and following a three-and-one-half-day fast, his symptoms cleared. Upon food challenge, with six out of twenty-four foods tested he experienced chest pain, gastrointestinal distress, sinusitis, headaches, and premature ventricular contractions. Challenge with 15-minute exposures to the ambient doses of natural gas, alcohol, chlorine, and insecticide produced sinusitis, general body aching, and headache. Challenge with phenol and formaldehyde produced severe chest pain, cardiac arrhythmias, numbness of the extremities, and headache. Immunological parameters were monitored during these challenges. No medication was necessary at the time of discharge. The patient, on appropriate dietary and environmental control, has remained asymptomatic for the past year. We feel that it is important to study all patients with unexplained cardiac arrhythmias and idiopathic heart disease to rule out environmental triggering.

8. *Vasculitis: Raynaud's Disease?*

This entity was originally described by Raynaud, and referred to any localized peripheral digital vascular spasm or collapse; it often leads to gangrene.[14] We have been able to identify triggering agents in ten patients. The following is an example.

CASE 10. A thirty-year-old, white female presented with a twenty-five-year history of severe recurrent headaches, sore throats, and kidney infections. She had been examined by a family practitioner in March, 1976, when she began to experience severe pain in her right index finger. A diagnosis of Raynaud's disease was made, and the patient was placed on vasodilators. The pain increased, requiring analgesics. During the next three weeks her condition rapidly deteriorated and she was referred to us. She entered the Environmental Unit with severe headaches, sore throat, and gangrene of the tip of the right index finger. Following a six-day fast her symptoms cleared completely and the color returned to her finger. Upon food challenge she experienced headache and sore throat with forty-five of sixty foods tested. Digital spasm was produced following challenge with watermelon and all of the ambient inhaled chemicals tested, including phenol, formaldehyde, methyl alcohol, insecticide, and chlorine. She was discharged and has remained relatively symptom-free for two and one-half years, unless she is inadvertently exposed to chemical inhalants, when her right index finger turns blue. It should be noted that this patient had a family history of severe vascular disease. Her father died of a cerebral hemorrhage at age forty, the latter's mother died at age thirty-nine, his mother's mother at age thirty-seven, and his brother at age forty-five, all with similar vascular symptoms.

9. *Vasculitis—Possibly Irreversible and Self-Perpetuating—Stages 3, 4, 5*

The potential of altering many vasospastic phenomena is exciting. Formerly, patients with these disorders had a progressive, downhill course and were quite miserable in the process. As the clinical picture has been well described in recent medical texts, attention will only be focussed on environmental factors.

Cutaneous Venulitis. According to most authors,[3,19] there are six major categories of necrotizing vasculitis. The first is cutaneous venulitis, in which postcapillary vessels are involved with a necrotizing inflammation. It is generally accepted that there are three main types.

a. The first is leukocytoclastic angiitis and involves mainly small vessel inflammation. It is distinguishable clinically from other forms by the presence of "palpable" purpura caused by exudation and hemorrhage around the involved vessel. The nuclei of neutrophils within the lesion disintegrate, producing basophilic drops that deposit in the involved vessel walls and are visible upon biopsy. Immune complexes commonly are present on the vessel wall. These complexes can activate the complement system, releasing chemotactic factors that attract neutrophils. This results in the release of proteolytic enzymes and other factors that cause vascular necrosis.

b. The second is hypersensitivity angiitis. This generally affects areas where immune complexes collect, i.e. kidney, joints, and skin. Eosinophilia occurs in approximately 20 percent of the patients. It is generally caused by drugs, heavy metals, and antisera, as well as other undefined agents, possibly foods and environmental chemicals.

c. The third is palpable purpura and closely resembles anaphylactoid, or Henoch-Schönlein purpura. Palpable purpura is present in the skin and mucosa throughout the body and is accompanied by abdominal pain and gastrointestinal bleeding. The etiology is unknown; it frequently is preceded by an upper respiratory tract infection.[19]

Periarteritis Nodosa. Next in the spectrum of vasculitis comes periarteritis nodosa (PAN). It generally follows a prodromal fever, arthralgia, and malaise; it may manifest itself as acute gastrointestinal distress, myocardial infarction, neuritis, muscle pain, and/or gangrene of the extremities. It generally presents in the muscular arteries involving all three layers of the arterial wall and adjacent veins. It usually is segmental. Biopsy of skin, subcutaneous nodules, or smooth muscle reveals acute healing vasculitis without giant cells. The infiltration process involves polymorphonuclear leukocytes, eosinophils, and edema followed by fibrinoid necrosis. The areas of fibrinoid necrosis are replaced by fibroblasts, and scar tissue is formed.

WEGENER'S GRANULOMATOSIS. Periarteritis nodosa is closely related to Wegener's granulomatosis, which is characterized by necrotizing granulomas in the respiratory tract, and vasculitis of the medium-size arteries, veins, arterioles, and venules. The onset may be acute or chronic. Though pathologically well defined, the etiology of the disease still is obscure. Our recent studies indicate that it is worthwhile looking for incitants. The following case is an example.

CASE 11—PERIARTERITIS NODOSA AND/OR GRANULOMATOUS DISEASE. This forty-five-year-old chocolate factory worker was admitted to the Environmental Unit complaining of excruciating leg pain, which rendered him unable to walk. Eleven years prior to admission he had experienced an episode of leg and chest pain with shortness of breath, necessitating hospitalization. Findings indicated heart failure accompanied by pulmonary infiltrates and eosinophilia. Steroids were required to bring the situation under control. Vessel biopsy revealed an inflammation compatible with periarteritis nodosa, or Wegener's granulomatosis. The patient had to retire from his job because of excruciating leg pain. For eleven years he had required morphine, 15 mg four-hourly, for relief of pain. He had barely been able to walk for five years and had developed paralysis of the left foot. On admission to the Environmental Unit he was unable to walk more than a few steps. His left foot was pulseless; the three smaller toes were paralyzed; he could not dorsiflex his feet. Light touch elicited extreme hyperesthesia with excruciating pain. During the first five days of environmental control, severe withdrawal symptoms occurred. However, on the sixth day peripheral pulses were noted, the toe paralysis disappeared, the color returned, and he was able to walk. No morphine was required after the fourth day. Random challenge with single, chemically less contaminated foods demonstrated the following sequence of reactions to four of the foods tested:

0 minutes	immediate repulsion at odor with nausea
5 minutes	a. itching in throat
	b. general malaise
	c. arms and legs aching
35 minutes	a. cyanosis of hands
	b. bloating
45 minutes	a. vomiting
	b. cyanosis of feet as well as of hands
50 minutes	pulse decrease in left foot, unable to walk, toe paralyzed, hyperesthesia

The four foods to which he reacted adversely were chocolate, sugar, figs, and dates; chocolate was the worst offender. Inhaled cigarette smoke produced similar symptoms. Challenge with 20 other foods resulted in no reactions.

ALLERGIC GRANULOMATOSIS OF CHURG AND STRAUSS. This represents the fourth type of necrotizing vasculitis. Asthma is common precurser and usually remits several years prior to the onset of the vasculitis. Granulomas develop on vessel walls with large numbers of giant cells, eosinophils, and plasma cells. Fever and multiple organ involvement are common. Congestive heart failure caused by myocardial damage is the most frequent cause of death.

TEMPORAL ARTERITIS. Temporal arteritis is part of the generalized vascular disorder characterized by granulomatous inflammation of the cranial arteries. The vessel wall commonly is infiltrated by monocytes, plasma cells, and giant cells.[4] There may be diffuse fibrotic thickening of the intima, with narrowing of the lumen occasionally resulting in thrombosis.

Intense headache and blindness are prominent features. There may be prodromal fever, joint stiffness, muscle pain, loss of weight, anorexia, and general malaise. The disease frequently is progressive unless treated with prednisone. Triggering agents can be identified in some cases.

CASE 12. This seventy-year-old, white female was admitted complaining of pain in her jaw and of difficulty in walking. Two years prior to admission she had developed a sharp pain in her eyes. A biopsy of the right temporal artery showed it to be completely occluded with classical temporal arteritis. During the next year her arthritic symptoms increased, and she developed sinusitis, tachycardia, and impaired vision. She was admitted to the Environmental Unit. Following a four-and-one-half-day fast her symptoms diminished, although they did not clear totally. Challenge with pork, wheat, potato, pears, yams, acorn squash, corn, pineapple, yellow squash, rice, carrots, egg, walnuts, soya beans, beef, broccoli, raisins, grape juice, millet, and goat reproduced all her admitting symptoms. Sixteen other foods caused no reactions. Later, challenge with commercial foods, phenol, formaldehyde, and natural gas also reproduced her admitting symptoms.

VASCULAR SPASM. Stage 4 vasculitis is represented in part by giant cell arteritis. It is characterized by necrotic inflammation of all layers of the involved vessels. Fibrosis or fibrinoid tissue generally is observed on biopsy. Initial clinical manifestations include severe headache, blurred vision, and gastrointestinal upsets. Patients with severe fibrinoid necrosis have been studied in the Environmental Unit. The etiological implications of food and chemicals are illustrated by the following case.

CASE 13. A forty-three-year-old, white female underwent a sudden onset of arterial occulusion of her left leg. Eventually, amputation was performed after an unsuccessful bypass. Microscopic sections of the leg showed that a nonarteriosclerotic fibrosis surrounded by severe inflammation with polymorphonuclear cells had occluded all arteries. Significant past history included two pulmonary emboli, recurrent phlebitis, sinusitis, recurrent gastrointestinal upset, and sensitivity to odors. Six months later her peripheral pulses disappeared and her remaining leg became cyanotic. An arteriogram showed severe spasm, and the patient developed pain at rest refractory to antispasmodics. Limb loss appeared imminent. Institutionalization in a relatively particle- and fume-free environment for five days resulted in restitution of 4+ dorsalis pedis pulse, and normal color and function of the limb. Challenge with numerous individual foods and chemicals entirely reproduced her initial symptoms. Three years later, the patient is on environmental control at home and is symptom-free.

10. Rheumatoid Arthritis

Diseases such as rheumatoid arthritis and systemic lupus erythematosus exhibit a variety of vascular manifestations and biopsy evidence of vasculitis. Although the etiology of these diseases is generally not known, we have found evidence of immune changes in patients with rheumatoid arthritis following food and chemical challenges. The following is an illustrative example.

CASE 14. A fifty-year-old, white female presented with a fifteen-year history of swelling of the hands and feet, with generalized polyarthritis, gastrointestinal distress, recurring diarrhea, hoarseness, sore throat, facial edema, sensitivity to noise, dyspnea, hypertension, dysuria, and frequency of micturition. The diagnosis of rheumatoid arthritis was made. The patient had a positive RA factor. She had been placed on prednisone 40 mg daily to relieve her symptoms. She was admitted to the Environmental Unit and taken off prednisone; after a five-day fast her symptoms began to clear. When challenged with foods, twenty were found to cause a return of her rheumatoid arthritis.

11. Systemic Lupus Erythematosus

Apparently, many foreign substances can trigger systemic lupus erythematosus. The following case report is an example of a patient whose symptoms were environmentally induced.

CASE 15. This thirty-six-year-old, white female developed recurrent bouts of vomiting at the age of five; these gave way to migraine at the age of eleven and the latter persisted. At the age of sixteen she developed a polyarthritis, and a diagnosis of systemic lupus erythematosus was made. Her disease progressed over the next several years, with further involvement of the gastrointestinal, genitourinary, respiratory, and vascular systems. Spontaneous bruising and petechiae occurred, together with peripheral edema. She eventually was placed on cortisone and cytotoxic drugs. Antinuclear antibodies and LE preparations were positive on numerous occasions. She was placed in the Environmental Unit, and all medications were discontinued. The stiffness and swelling of her joints gradually disappeared. Her sedimentation rate fell from 63 to 15 mm in one week. This was the lowest it had been for many years. The circumference of her fingers diminished by 1.5 to 2 cm while fasting, reflecting the massive loss of edema. She was able to open and close her hands for the first time in many years. Challenges with foods indicated that twenty precipitated a return of her symptoms; ten did not. The inhalation of chemicals such as perfume, phenol, and natural gas also triggered symptoms.

TREATMENT

The first item and cardinal rule in treatment of vasculitis should be elimination of incitants. This includes drinking a water proven by oral challenge to be safe, eating less chemically contaminated foods, and using a rotary diversified diet, not eating any one food more frequently than once every four to seven days, preferably the latter. Many of our most difficult patients have eaten only one meal per day for two to three years so as to lengthen their food rotation. This sometimes will allow them to eat the same food only once in two to four weeks. This often will decrease the severity of the incitant reaction sufficiently to make it relatively innocuous.

The home environment must be tailored to eliminate most of the fuming petrochemicals as well as particulate matter. This includes the elimination of all gas heating and cooking units, and synthetic carpets, bedding, drapery, and clothes. Meticulous efforts must be made to keep this environment as clean as possible. The home environment is judged clean only if the patient rapidly clears his symptoms after entering.

Drinking a tested, safe water also is necessary. Care should be taken that the water is not contaminated by chlorine, fluoride, or synthetics. Containers should always be made of glass. Various spring waters appear to be the safest water. Once an inadvertent overload occurs, emptying the gastrointestinal tract with a laxative, abstaining from eating, and retreating to a good environment usually clear symptoms rapidly. Laxatives used should be nontoxic to the individual, and can be determined only by testing. The safest laxatives appear to be milk of magnesia, Epsom salt, phosphates mixed with the patient's own drinking water, or potassium bicarbonate.

Indocin and salicylates have been recommended to counteract the instant reactions that trigger prostaglandins. However, their value is short-lived, for the patient who most needs them often becomes sensitive to them. They may be used for short bursts, while repetive, chronic use is to be avoided.

Trialkali Salts—This is a combination of three parts sodium bicarbonate, two parts potassium bicarbonate, and one part calcium carbonate. One tablespoonful in a glass of water after an adverse reaction will frequently markedly decrease the duration and severity of the reaction.

Nasal Oxygen frequently will relieve the vasospasm that occurs when an incitant affects a blood vessel. This can be given until symptoms are relieved.

Oral Cromoglycate occasionally will obscure some symptoms in this type of patient; however, the patient may become sensitive to this substance. Therefore, its use appears limited. Initially, it may be tried but should be considered only for short-term prophylaxis.

Immunotherapy for pollen, dusts, molds, and foods should be used when indicated. An optimum starting dose based on dilution titration and/or RAST score and/or neutralization is desirable to obtain maximal effect as soon as possible. Most chemically sensitive patients appear to be very mold sensitive and, when properly treated with nonphenolated aqueous extracts, respond well to immunotherapy.

Unfortunately, there are patients who do not have immediate or even delayed (24– or 48-hour) skin responses to these inhalants. Some patients with severe vasculitis are obviously sensitive to molds, proven by provocation, but have negative skin tests, though the injection of mold extract may cause signs and symptoms that persist for 24 to 48 hours. In such patients injection therapy is very inconsistent and frequently impossible. Most patients with vasculitis are very sensitive to preservatives in extracts. For this reason, aqueous nonglycerinated, nonphenolated extracts are preferred.

Immunotherapy with food extracts is frequently necessary, particularly in those patients who still react to most foods, even when on a rotary diet. We prefer to initially "neutralize" the patient on the lines suggested by Miller,[32] and then to give an injection of the food extract daily for one to two weeks. The injections are then spread out to once every three to four days. However, if the patient develops symptoms after a meal, he may safely be given another injection. Contents of the food extracts can vary, but usually contain the foods to which the patient reacts mildly or moderately. Foods to which he has extreme reactions should be excluded from the extract and the diet for several months, since even in minute doses, they may cause a return of the vasculitis. Foods to which reactions are less severe may be included in the extract, but should be left out of the diet. Care should be taken to make sure that even the small amount of food in the extract does not precipitate a return of symptoms. Reactions have been observed with food injection in extreme reactors.

Steroids may be needed for the treatment of advanced cases of vasculitis. However, efforts should be made to rapidly reduce and eliminate them; long-term use may further damage vessel walls. In stage 3 through 5 patients whom we have encountered, once the environmental load has been reduced, steroids can be tapered or discontinued. Emphasis on reducing the incitant load should constantly be stressed in these diseases.

Vitamins frequently are effective in reducing body reactivity to many incitants. *Vitamin C* is particularly well known as an antioxidant, and apparently aids the body in fending off pollutants in addition to aiding production of the ground substance of the vessel. Careful administration of 4 to 10 grams of ascorbic acid powder daily helps some patients. Little to no toxicity has been reported from the use of this vitamin at any dosage. However, extreme care must be taken that the patient is not sensitive to, or does not become sensitive to, the corn from which most preparations of vitamin C are made.

Zinc apparently is another substance in which many individuals are deficient, and up to 150 mg/24 hours may be used. This is frequently ineffective unless vitamin B_6 is also administered; we have given up to 800 mg daily of the powdered form without ill effects. Care again must be taken to be sure that the patient is not sensitive to any of the excipients.

Other B vitamins also may be needed, and the same precautions should be used. The preterminal, far-advanced chronic vasculitis may become progressive at some point, and all efforts at treatment are to no avail.

Experimentally, transfer factor and antimetabolite cytotoxic agents have been tried without much effect.

CONCLUSION

Our environment is steadily becoming more contaminated by synthetic chemicals. It is important to recognize their influence in causing disease. If one is not aware of the environment's effect on the individual, the disease will progress relentlessly. However, the effect of the chemical environment is lessened, and recovery can occur if the patient is able to withdraw to an environmentally sound, less chemically contaminated home. Sensitivities will then gradually subside, and the patient will be able to return to and function in the outside world.

The spectrum of inflammatory vascular disease is vast. The effects on the body can be as minor as a little urticaria or as major as organ necrosis with resultant loss of life. These diseases tend to become chronic and may persist for years, making the individual extremely uncomfortable and often incapacitated. We feel that it is important to recognize that any substance taken into the body can cause the varieties of vascular inflammation described, and that the elimination of incitants will lead to recovery. Furthermore, realization that the incitant load is multifaceted is important in understanding how to deal with these entities. Understanding these concepts should enable us not only to better manage but also to prevent the development of inflammatory vascular disease.

REFERENCES

1. Adolph, E.F.: General and specific characteristics of physiological adaptations. *Am J Physiol, 184*:8, 1956.
2. Austen, K.F.: Periarteritis Nodosa (Polyarteritis Nodosa). In Beeson, P.B. and McDermott, W. (Eds.): *Textbook of Medicine,* 14th ed. Philadelphia: Saunders, 1975, p. 139.
3. ———: Introduction to Connective Tissue Diseases ("Collagen Diseases") Other than Rheumatoid Arthritis. In Beeson, P.B. and McDermott,

W. (Eds.): *Textbook of Medicine,* 14th ed. Philadelphia: Saunders, 1975, p. 123.

4. Beeson, P.B.: Polymyalgia Rheumatica and Cranial Arteritis (Temporal Arteritis, Giant Cell Arteritis, Polymyalgia Arteritica). In Beeson, P.B. and McDermott, W. (Eds.): *Textbook of Medicine,* 14th ed. Philadelphia: Saunders, 1975, pp. 175-176.
5. Belkin, G.A.: Cocktail purpura: An unusual case of quinine sensitivity. *Ann Intern Med, 66:*583, 1967.
6. Bell, I.R.: A kinin model of mediation for food and chemical sensitivities: Biobehavioral implications. *Ann Allergy, 35:*206, 1975.
7. ———: *A Unified Theory of Mechanism for Disease Caused by Maladaptation to Exogenous Substances.* Ph.D. thesis. Stanford U Pr, 1977.
8. Blackwell, B.: Hypertensive crisis due to monoamine-oxidase inhibitors. *Lancet, 2:*849, 1963.
9. Booth, D.F.: Acute anaphylaxis from orally administered penicillin G. *JAMA, 85:*1367, 1972.
10. Boxer, R.W.: Cardiac Arrhythmias due to Foods. In Dickey, L.D. (Ed.): *Clinical Ecology.* Springfield: Thomas, 1976, p. 193.
11. Brown, T.R.: Role of diet in etiology and treatment of migraine and other types of headache. *JAMA, 77:*1396, 1921.
12. Buisseret, P.D., Youlten, L.J.F., Heinzelmann, D.L., and Lessof, M.H.: Prostaglandin-synthesis inhibitors in prophylaxis of food intolerance. *Lancet, 1:*906, 1978.
13. Churg, J. and Strauss, L.: Allergic granulomatosis, allergic angiitis and periarteritis nodosa. *Am J Pathol, 27:*277, 1951.
14. Coffman, J.D.: Diseases of the Peripheral Vessels. In Beeson, P.B. and McDermott, W. (Eds.): *Textbook of Medicine,* 14th ed. Philadelphia: Saunders, 1975, p. 1076.
15. Creech, J.L. and Makk, L.: Liver disease among polyvinyl chloride production workers. *Ann NY Acad Sci, 246:*88, 1975.
16. Dalton, K.: Food intake prior to a migraine attack—study of 2,313 spontaneous attacks. *Headache, 15(3):*188, 1975.
17. Daughters, D., Zackheim, H., and Maibach, H.: Urticaria and anaphylactoid reactions. *Arch Dermatol, 107:*429, 1973.
18. Dickey, L.D.: Personal communication.
19. Gilliam, J.N. and Smiley, J.D.: Cutaneous necrotizing vasculitis and related disorders. *Ann Allergy, 37:*328, 1976.
20. Glaze, W.E.: North Texas State University, Environmental Division. Personal communication.
21. Grant, E.C.G., Albuquerque, M., Steiner, T.J. and Rose, F.C.: Oral Contraceptives, Smoking and Ergotamine and Migraine. In Greene, R. (Ed): *Current Concepts in Migraine Research.* New York: Raven, 1978, p. 97.

22. Hanington, E.: Preliminary report on tyramine headache. *Br Med J*, 2:550, 1967.
23. ———: Tyramine and Other Factors. In Hanington, E. (Ed.): *Migraine*. London: Priory, 1975.
24. Hare, F.: *The Food Factor in Disease*, vol. I. London: Longmans, 1905, p. 274.
25. Harkavy, J.: *Vascular Allergy and its Systemic Manifestations*. Washington: Butterworths. 1963, p. 93.
26. Klotz, S.D.: Drug Allergy. In Frazier, C.A. (Ed.): *Annual Review of Allergy*. Flushing: Medical Examination Publishing Co., 1974, p. 349.
27. Lichtwitz, L.: Pharmacotherapy of anomalies of function of smooth musculature. *Klin Wschr, 4*:2353, 1925.
28. Lord, G.D.A., Duckworth, J.W., and Charlesworth, J.A.: Complement activation in migraine. *Lancet, 1*:781, 1977.
29. Mackarness, R.C.: *Not all in the Mind*. London: Pan Books, 1976.
30. Man, P.L. and Chen, C.H.: Severe shock caused by chlorpromazine hypersensitivity. *Br J Psychiatry, 122*:185, 1973.
31. Marquez-Julio, H.J.: A phenylethylamine oxidizing defect in migraine. *Nature, 250*:335, 1974.
32. Miller, J.B.: *Food Allergy: Provocative Testing and Injection Therapy*. Springfield: Thomas, 1972.
33. Mining Safety Products Co., Dallas, Texas.
34. Nachman, R.L.: Hemorrhagic Disorders: Disorders of Primary Hemostasis. In Beeson, P.B. and McDermott, W. (Ed.): *Textbook of Medicine*, 14th Ed. Philadelphia: Saunders, 1975, pp. 1557-1560.
35. Nour-Eldine, F.: Uptake of phenol by vascular and brain tissue. *Microvasc Res, 2*:224, 1970.
36. Parish, W.E.: Studies in vasculitis, immunoglobulins, Blc, C-reactive proteins and bacterial antigens in cutaneous vasculitis lesions. *Clin Allergy, 1*:97, 1971.
37. Postlethwaite, A.E.: Mechanisms of vasculitis. *Cutis, 15*:930, 1975.
38. ———: Vasculitis: A Consideration of Causes and Mediators. In Frazier, C.A. (Ed.): *Annual Review of Allergy*. Flushing: Med Exam, 1974, p. 336.
39. Quick, A.J.: *Bleeding Problems in Clinical Medicine*. Philadelphia: Saunders, 1970, p. 133.
40. Randolph, T.G.: Specific adaptation syndrome. *J Lab Clin Med, 48*: 934, 1956.
41. ———: *Human Ecology and Susceptibility to the Chemical Environment*. Springfield: Thomas, 1962.
42. ———: Ecologic orientation in medicine: Comprehensive environment control in diagnosis and therapy. *Ann Allergy, 23*:7, 1965.
43. Rapp, D.: Personal communication.

44. Rea, W.J., Bell, I.R., Suits, C.W., and Smiley, R.E.: Food and chemical susceptibility after environmental chemical overexposure: Case histories. *Ann Allergy, 41*:101, 1975.
45. Rea, W.J.: Environmentally triggered small vessel vasculitis. *Ann Allergy, 38*:245, 1977.
46. ———: Environmentally triggered large vessel vasculitis. to be published.
47. Rinkel, H.J., Lee, D.H., Brown, D.W., Willoughby, J.W., and Williams, J.R.: The diagnosis of food allergy. *Arch Otolaryngol, 79*:71, 1964.
48. Rosenfeld, I., Silverblatt, M.L. and Grishman, A.: Allergic shock in humans: Report of two cases with electrocardiographic findings. *Am Heart J, 53*:463, 1957.
49. Rowe, A.H. and Rowe, A.: *Food Allergy: Its Manifestations and Control and the Elimination Diets: A Compendium.* Springfield: Thomas, 1972.
50. Sandberg, D.H., Burnstein, C.W., McIntosh, R.M., Carr, R., and Strauss, J.: Severe steroid-responsive nephrosis associated with hypersensitivity. *Lancet, 1*:388, 1977.
51. Selby, G. and Lance, J.W.: Observations on 500 cases of migraine and allied vascular headache. *J Neurol Neurosurg Psychiatry, 23*:23, 1960.
52. Selye, H.: The general adaptation syndrome and disease of adaptation. *J Allergy, 17*:231, 1946.
53. Shookhoff, C. and Lieberman, D.L.: Angina pectoris syndrome activated by ragweed sensitivity in a patient with coronary vessel sclerosis: Case report. *J Allergy, 4*:513, 1933.
54. Shookhoff, C. and Lieberman, D.L.: Hypersensitiveness to acetylsalicylic acid expressed by angina pectoris syndrome with and without urticaria. *J Allergy, 4*:506, 1933.
55. Siroty, R.R.: Purpura on the rocks—with a twist. *JAMA, 235*:2521, 1976.
56. Speer, F.: *Migraine.* Chicago: Nelson-Hall, 1977.
57. Speizer, F.E., Wegman, D.H., and Ramirez, A.: Palpitation rates associated with fluorocarbon exposure in a hospital setting. *N Engl J Med, 292*:624, 1975.
58. Stewart, R.D. and Hake, C.L.: Paint remover hazards. *JAMA, 235*:398, 1976.
59. Taylor, G.J. and Harris, W.S.: Cardiac toxicity of aerosol propellants. *JAMA, 214*:81, 1970.
60. Theorell, H., Blombock, M., and Lockum, C.: Demonstration of reactivity to airborne and food antigens in cutaneous vasculitis by variations in fibrino-peptide A and other blood coagulation, fibrinolysis and complement parameters. *Thromb Haemost (Stuttz), 36*:593, 1976.
61. Vaughn, W.T.: Allergic migraine. *JAMA, 88*:1383, 1927.

62. Von Pirquet, C.E.: Allergie. *Klin Wochenschr, 53*:1457, 1906.
63. Werley, G.: Is allergy a factor in angina pectoris and cardiac infarct. *J Allergy, 4*:65, 1932.
64. Whitby, K. and Willeke, K.: Atmospheric aerosols: Size distribution interpretation. *J Air Pollut Control Assoc, 25*:529, 1975.
65. Yevick, P.: Personal communication.
66. Zeek, P.M.: Periarteritis nodosa and other forms of necrotizing angiitis. *N Eng J Med, 248*:764, 1953.

Chapter 6

RENAL DISEASE RELATED TO HYPERSENSITIVITY TO FOODS

DOUGLAS H. SANDBERG, THOMAS F. McLEOD, AND JOSE STRAUSS

AN IMMUNOLOGICAL basis for certain renal diseases has been suspected for many years. The improved techniques of modern immunology have subsequently provided abundant evidence both in animals and man confirming this hypothesis.[12,21,34,35] Although immunologically mediated injury appears to be causally related to some renal disorders, the mechanisms involved have only partially been elucidated. Hypersensitivity to specific antigens has been reported to be an etiological factor in certain kidney diseases, but the frequency of occurrence is not known.[21,34,49] Antigens that have been reported to be involved include bacterial and viral antigens, pollen, drugs, toxins, insect stings, and foods.[49] Hypersensitivity mechanisms for renal injury proposed include classical immunoglobulin E–mediated allergy,[44,58] delayed hypersensitivity,[60] immune complex disease,[34] and more recently, direct cytotoxicity.[9]

It is not the purpose of this paper to discuss fully immunologically mediated renal disease; rather, we shall endeavor to describe some evidence presently available concerning the role of hypersensitivity to external environmental agents and, in particular, foods.

Acute post-streptococcal glomerulonephritis has been considered to be related to hypersensitivity to antigenic determinants of the streptococcus itself, which may cross-react with a component or components of human glomerular basement membrane.[33,59] Serum sickness also has been shown to be associated with glomerular abnormalities and proteinuria in animals and man.[59] The glomerular lesion of serum sickness was shown to be related to presence of circulating immune complexes, and these complexes have been found localized in the glomerulus. Development of glomerulonephritis in animal models with serum sickness has been shown experimentally to be related to clearance of antigen from serum as well as to the nature of specific antibody response, size of complexes, etc. Other factors have also been shown to be of importance. Vascular permeability changes due to release of mediators such as histamine or serotonin have been postulated to be of importance with regard to localization of complexes in blood vessels.[3,4] The mechanisms whereby immune complexes cause glomerular injury appear in some instances to be associated with their ability to fix complement.[18,23] Complement activation results in release of a variety of substances that mediate an inflammatory response. In addition to these humoral mechanisms there has been some recent evidence suggesting that renal damage may be due to cellular hypersensitivity mechanisms.[25,50] Certainly some renal diseases such as lupus nephritis and rapidly progressive nephritis often have significant infiltrates of mononuclear cells present in the renal cortex.[55] The migration inhibition assay has been used to demonstrate that abnormal cellular hypersensitivity mechanisms were present in some patients with glomerulonephritis. Also, Zabriskie et al. have shown *in vitro* cellular hypersensitivity to the glomerular basement membrane and to the streptococcus in patients with glomerulonephritis.[7,11]

THE NEPHROTIC SYNDROME

Of all the renal disorders recognized to be related to immunological mechanisms, the nephrotic syndrome in some patients has perhaps been most clearly identified with classical allergens as etiologic factors.[13,17,58] This association has been considered to be present in only a small minority of patients with regard to pollens and other inhalant allergens. Recently, evidence for a role in childhood nephrosis for food hypersensitivity has been reported by Matsumura et al.[29,31] This sensitivity does not appear to be IgE mediated, although it may occur in atopic individuals.[27,45] Evidence for presence of circulating immune complexes in nephrosis has been presented.[26,54] These complexes were not detected, however, by the Clq binding assay; the lack of evidence of deposition of complexes in the glomerulus,[27,45] as well as the normal serum concentration of complement, suggests that neither the complexes nor the complement is significantly involved in the glomerular injury. There is evidence for involvement of cellular immune mechanisms in minimal change nephrosis with the report by Moorthy et al. that plasma from patients with that disorder inhibited the blastogenic response of lymphocytes to PHA and to allogenic lymphocytes in mixed lymphocyte culture.[37] In addition, Eyres et al. have shown that lymphocytes from patients with minimal change nephrotic syndrome demonstrated direct lymphocytotoxicity against an epithelial cell culture from human kidney.[9]

POSTURAL PROTEINURIA

Although postural proteinuria is a separate entity from childhood nephrosis, Matsumura and his colleagues have demonstrated that sensitivity to foods may be a significant factor in that disorder as well as in nephrosis.[15,30] He studied both orthostatic and lordotic proteinuria. In this disorder the upright or exaggerated lordotic positions produce compression of renal veins and inferior vena cava. This results in transient venous compression of the kidney, causing increased protein excretion. Postural proteinuria is often associated with symptoms related to other organ systems, i.e. fatigue, gastrointestinal complaints, etc., which occur commonly in children with food sensitivities.[28] Detection of food sensitivity in their patients was accomplished by history, food diaries, elimination diets, and subsequent trials of suspected foods. Matsumura and his group found in almost all individuals that a single feeding of a food was enough to produce postural proteinuria (see Fig. 6-1). In thirty-six patients they found seventy-two instances in which foods produced postural proteinuria. In order of frequency, milk was a cause in thirty patients, eggs in twenty cases, soybeans in seventeen instances, and pork, red beans, and tuna in a few individuals. Disappearance of postural proteinuria was demonstrated when the specific foods were eliminated from the diet. Of interest with regard to the quantity of food required to produce proteinuria was the observation that six of the thirty-six

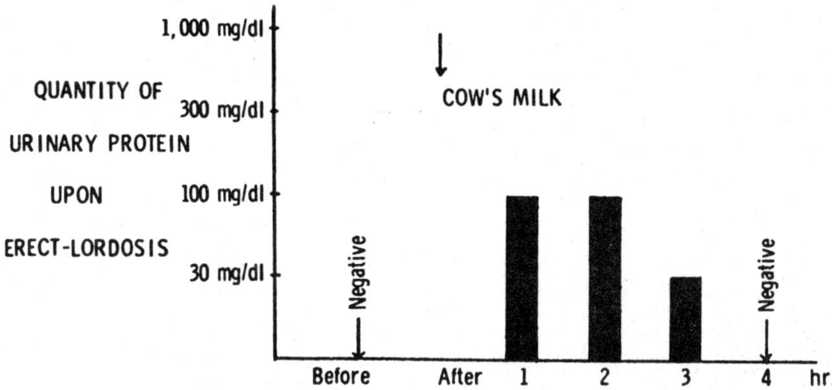

Case of a single administration of the usual amount of allergenic food.

Figure 6-1. Lordotic proteinuria resulting from administration of a single feeding of cow's milk. From L. Dickey (Ed.), *Clinical Ecology,* 1976. Courtesy of Charles C Thomas, Publisher, Springfield, Illinois.

patients had lordotic proteinuria with ingestion of minute amounts of soy, milk, chicken, or red beans (see Table 6-I). The authors also noted that after proteinuria was provoked by ingestion of a food such as cow's milk or egg, they were able to detect the food antigen in the urine specimens containing increased concentrations of proteins. Matsumura's studies provide considerable evidence that food sensitivity may play an important role in etiology of postural proteinuria.

Table 6-I

LP DUE TO MINUTE AMOUNT OF ALLERGENIC FOODS*

Case No.	*Name*	*Age*	*Allergenic Foods*	*Amount of Foods*	*Protein in Urine*
1	H.T.	5 yrs.	Soybean	Several Pieces of Rice - biscuits Baked with Soybean - Oil	100 mg/dl
2	Y.K.	12 "	Egg	Several Chopped Chicken	30 mg/dl
3	T.N.	16 "	Milk	A few Pieces of Biscuit	30 mg/dl
4	K.T.	11 "	Milk	A small Piece of Chocolate	100 mg/dl
5	K.K.	12 "	Milk	A little Butter	30 mg/dl
6	M.T.	15 "	Red Bean	A spoonful of Red Bean Jam	300 mg/dl

* From T. Matsumura in L. Dickey (Ed.), *Clinical Ecology,* 1976. Courtesy of Charles C Thomas, Publisher, Springfield, Illinois.

MEMBRANOUS GLOMERULOPATHY

Membranous glomerulopathy (MG) is a type of glomerular disease characterized pathologically by minimal mesangial proliferation and diffuse thickening of glomerular capillary walls and epithelial cell hypertrophy.[44]

The capillary wall thickening is due to presence of abnormal deposits located subepithelially. The pattern of these deposits on immunofluorescent staining is related to presence of granules fixing immunoglobulin G and less frequently immunoglobulins A and M. Deposits of C3 also occur commonly, and occasionally one may find other complement components, i.e. Clq and C4.

Membranous glomerulopathy usually presents with proteinuria and hematuria. In most patients the proteinuria is sufficiently marked to be classified as a nephrotic syndrome. This nephrotic syndrome is often relatively mild, although some degree of generalized edema is present in approximately one-third of the patients. The disease process is much more common in adults than in children. Membranous glomerulopathy has been found in about 20 percent of adults with nephrosis, and in only 6 percent of children with the nephrotic syndrome.[37]

The glomerular lesions are believed to result from deposition of small immune complexes along the epithelial side of the glomerular basement membrane. A number of antigens have been demonstrated in a small number of patients in whom the renal lesion was associated with other disease processes. Malignancy has been the disorder most frequently present. Carcinomas and lymphoid cell line tumors have been the most common of these. In some instances a tumor antigen was detected in the glomerular deposits.[6,57]

This same renal lesion has also been found in patients with circulating HB_sA_g, with or without clinical hepatitis.[5,42,39] This antigen has been detected in glomerular deposits and in cryoglobulins in some patients. Membranous glomerulopathy has also been present in patients with systemic lupus erythematosus,[14] idiopathic thrombocytopenic purpura,[22] syphilis,[56] sickle cell disease,[53] and streptococcal infections.[42] In addition, the same lesion has been associated with certain drugs, i.e. penicillamine, gold, and trimethadione.[2,8,52] In fact, penicillamine, gold, and mercury compounds have been used experimentally to produce a lesion apparently identical to MG.[20,38,49] The antigens so far reported to be associated with MG are derived from infectious agents or drugs. Until recently, foods or common inhalant allergens had not been considered to be causally related to the renal disease accompanied by this histological abnormality.

ANAPHYLACTOID PURPURA NEPHRITIS

Anaphylactoid purpura (Henoch-Schönlein disease) nephritis has been reported to be associated with hypersensitivity to such agents as drugs, insect bites, and even foods.[1,19,49,51] Nephritis occurs in approximately 25 percent of patients with anaphylactoid purpura.[16] The renal lesion is a focal nephritis involving some glomeruli and sparing others. There are no characteristic changes in the glomerular basement membrane. There is deposition of immunoglobulins G and A as well as C3 in the mesangium of the glomerulus consistent with presence of immune complexes. The site of deposition may be related to clearing of complexes from the circulation and the mesangium with resulting, usually mild, nephritis. The skin lesions seen in anaphylactoid purpura are histologically those of a vasculitis. They resemble Arthus's reaction, which has been demonstrated to be the result of immune complex–mediated injury. However, deposition of immunoglobulins and/or complement around involved blood vessels has not been demonstrable, and in general, serum complement component concentrations have been reported to be in the normal range.[16]

The syndrome of benign recurrent hematuria is also associated with focal nephritis and probably can be considered to be a variant of anaphylactoid purpura nephritis.[10] In this disorder, deposits of immunoglobulins A and G have been detected both in the mesangium and along the epithelial side of the basement membrane. No definite relationship to food sensitivity has been reported, although some authors have described patients with food sensitivity and chronic hematuria.[44]

We would like to devote the remainder of this article to a summary of results of our own studies of hypersensitivity in the nephrotic syndrome. We have studied patients with childhood nephrosis, both steroid responsive and steroid resistant, membranous glomerulopathy, and anaphylactoid purpura nephritis.

MINIMAL CHANGE DISEASE NEPHROSIS

Our initial studies of six patients with milk-sensitive, frequently relapsing, steroid-responsive, minimal change disease (MCD) nephrosis were reported in 1977.[47] We have now studied nineteen children with MCD.[48] Investigation of the first six patients demonstrated that all were sensitive to cow's milk, and in five of the six, relapse with proteinuria and edema occurred following milk ingestion (see Table 6-II). For these studies, patients were admitted to the Clinical Research Center of the University of Miami in relapse after prednisone therapy had been discontinued. Proteinuria decreased on an elemental diet (Vivonex,® Eaton Laboratories), and recurred when milk was added to the diet (see Fig. 6-2). Severity and duration of the induced relapses varied in different individuals and appeared to be related to overall severity of the disease process. Relapses included increased protein excretion with peak values ranging from 2 to 29 gm/24 hr. fluid retention, and decreased urine output. These six patients all had positive intradermal skin tests to cow's milk using the technique described by Lee[43] and by Miller,[36] and all showed acute alteration of plasma C3 complement component following ingestion of 1 ounce of milk.[32,46] None of this group of patients were selected for investigation based on a positive history of atopic disease. However, on questioning, five had a history of asthma or eczema. In the one patient without any history of allergic disorders, his parents later reported that they had noticed, before these studies were done, that ingestion of pork appeared to cause increased proteinuria and edema.

Since that initial report, we have studied thirteen more patients with frequently relapsing MCD and have carried out further studies in three of the six original patients. All nineteen patients included in the investigation had persistent disease requiring repeated courses of or continuous prednisone therapy; in nine, treatment with cytotoxic agents was considered necessary because of poor control of the nephrosis with prednisone. In two of the nineteen patients it has not been possible to control their

TABLE 6-II

CLINICAL DATA IN
NINETEEN PATIENTS WITH MINIMAL CHANGE
DISEASE NEPHROSIS

PTS	*AGE*	*SEX*	*AGE AT ONSET (yr.)*	*HISTORY OF ATOPIC DISEASE*	*PREVIOUS TREATMENT*	*DURATION OF TREATMENT (yr.)*	*INITIAL STUDY*
1.	13	M	8	ASTHMA	PREDNISONE	5	1974
2.	10	F	2	ECZEMA	PREDNISONE	8	1974
3.	10	M	3	ASTHMA ECZEMA	PREDNISONE CYCLOPHOSPHAMIDE	7	1974
4.	12	M	3	NONE	PREDNISONE VINCRISTINE	9	1974
5.	10	M	4.5	ASTHMA	PREDNISONE	5.5	1974
6.	13	F	3.5	ECZEMA	PREDNISONE	9.5	1974
7.	4.5	M	3.5	ECZEMA	PREDNISONE	1	1976
8.	9.5	F	1.5	NONE (HEADACHE)	PREDNISONE CYCLOPHOSPHAMIDE	8	1977
9.	6	M	3	ALLERGIC RHINITIS	PREDNISONE CYCLOPHOSPHAMIDE	2.5	1976
10.	9.5	M	5	ASTHMA	PREDNISONE CYCLOPHOSPHAMIDE	4.5	1978
11.	15	M	10	NONE (HEADACHE)	PREDNISONE CHLORAMBUCIL	5	1978
12.	13	F	12	NONE (HEADACHE)	PREDNISONE CYCLOPHOSPHAMIDE	1	1975
13.	10	M	1.5	NONE	PREDNISONE CYCLOPHOSPHAMIDE	8	1975

TABLE 6 — continued

PTS	AGE	SEX	AGE AT ONSET (yr.)	HISTORY OF ATOPIC DISEASE	PREVIOUS TREATMENT	DURATION OF TREATMENT (yr.)	INITIAL STUDY
14.	9	M	3.5	INSECT HYPERSENSITIVITY	PREDNISONE	5.5	1976
15.	6	M	5.5	NONE	PREDNISONE	0.5	1976
16.	2	M	1.3	ASTHMA	PREDNISONE (NO RESPONSE)	0.2	1978
17.	13	M	3	ASTHMA	PREDNISONE CYCLOPHOSPHAMIDE	10	1978
18.	5.5	F	1.5	CHRONIC URTICARIA	PREDNISONE	4	1978
19.	6.5	M	4.5	ASTHMA	PREDNISONE	2	1978

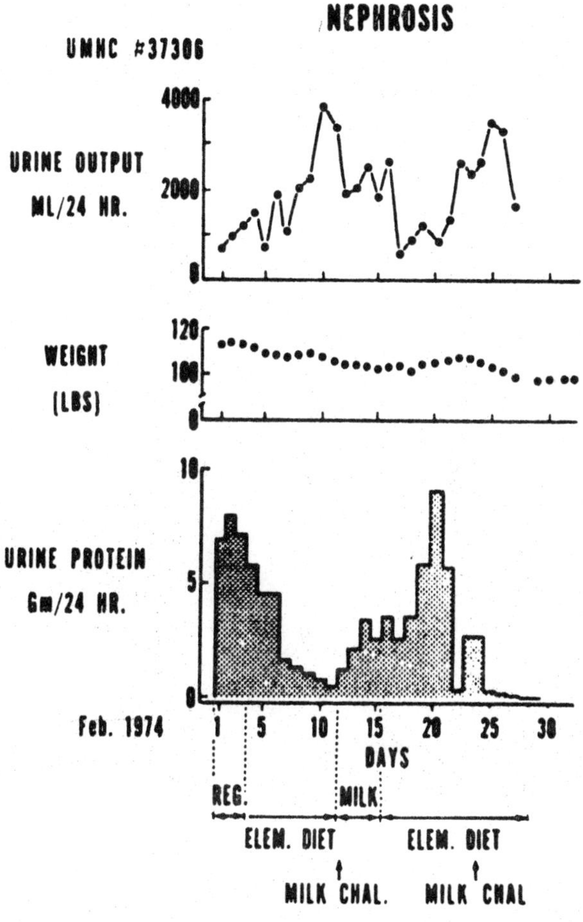

Figure 6-2. Changes in urine output, weight, and protein excretion during dietary changes in a patient with nephrosis.

disease adequately to demonstrate unequivocally that hypersensitivity to foods was an etiologic factor in their illness. In the other seventeen patients, sensitivity to one or more foods was clearly demonstrated. Thirteen of fifteen tested showed alteration of plasma C3 when challenged orally with one or more foods[46] (see Fig. 6-3). Thirteen patients have been skin tested with positive skin tests to one or more foods.

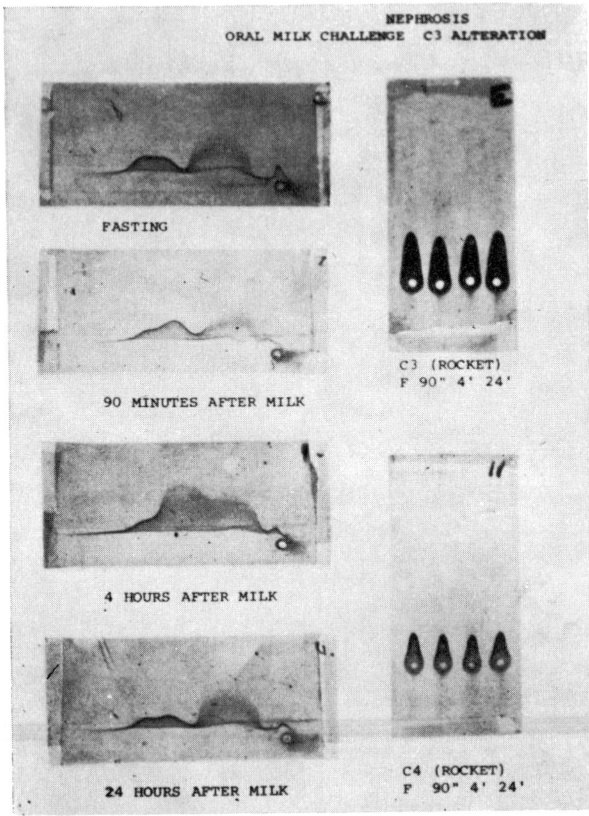

Figure 6-3. Serum C3 and C4 complement components measured by crossed immunoelectrophoresis and by one-dimensional immunoelectrophoresis at intervals before and after ingestion of 1 ounce of cow's milk in a child with MCD nephrotic syndrome.

One patient with MCD had been unresponsive to prednisone therapy. He had a history of almost continuous edema and proteinuria. However, he responded to diet manipulation in a manner similar to that of patients who had been steroid responsive.

In fourteen of the nineteen patients in whom serial values were obtained, relapse was associated with decreased concentrations of immunoglobulin G. Five of nineteen patients had elevated serum concentrations of immunoglobulin M during relapse. Serum total immunoglobulin E concentrations were variable, but in ten of thirteen patients, values were over one standard deviation above the mean for age. In one patient studied recently, serum histamine measured by a radioenzymatic assay increased during relapse induced by a single feeding of 8 ounces of cow's milk. With the exception of two patients included in the original report on milk sensitivity and two patients in whom control of the nephrosis has not been sufficient to carry out an adequate evaluation, all patients have been found to be sensitive to more than one food. In most patients ingestion of several to many foods was related to increased proteinuria.

In an attempt to increase the efficiency of diagnosis of specific food sensitivities present in each patient we attempted to use the fasting and individual food challenge technique developed by Rinkel and Randolph[41] to study 3 patients. However, once precipitated, proteinuria tended to persist for a period of days, which made this approach to diagnosis slow and cumbersome.

Four patients reacted to the elemental diet itself with increased proteinuria, and the increased protein excretion subsided when the diet was changed to another type of limited diet or spring water (see Fig. 6-4).

Although this group was too small to draw conclusions regarding response to treatment, some of these children with severe MCD appeared to be significantly improved by therapy directed at control of food sensitivities. Two of the original six patients moved out of town and were lost to follow-up. One patient who had had many relapses over several years did not relapse when prednisone was discontinued and has not relapsed since that time. However, since she was demonstrated to react to milk with *in vivo* plasma C3 alteration and a positive intradermal skin test to milk, she has limited her intake of milk products. The other three patients in the original report have been either free of relapses or have had only occasional brief relapses associated with acute infectious diseases over the past four years. Two other children evaluated more recently have had significantly less relapses since institution of treatment three or more years ago. These five patients are now on no prednisone therapy. Three other patients were not

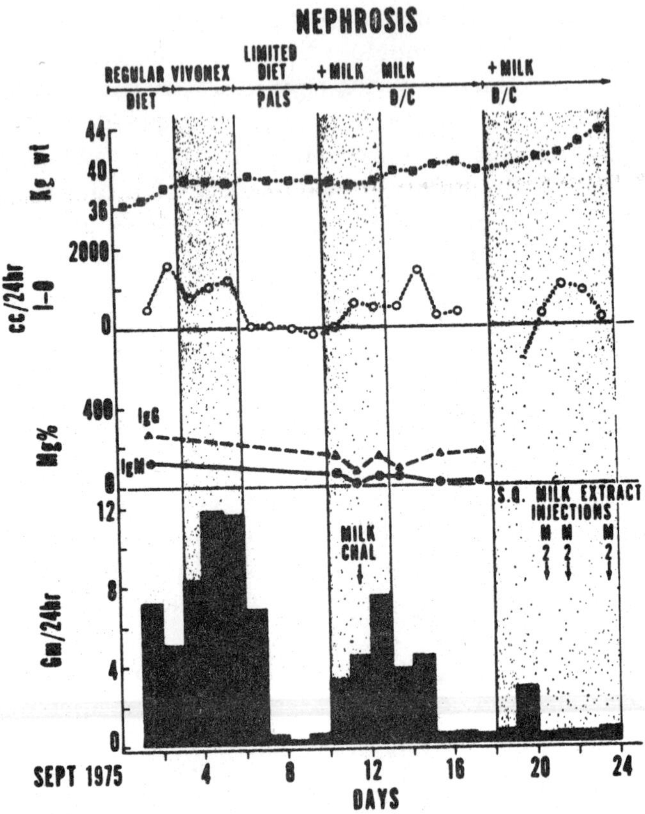

Figure 6-4. Proteinuria resulting from ingestion of milk in a 9-year-old boy with MCD nephrotic syndrome. This patient also developed increased proteinuria with feedings of an elemental diet, Vivonex. M2 represents S.Q. milk extract injections of a 1:250 dilution.

able to follow the necessary dietary restrictions although they were improved and have reverted to standard management with prednisone and continued some form of limited diet. Three other patients have been improved as a result of treatment for their food sensitivities, but have required a low dose of prednisone intermittently for adequate control of their nephrosis. The one patient with MCD unresponsive to prednisone has been markedly improved by a limited diet and food extract injection therapy. More recently he was also tested for some inhalant allergens and is receiving immunotherapy with those extracts giving positive skin tests. Two patients have not been on treatment long enough to evaluate response to therapy. Adequacy of response to the limited diets and food extract therapy appeared to be related to overall severity of the disease process. That is, patients with the most severe disease have had more widespread sensitivities and have been more difficult to control. It is likely that some of this difficulty is related to associated chemical sensitivities, the control of which demands even more alteration of life-style and stringent measures for environmental control of such exposures. This question of the role of chemical sensitivities is presently under investigation.

Eleven patients have been treated with food extract injection or sublingual therapy. This technique has been a major addition to their management, since it has allowed them much more flexibility with the diet, particularly with regard to use of so-called "hidden foods" such as milk, wheat, corn, etc. Provocative intradermal testing confirmed the multiple food sensitivities in these patients. The extent of skin testing and food extract treatment has varied depending on the individual patient and his circumstances. It should be noted that accurate testing may be more difficult in patients with appreciable water retention since there is excess water in the skin, which tends to disperse the injected extract more rapidly than in normal skin. Thus, it is preferable to have patients free of edema before testing.

Some patients have also been tested and treated for those inhalant allergens to which they were sensitive. However, it has not appeared that this additional therapeutic effort has produced any remarkable effect. It is possible, however, that it may stabilize the treatment doses of food extracts and thus minimize changes in those doses.

During initial management, those foods shown to cause relapse have been carefully excluded from the diet. Subsequently, they were often returned to the diet after skin testing and addition of the proper treatment dose to the food extract treatment mixture. This mixture was then given either by subcutaneous injection at intervals of one to three days or by sublingual administration daily. A rotary diversified diet alone produced a good therapeutic response in two patients, although use of food extract therapy later allowed resumption of a more normal diet.

MEMBRANOUS GLOMERULOPATHY

Three patients ages thirteen to fifteen years with the nephrotic syndrome associated with MG have also been studied (see Table 6-III). Although unselected for a positive history of allergy, all had had asthma and one had eczema. All three were shown to be sensitive to multiple foods. Figure 6-5 shows results of a study of sensitivity to milk in one patient. Although glomerular pathology is histologically quite different in MG from that seen in MCD, these patients have appeared remarkably similar to patients with MCD as far as their food sensitivity was concerned. One patient had decreased concentrations of plasma C3 complement component. Two had decreased serum immunoglobulin G concentrations; only one patient was found to have an increase in serum immunoglobulin M levels. All showed elevated serum total immunoglobulin E concentrations. Positive acute *in vivo* alteration of plasma C3 following oral milk challenge as well as positive intradermal skin tests to milk using the titration technique were demonstrated in all three children. Response to therapy directed at control of the hypersensitivity has been excellent in two patients with apparent complete control of proteinuria and edema and normalization of serum levels of immunoglobulins, total protein, and cholesterol. One patient was significantly improved with control of edema and increase in serum proteins, although she continued to have proteinuria in the range of 3 to 6 gm/24 hr. Her disease process was much more severe from onset than that of the other two patients. Recently, after approximately two years follow-up on treatment during which time her disease appeared to be stable, she had a sudden worsening of her renal disease with appearance of hypertension, increased serum urea nitrogen and creatinine, and decreased glomerular filtration rate. This appeared to follow administration of an influenza vaccine booster and removal of wisdom teeth under meperidine analgesia, at which time she developed transient acute severe hypertension. Whether these events were responsible in part for the acute de-

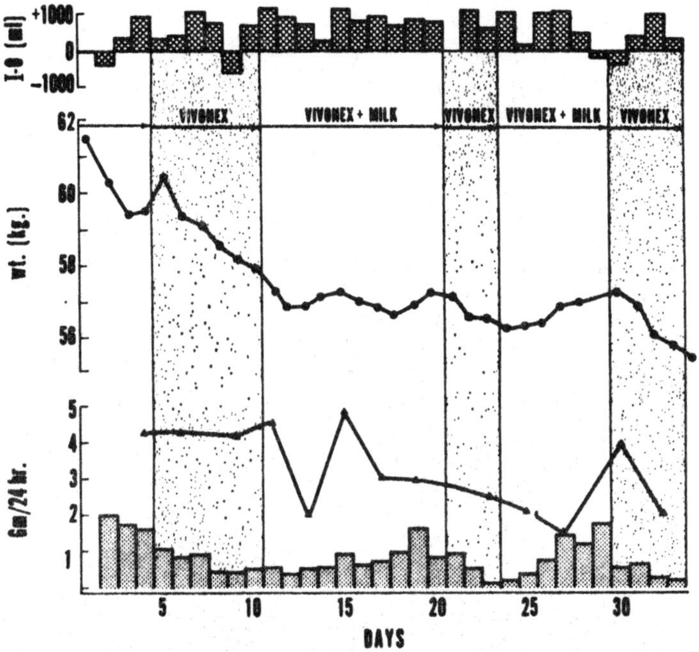

Figure 6-5. Changes in weight, net water balance, and protein excretion during dietary changes in a patient with the nephrotic syndrome associated with MG.
I − 0 = 24 hr fluid intake minus urine output.
Gm/24 hr = Protein excretion during a 24-hr period.

●———● = Changes in body weight in Kg.

▲———▲ = Changes in red blood cell sedimentation rate.

terioration of renal function is not known. A renal biopsy at that time showed approaching end-stage renal disease, so that it seems clear that the patient's disease process was progressive even before the acute deterioration. It is possible that this girl's course was the result of chemical sensitivities that were not treated, or alternatively that a chronic viral infection could have contributed to the persistent disease process.

This disorder is of particular interest because it is considered

TABLE 6-III

CLNICAL DATA IN THREE PATIENTS
WITH NEPHROSIS DUE TO MEMBRANOUS GLOMERULOPATHY

PATIENTS	AGE	SEX	AGE AT ONSET (yr.)	HISTORY OF ATOPIC DISEASE	PREVIOUS TREATMENT	BIOPSY LM	BIOPSY IH	INITIAL STUDY
1.	15	M	14	ASTHMA	NONE	STAGE II MG	IgG 3+ C3 3+	1975
2.	14	F	13	ASTHMA	NONE	STAGE II MG	IgG 3+ C3 3+ IgA 1+ IgM 1+	1975
3.	13	F	13	ASTHMA ECZEMA	NONE	STAGE II MG	IgG 3+ C3 3+ G4 3+ IgA 1+ IgM 3+ C4 3+	1977

to be unresponsive to adrenal cortocosteroid therapy; therefore, these patients had not received prednisone therapy.

ANAPHYLACTOID PURPURA NEPHRITIS

Two children whose chronic nephritis and nephrotic syndrome developed following occurrence of typical Henoch-Schönlein purpura also have been studied[48] (see Table 6-IV). Renal biopsy was performed in both patients. Histopathological characteristics found were consistent with the diagnosis of anaphylactoid purpura nephritis of moderately severe degree. The first patient was a five-year-old, white male who has been followed for over three years in our clinic. His initial presentation was that of typical, though severe, purpura with abdominal pain. This was followed by development of chronic nephritis, hypertension, and then a typical nephrotic syndrome. Renal biopsy showed focal and segmental glomerulonephritis with immune deposits and "crescent" formation categorized as class IV histological changes. He was admitted to the Clinical Research Center for study six months after onset of the disease. Laboratory results included a normal blood urea nitrogen (BUN) (8 mg/dl) and creatinine (0.3 mg/dl); serum IgG (350 mg/dl) was decreased and serum total IgE (325 U/ml) increased for age; serum cholesterol (334 mg/dl) was elevated, and serum total protein/albumin (3.3/1.6 gm/dl) was low; C_{cr} = 79 ml/min/1.73 m^2; protein excretion ranged from 2–3 gm/24 hr., and on microscopic examination of the urine there were 50–60 RBC/hpf and 5–8 WBC/hpf. An Addis count was abnormal with 76 × 10^6 RBC, 43 × 10^6 WBC and 13 × 10^6 casts/12 hr urine collection. The patient was fed a control diet during an initial period when baseline laboratory studies were carried out. He was then put on a gluten free, rotary diet with no food eaten more often than once in four days. Using this basic diet with addition and removal of foods, he was demonstrated to have increased proteinuria following ingestion of lima beans, milk, and eggs. Subsequently, he has been found to be sensitive to a number of other foods and some "inhalant" allergens as well as environmental chemicals such as household cleaning solutions and insecticides. With a management program including a limited rotary diet, environmental control measures, and food and inhalant extract in-

TABLE 6-IV

CLINICAL DATA IN TWO PATIENTS WITH NEPHROSIS DUE TO ANAPHYLACTOID PURPURA NEPHRITIS

PATIENTS	*AGE*	*SEX*	*ONSET (yr.)*	*HISTORY OF ATOPIC DISEASE*	*PREVIOUS TREATMENT*	*IM*	*IH*	*INITIAL STUDY*
1.	5	M	5	NONE	NONE	FOCAL & SEGMENTAL GLOMERULO-NEPHRITIS, CLASS IV	IgA 2+ C3 3+ C4 1+ GRANULAR & FOCAL DEPOSITS	1975
2.	5	F	4.5	NONE	NONE	DIFFUSE PROLIFER-ATIVE GLOMERULO-NEPHRITIS	IgG 3+ C3 3+	1978

jection therapy using the method described by Miller,[36] the Addis count, protein excretion, blood chemistry, and immunoglobulin values became normal within six months and have remained so. However, it has still been necessary for him to continue a strict, limited rotary diet and careful environmental control measures, avoiding chemical exposures.

The second patient was a five-year-old, white female who also had onset of nephritis following a typical episode of anaphylactoid purpura. She then developed a nephrotic syndrome of moderate severity. Renal biopsy showed extensive electron-dense deposits and some "crescent" formation. Six months after onset of her disease she was admitted to the Clinical Research Unit with an active nephrotic syndrome. During the initial control period on a regular diet, protein excretion was 2.7 gm/24 hr. Serum total protein/albumin was 5.0/3.2 gm/dl; cholesterol (276 mg/dl), IgM (145 mg/dl), and IgE (18 U/ml) were all normal; serum IgG (280 mg/dl) was decreased. The Addis count was abnormal with RBC and WBC too numerous to count and 3×10^3 casts/12 hr urine specimen. When she was fed only Vivonex, an elemental or chemically defined diet, 1800 cal/24 hr, protein excretion decreased to 600 mg/24 hr, serum IgG concentration rose to 355 mg/dl, C3 to 138 mg/dl, and serum total protein/albumin to 5.3/3.3 gm/dl. Cholesterol and BUN did not change significantly. When cow's milk was added to the diet, protein excretion increased with a peak value of 2.4 gm/24 hr and then decreased when milk was removed from the diet. Oral challenge with 1 ounce of milk did not produce any acute change in plasma C3 as measured by crossed immunoelectrophoresis of C3 and its breakdown products. Serum cryoglobulins were negative before, two, and four hours after milk challenge. Milk was added to the diet a second time three days later, and this resulted again in increased protein excretion with a peak of 5.4 gm/dl; as before, this decreased when she was fed Vivonex. Concentrations of serum proteins gradually increased with some fluctuations over the period of hospitalization to values for total protein/albumin of 7.8/5.0 gm/dl, while cholesterol decreased to 211 mg/dl. Blood urea nitrogen and creatinine remained in the normal range throughout. Serum IgG remained below normal (350 mg/dl), and serum total IgE was unchanged during hospitalization. Body weight increased with visible edema in association with the periods of milk ingestion and decreased when she was taken off milk. Urine RBC excretion also increased with milk feeding and decreased when the patient was taking only Vivonex. Subsequently, the patient was found also to be sensitive to other foods as well as some airborne allergens and is clinically improved on a limited diet and food and inhalant injection therapy. Follow-up of this patient has been carried out for just a few months; thus, conclusions about therapy are only tentative.

None of the patients with MCD, MG, or anaphylactoid purpura nephritis have had another renal biopsy since beginning treatment for their food sensitivities, except for the girl with very severe MG and progressive renal disease. Such information will be important for evaluation of therapy, particularly in those disorders with definite histological abnormalities and immune deposits.

The similar response to diagnostic testing and management of hypersensitivity to foods in a group of patients with the nephrotic syndrome associated with three distinctly different histological lesions raises many questions. The demonstration of a significant role for hypersensitivity in a patient with MCD unresponsive to prednisone is also of great interest. It would appear that this group of patients has an unusual degree of sensitivity to environmental agents. This may initiate a chain of biochemical events that diverges in different individuals, eventually producing distinct clinical disorders with the common elements of proteinuria, hypoproteinemia, and edema, collectively known as the nephrotic syndrome.

SUMMARY

There is appreciable evidence implicating hypersensitivity reactions in pathogenesis of certain types of renal disease. The data presented above strongly suggest that sensitivity to foods may be an important component of the multifactorial etiology of renal injury in such patients. Use of newer techniques for diagnosis and treatment of food hypersensitivity promises to be helpful for better management of these chronic diseases.

REFERENCES

1. Ackroyd, J.F.: Allergic purpura, including pupura due to foods, drugs and infections. *Am J Med, 14*:605, 1953.
2. Bar-Khayim, Y., Teplitz, C., Garella, S., and Chazan, J.A.: Trimethadione (Tridione®)-induced nephrotic syndrome. *Am J Med, 54*:272, 1973.
3. Cochrane, C.: Studies on the localization of circulating antigen-antibody complexes and other macromolecules in vessels. *J Exp Med, 118*:489, 1963.
4. Cochrane, C. and Hawkins, D.: Studies on circulating immune complexes. *J Exp Med, 127*:137, 1967.
5. Combes, B., Stastny, P., and Shorey, J.: Glomerulonephritis with deposition of Australia antigen-antibody complexes in glomerular basement membrane. *Lancet, 2*:234, 1971.
6. Couser, W.G., Wagonfield, J., Spargo, B.J., and Lewis, E.J.: Glomerular deposition of tumor antigen in membranous nephropathy associated with colonic carcinoma. *Am J Med, 57*:962, 1974.
7. Dardenne, M., Zabriskie, J., and Bach, J.F.: Streptococcal sensitivity in chronic glomerulonephritis. *Lancet, 1*:126, 1972.
8. Dische, F.E., Swinson, D.R., Hamilton, E.B., and Parsons, V.: Immunopathology of penicillamine induced glomerular disease. *J Rheumatol, 3*:145, 1976
9. Eyres, K., Mullick, N.P., and Taylor, G.: Evidence for cell-mediated immunity to renal antigens in minimal-change nephrotic syndrome. *Lancet 1*:1158, 1976.
10. Ferris, T.F.: Recurrent hematuria and focal nephritis. *N Engl J Med,* 276:770, 1967.
11. Fillit, H.M., Read, S.E., Sherman, R.L., Zabriskie, J.B., and deRijn, I.V.: Cellular reactivity to altered glomerular basement membrane in glomerulonephritis. *N Engl J Med, 298*:861, 1978.
12. Fish, A.J., Michael, A.F., and Good, R.A.: *Pathogenesis of Glomerulonephritis.* In Strauss, M.B. and Welt, L.G. (Eds.): *Diseases of the Kidney,* 2nd ed. Boston: Little, 1963.
13. Fontana, V.J., Spain, W.G., and DeSanctis, A.: The role of allergy in nephrosis. *NY State J Med, 56*:3907, 1956.
14. Friend, P.S., Kim, Y., Michael, A.F., and Donadio, J.V.: Pathogenesis of membranous nephropathy in systemic lupus erythematosus: Possible role of non-precipitating DNA antibody. *Br Med J, 1*:25, 1977.
15. Fukushima, I. and Kuroume, T.: Significance of food allergy in the etiology of orthostatic albuminuria found in healthy school children. *Jap J Allergy, 16*:609, 1967.
16. Habib, R., Broyer, M., and Levy, M.: Schönlein-Henoch Purpuro Glomerulonephritis in Children. In Strauss, J. (Ed.): *Pediatric Neph-*

rology: Current Concepts in Diagnosis and Management, vol. 3. New York: Plenum Pub, 1976, p. 155.

17. Hardwicke, J., Soothill, J.F., Squire, J.R., and Holti, G.: Nephrotic syndrome with pollen hypersensitivity. *Lancet, 1*:500, 1959.
18. Henson, P.M. and Cochrane, C.G.: Acute immune complex disease in rabbits. *J Exp Med, 133*:554, 1971.
19. Jensen, B.: Schönlein-Henoch's purpura. Three cases with fish or penicillin antigen. *Acta Med Scand, 152*:61, 1955.
20. Kelchner, J., McIntosh, R., and Boedecker, E.: Experimental autologous immune deposit nephritis in rats associated with mercuric chloride administration. *Experentia, 32*:1204, 1976.
21. Klassen, J.: Experimental Immunological Rental Disease. In Rubin, M.I. and Barratt, T.M. (Eds.): *Pediatric Nephrology.* Baltimore: Williams and Wilkins, 1975, p. 241.
22. Kleinknecht, M.D., Levy, M., Gubler, M.C., and Habib, R.: Membranous glomerulonephritis. In Strauss, J. (Ed.): *Pediatric Nephrology: Current Concepts in Diagnosis and Management.* New York: Plenum Pub, 1977.
23. Kniker, W.T. and Cochrane, C.G.: Pathogenic factors in vascular lesions of experimental serum sickness, *J Exp Med, 122*:83, 1965.
24. Kohler, P.F., Cronin, R.E., and Hammond, W.S.: Chronic membranous glomerulonephritis caused by hepatitis B antigen-antibody immune complexes. *Ann Intern Med, 81*:448, 1974.
25. Lagrue, G., Xheneumont, S., Branellec, H., and Weil, B.: Lymphokines and nephrotic syndrome. *Lancet, 1*:271, 1975.
26. Levinsky, R.J., Malleson, P.N., Barrett, T.M., and Soothill, J.F.: Circulating immune complexes in steroid-responsive nephrotic syndrome. *N Engl J Med, 298*:126, 1978.
27. Lewis, E.J., Kallen, R.J., and Rowe, D.S.: Glomerular localisation of IgE in lipoid nephrosis. *Lancet, 1*:1395, 1973.
28. Matsumura, T.: Postural Proteinuria. In Dickey, L. (Ed.): *Clinical Ecology.* Springfield: Thomas, 1976, p. 233.
29. Matsumura, T. and Kuroume, T.: The role of allergy in the pathogenesis of the nephrotic syndrome. *Jap J Pediatr, 14*:921, 1961 (in Japanese).
30. Matsumura, T., Kuroume, T., and Fukushima, I.: Significance of food allergy in the etiology of orthostatic albuminuria. *J Ashma Res, 3*: 325, 1966.
31. Matsumura, T., Kurome, T., Matsui, A., Fukazawa, T., Kimura, S., and Tamura, H.: Therapy of the nephrotic syndrome by eradication of foci and elimination diets. Proc. *13th Int Cong Pediatr,* 1971, p. 41.
32. Matthews, T.S. and Soothill, J.F.: Complement activation after milk feeding in children with cow's milk allergy. *Lancet, 2*:893, 1970.

33. McCluskey, R.T.: Evidence for immunologic mechanisms in several forms of human glomerular diseases. *Bull NY Acad Med, 46*:769, 1970.

34. McIntosh, R.M., Griswold, W.R., Chernack, W., and Koss, M.N.: The Glomerulonephropathies-Etiopathogenesis. In Strauss, J. (Ed.): *Pediatric Nephrology:* Current Concepts in Diagnosis and Management, vol 1. Miami: Symposia Specialists, 1974, p. 89.

35. McIntosh, R.M. and Ozawa, T.: Immunologically Mediated Cell Injury. In Strauss, J. (Ed.): *Pediatric Nephrology:* Epidemiology, Evaluation and Therapy, vol. 2. Miami: Symposia Specialists, 1976, p. 161.

36. Miller, J.B.: *Food Allergy: Provocative Testing and Neutralization Therapy.* Springfield: Thomas, 1972.

37. Moorthy, A.V., Zimmerman, S.W., and Burkholder, P.M.: Inhibition of lymphocyte blastogenesis by plasma of patients with minimal-change nephrotic syndrome. *Lancet, 1*:1160, 1976.

38. Nagi, A.H., Alexander, F., and Barabas, A.L.: Gold nephropathy in rats. Light and electron microscopic studies. *Exp Mol Pathol, 15:* 354, 1971.

39. Ozawa, T., Levisohn, P., Orsini, E., and McIntosh, R.M.: Acute immune complex disease associated with hepatitis. *Arch Pathol Lab Med, 100*:484, 1976

40. Pollak, V.E., Pirani, C.L., and Clyne, D.H.: The natural history of membranous glomerulo-nephropathy. In Kincaid, Smith, P., Mathew, T.H., and Becker, E.L. (Eds.): *Glomerulonephritis,* part 1. New York: Wiley, 1973, p. 429.

41. Randolph, T.G.: Hospital Comprehensive Environmental Control Program. In Dickey, L. (Ed.): *Clinical Ecology.* Springfield: Thomas, 1976, p. 70.

42. Richet, G., Fillastre, J.P., Morel-Maroger, L., and Bariety, J.: Change from diffuse proliferative to membranous glomerulonephritis: Serial biopsies in four cases *Kidney Int, 5*:57, 1974.

43. Rinkel, H.J., Lee, C., Brown, D.W., Willoughby, J.W., and Williams, J.M.: The diagnosis of food allergy. *Arch Otolaryngol, 79*:71, 1964.

44. Rowe, A.H.: Diagnosis and Control of the Causes of Hematological Allergy. In Rowe, A.H.: *Food Allergy.* Springfield: Thomas, 1972, p. 426.

45. Roy, L.P., Westberg, N.G., and Michael, A.F.: Nephrotic syndrome—no evidence for a role for IgE. *Clin Exp Immunol, 13*:553, 1973.

46. Sandberg, D.H. and Bernstein, C.W.: Alteration of plasma C'3 complement component following challenge with food antigens in the sensitive patient. *Pediatr Res, 6*:83, 1972.

47. Sandberg, D.H., McIntosh, R.M., Bernstein, C.W., Carr, R., and Strauss, J.: Severe steroid-responsive nephrosis associated with hypersensi-

tivity. *Lancet, 1*:388, 1977.
48. Sandberg, D.H., McLeod, T.F., and Strauss, J.: Food hypersensitivity and the nephrotic syndrome of anaphylactoid purpura. *Pediatr Res (Abstract).* In press.
49. Schreiner, G.E.: *The nephrotic syndrome* In Strauss, M.B. and Welt, L.G. (Eds.): *Diseases of the Kidney,* 2nd ed. Boston: Little, 1971, p. 503.
50. Shalhoub, R.J.: Pathogenesis of lipoid nephrosis: A disorder of T cell function. *Lancet, 2*:556, 1974.
51. Siegel, J.M., Brown, H.E., and DiLeo, L.W.: Purpura as a result of insect allergy: Treatment with cortisone. *Postgrad Med, 15*:46, 1959.
52. Silverberg, D.S., Kidd, E.G., Shnitka, T.K., and Ulan, R.A.: Gold nephropathy. A clinical and pathologic study. *Arthritis Rheum, 13*:812, 1970.
53. Strauss, J., Pardo, V., and Koss, M.N.: Nephropathy associated with sickle cell anemia: An autologous immune complex nephritis. *Am J Med, 58*:382, 1975.
54. Stuhlinger, W.D., Verrouse, P.H., and Morel-Maroger, L.: Detection of circulating soluble immune complexes in patients with various renal diseases. *Immunology, 30*:43, 1976.
55. Thaler, M.S., Klausner, R.D., and Cohen, H.J.: Immune Complexes and Immune Complex Disease. In *Medical Immunology.* Philadelphia: Lippincott, 1977, p. 139.
56. Tourville, D.R., Byrd, L.H., and Kim, D.U.: Treponemal antigen in immunopathogenesis of syphilitic glomerulonephritis. *Am J Pathol, 82*:479, 1976.
57. Weksler, M.E., Carey, T., and Day, N.: Nephrotic syndrome in malignant melanoma. Demonstration of melanoma antigen-antibody complexes in kidney. *Kidney Int, 6*:112A, 1974.
58. Wittig, H.J., and Goldman, A.S.: Nephrotic syndrome associated with inhaled allergens. *Lancet, 1*:542, 1970.
59. Zabriskie, J.B.: The role of streptococci in human glomerulonephritis. *J Exp Med, 134*:1085, 1971.
60. Zaldivar, N.M. and Glade, P.R.: The Possible Role of Cell-Mediated Immunity in Renal Diseases. In Strauss, J. (Ed.): *Pediatric Nephrology:* Epidemiology, Evaluation and Therapy, vol. 2. Miami: Symposia Specialists, 1976, p. 186.

Chapter 7

NOCTURNAL ENURESIS

John W. Gerrard

Nocturnal enuresis is an all too common problem that, in its care and management, has taxed the ingenuity of family physicians, pediatricians, psychologists, and urologists. It has given rise to much speculation, but its pathogenesis still remains obscure. Data derived from studies and surveys in children with nocturnal enuresis do, however, reveal the following:

1. Nocturnal enuresis is a disorder of the growing child, and while 50 percent of childen are wet at night at the age of two, only 10 to 15 percent are wet at four, and less than 5 percent are still wet at twelve.[17]
2. Boys are more frequently affected than girls and, in the United States, blacks more than whites, and children with low birth weights more than those with normal birth weights.[17]
3. In girls, nocturnal enuresis predisposes to the development of urinary tract infections; the more frequently the child wets the bed the more likely is she to have or to develop a urinary tract infection.[2,5,11]
4. There is a strong genetic component toward developing nocturnal enuresis.[1,23]
5. Nocturnal enuresis is nearly always associated with a small bladder capacity.[10,16,19,21,24]
6. The acquisition of continence and the ability to sleep through the night without voiding is associated with an increase in bladder capacity.[6,20]

In what follows, the author will first draw attention to the familial nature of nocturnal enuresis and then enlarge on the importance and significance of the associated small bladder capacity.

THE FAMILIAL NATURE OF ENURESIS

Bakwin,[1] studying the genetic basis of behaviour disorders in 338 twin pairs, noted that concordance for enuresis was greater in monozygous (68%) than in dizygous twins (36%) and that if one twin was enuretic there was a 25 percent chance that siblings would also be enuretic. In these same families there was further evidence of the familial incidence of nocturnal enuresis, for when both parents had been enuretic, 77 percent of the children were enuretic; when one parent had been enuretic, 43 percent of the children were enuretic; when neither parent had been enuretic, only 15 percent of the children were enuretic.

Zaleski et al[23] have also studied the familial incidence of enuresis in 176 families, and with very similar findings. Our data and Bakwin's are combined in Table 7-I.

TABLE 7-I

THE PREVALENCE OF NOCTURNAL ENURESIS IN THE OFFSPRING OF ENURETIC AND NONENURETIC PARENTS

	Neither parent enuretic		*One parent enuretic*		*Both parents enuretic*	
	Dry	Enuretic	Dry	Enuretic	Dry	Enuretic
Children	1170	183	84	64	7	19
Percentage enuretic	13		43		73	

Zaleski et al. also studied the prevalence of enuresis in parents and siblings in two groups of eighty-four families.[23] In the first, the proband was enuretic; in the second, matched for age and socioeconomic status, the proband was dry (Table 7-II). Not only are enuretic parents prone to have enuretic children, but enuretic children frequently have parents who at one time were enuretic.

TABLE 7-II
PREVALENCE OF ENURESIS IN PARENTS AND SIBLINGS OF ENURETIC AND NONENURETIC CHILDREN

	Proband		
	Enuretic (n = 84)	*Dry (n = 84)*	*P**
Fathers enuretic	24	3	<.001
Mother enuretic	26	4	<.001
Siblings	38 (n = 249)	19 (n = 231)	.025

*P indicates the significance of the differences.

THE SIGNIFICANCE OF THE SMALL BLADDER CAPACITY

There is now overwhelming evidence that a small bladder capacity is the hallmark of nocturnal enuresis,[10,16,19,21,24] and that it is because bladder capacities are small that enuretics are unable to go through the night without voiding. Our data are given in Table 7-III and illustrated in Figure 7-1. For the same reason, unless their fluid intake is reduced, enuretics pass urine frequently during the daytime. Some children, day dribblers, are also incontinent during the daytime; these children usually have very obvious urgency and frequency. They pass, on average, smaller volumes of urine at a time than do those who are wet only at night.[24] Their maximum bladder capacities are often, though not

TABLE 7-III
MAXIMUM BLADDER CAPACITIES (ML) IN 223 NORMAL CHILDREN AND 75 ENURETICS

	Normals			*Enuretics*		
Age in Years	*N*	*Mean*	*SD*	*N*	*Mean*	*SD*
4	19	234.0	61.2	8	118.1	46.1
5	25	255.3	90.2	9	158.9	40.8
6	22	318.4	92.9	9	136.1	28.7
7	25	305.2	72.3	9	176.7	49.4
8	20	390.0	98.1	12	233.3	99.2
9	28	375.8	107.1	9	278.9	102.8
10	38	407.0	103.7	7	275.7	114.0
11	24	427.3	100.0	7	322.9	173.5
12-14	22	450.1	122.3	5	358.0	167.3
Totals	223			75		

always,[2] smaller than those of similar-aged children who are wet only at night. A small bladder capacity is not an invariable accompaniment of nocturnal enuresis, but it is present in the vast majority; of the last 107 enuretics studied by us, for example, only four had maximum bladder capacities that fell within the normal range. The bladder is small functionally but not anatomically; it can enlarge under the influence of drugs, such as imipramine, and occasionally with the exclusion of foods such as cow's milk from the diet (Fig. 7-2). It is small in most if not in all instances because the bladder is in spasm. That this is the probable explanation has been shown by cystometric findings in enuretics.[13,22] In the normal individual the bladder contracts rhythmically, and as it fills it relaxes repeatedly, due to inhibition of detrusor contraction, until the detrusor muscle has been fully stretched, when it contracts and voiding follows.

Cystometric studies indicate that frequently, in 45 percent of seventy-nine patients studied by Linderholm,[13] and in 76 percent of patients studied by Whiteside,[22] the enuretic's detrusor muscle

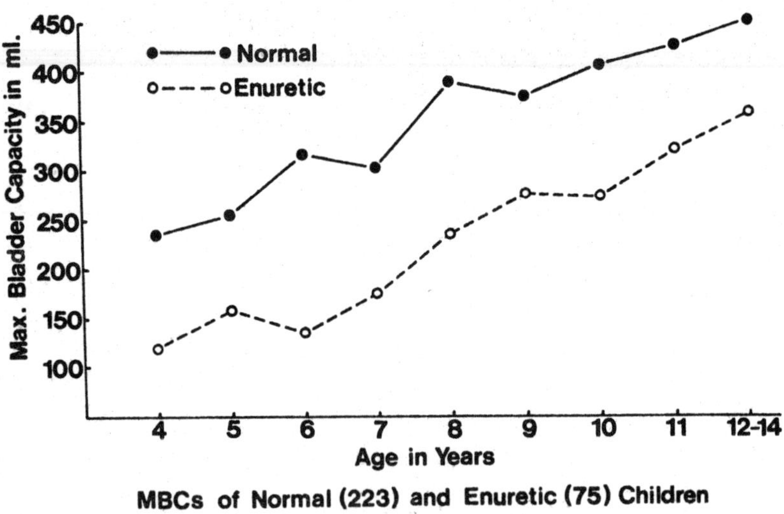

Figure 7-1. Mean maximal functional bladder capacities in 223 normal children and in 75 enuretics. From Zaleski: et al.[24] Courtesy of J.B. Lippincott Company.

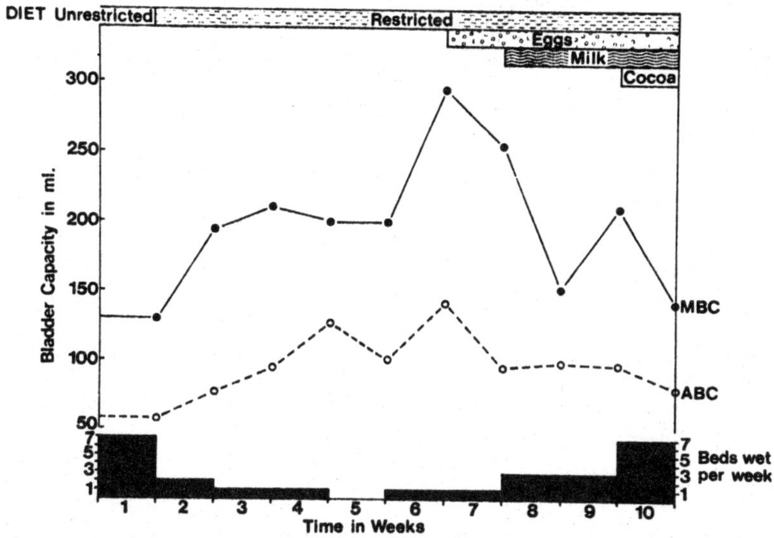

Figure 7-2. Illustrates the increase in bladder capacity and cessation of enuresis with dietary restriction, and the converse on an unrestricted diet.

does not relax as the bladder fills, i.e. it is "uninhibited"; filling of the bladder leads to contraction and not to relaxation. The bladder is unable to relax to accommodate more urine, and when the latter enters the bladder there is a prompt increase in intravesical pressure due to detrusor contraction, and voiding follows. These features are characteristic both of the adult and of the child, and though Whiteside found the "uninhibited" bladder only in those with diurnal enuresis, Linderholm also found it in those with only nocturnal enuresis. It was always associated with a small bladder capacity; it could be modified by anticholinergic drugs such as Pro-Banthine®. The author suspects that imipramine would have a similar effect. The urethra does not have a sphincter comparable, for example, to the pyloric sphincter, but continence is assured by the walls of the proximal urethra falling together when the detrusor muscle relaxes. When the detrusor contracts, muscle fibres in the proximal urethra are drawn apart, the urethra opens, and voiding occurs.[12] It is for this reason that detrusor contraction is associated with urgency and incontinence.

Three reasons have been put forward to explain the uninhibited detrusor contraction; the first is that it is due to a selective delay in autonomic control, a maturational delay. McKeith[14] felt that this was an unsatisfactory explanation, for it could neither be proved nor disproved. The second, put forward by Rutter,[18] is that the small bladder is a developmental anomaly, arising from the frequency with which the enuretic voids—the bladder never having had a chance to be stretched. If this were the correct explanation, it should be easy, by encouraging the child to void infrequently, to stretch the bladder and so facilitate continence at night. Bladder exercises sometimes help marginally, as breathing exercises may help the asthmatic, but the almost universal recourse to other forms of treatment, as in the asthmatic, attests to their relative uselessness. The third suggestion is that the spasm manifested by the "uninhibited" bladder is the end result of an allergic reaction. It is analagous in this respect to the bronchospasm that accompanies asthma.

Bray,[3] in 1931, was the first to suggest that enuresis might sometimes be allergic in origin. He suggested this because three asthmatic children with enuresis, and a fourth with urticaria and enuresis, when treated by him lost not only their asthma and urticaria but also their enuresis. The first child had to avoid wheat products; the second feathers and rabbit fur; the third feathers, horse hair, egg, pork, potato, and rice; and the fourth pork and pork products. Enuresis was caused by foods alone in two, by inhalants alone in one, and by both in a fourth. These children were unusual in that the enuresis was associated with asthma and urticaria and that the allergens were relatively easy to identify, for prick skin tests to all were markedly positive.

The author stumbled across the association of enuresis and allergy through an interest in cow's milk allergy. Cow's milk is a very common and often unrecognized cause not only of diarrhea and vomiting in infancy but also of recurrent rhinorrhea and bronchitis. Sensitivities to cow's milk tend to run in families, but the manifestations, though sometimes the same, often differ in different members of the same family. One parent, for example, may have migraine, a daughter vomiting, and a son bronchitis—all due to cow's milk. In searching for a common denominator to the systems involved in cow's milk allergy, it seemed to me that the one common feature shared by the vascular system and the gastrointestinal and respiratory tracts was that they were all under autonomic control. If this were an important common factor, the function of other tissues under autonomic control, viz., the urinary bladder, might also be expected to be disturbed by allergens, cow's milk included.

By chance, the author was asked to see a family in which a baby vomited when given cow's milk. An older sister in this family had earlier been seen on account of her enuresis. In spite of reassuring her that her nocturnal enuresis was only a developmental problem and that she would grow out of it, she had failed to do so. After seeing the baby brother who could not tolerate cow's milk, it crossed the author's mind that his older sister might also be sensitive to cow's milk, but he was reluctant to suggest that she should avoid cow's milk. (The author's apparent eagerness to blame cow's milk for a multitude of problems is well known locally, and he did not want to add fuel to the fire.) However, in looking for a possible explanation, a sensitivity to cow's milk appeared to be a real possibility, for the child herself was very fond of cow's milk and drank a great deal, while the mother, as often happens when one of her offspring is sensitive to cow's milk, was free from allergies but hated cow's milk and never drank it. After waiting a year, and discovering that the child's enuresis persisted and that it had resulted in, in this instance, an unnecessary cystoscopy and intravenous pyelogram, the author suggested to the mother that the daughter should surreptitiously be taken off cow's milk and all dairy products. To the surprise of the author and the mother, she quickly became dry. A few weeks later the mother, again surreptitiously, offered the child cow's milk. She refused it, but when offered ice cream took it and promptly wet the bed, earning a thrashing from her father, for he asserted that she could "easily be dry at night if she wanted." This and several similar, subsequent experiences initiated bladder capacity studies in normal children, enuretics, and girls with urinary tract infections.

Quite independently, Breneman[4] had earlier suggested that enuresis might be allergic in origin. Of sixty consecutive cases reported by him, all had responded to the elimination of foods from their diets. The foods incriminated, in order of frequency, were as follows:

Milk	24	Pork	3	Berries	2
Wheat	20	Tomato	3	Peas	2
Egg	17	Peanut	2	Chocolate	2
Corn	13	Beef	2	Rye	1
Chicken	4	Apple	2	Cauliflower	1
Orange	4	Fish	2		

He had also, in cases not responding to dietary treatment, prescribed a medication containing scopolamine methyl nitrate 2.4 mg, ephedrine sulfate 10 mg, and chlorpheniramine 2 mg, made up to 5 ml, and had found this useful in the management of nocturnal enuresis.

When studying bladder capacities, maximum bladder capacities were initially compared after a water load test with those measured during the course of a week in which all volumes of urine passed were measured; the maximum bladder capacities passed during the course of a normal week were significantly greater than those passed after a water load test. This was probably because water load tests are carried out under supervision in a hospital or clinic setting, and the child knows that as soon as the test is over he or she may go home, and possibly also because bladders that fill slowly are less likely to demand emptying than those which fill rapidly. The bladder capacity studies confirmed previous studies and emphasized the importance of small bladder capacities (Table 7-III, Figure 7-1) in the etiology of nocturnal enuresis.

The study of normal children showed a surprising variation in the volumes of urine passed and the frequency with which urine was passed. Two perfectly normal girls, for example, emptied their bladders only once a day, and then passed 900 ml at a time. We found as much or more variation in bladder habits as in bowel habits, but children who wet the bed at night or who could not go through the night without getting up to pass urine had significantly smaller maximum bladder capacities than did normals. These same children, teachers often noted (some studies were carried out on school children), were the children who frequently had to leave the classroom to visit the toilet. Enuresis might well be called "urinary diarrhea"; conversely, diarrhea could equally well be renamed "bowel frequency."

The fundamental question is not why the child is enuretic, but why his bladder capacity is so small. The reasons for suggesting that nocturnal enuresis may be allergic in origin include the following: first, in approximately one-quarter of the children seen by us, nocturnal enuresis subsides and bladder capacities normalize when the child is taken off a few simple foods—cow's milk in any shape or form, the fruits included in Feingold's K-P diet, and chocolate and foods containing additives, this includes sugar and honey.

Other foods, as Bray and Breneman have shown and the author has noted, as well as inhalants can also cause enuresis. In seventy-nine instances bladder capacities have been measured, both before and while the child has been on a restricted diet; maximum bladder capacities have increased by 50 percent or more in thirteen (16%), by between 25 and 50 percent in thirteen (16%), while remaining relatively unchanged in the remaining fifty-three (66%). Whether diet does or does not lead to dryness depends on the initial bladder capacity. To give examples, a four-year-old boy who was wet six nights out of seven had an initial maximum bladder capacity of 98 ml. This rose to 184 ml on a restricted diet, but he continued to wet the bed six nights out of seven. The diet had not helped him to be dry at night, even though it had doubled his bladder capacity. Imipramine also did not help him to become dry, but a combination of both did. In a few instances, dietary changes have aggravated enuresis. McKendry[15] does not recommend dietary restriction, since he finds it rarely leads to dryness. In his study, children were treated randomly by diet, imipramine, and the equivalent of a wet alarm, a "Mozes detector," which the child wears at night. The diet consisted of the elimination of cow's milk and dairy products, egg, citrus and tomato products, and chocolate; apple juice and ginger ale were the prescribed fluids. Sixty-four completed dietary treatment; one became dry; thirty-four improved, i.e. had a 50 percent or greater reduction in wet beds; and seven were worse. Sixty-two completed treatment with imipramine; thirteen were cured, twenty-eight were improved, and only one was worse. Forty-three completed treatment with the "Mozes detector"; twenty-three were cured and sixteen were better, none were worse. The study showed that modifying the diet can influence the pattern of nocturnal enuresis, and just as the elimination of some foods can lead to dryness, so the introduction of others can lead to an increase in wetness; we would suspect that apple juice may have interfered with the possible benefits of McKendry's restricted diet. His findings are summarized in Table 7-IV.

TABLE 7-IV
RESULTS OF TREATMENT WITH DIET, IMIPRAMINE AND "MOZES DETECTOR"*

Enuresis	*Dry*		*Drier*		*Unchanged*		*Worse*	
Treatment	*n*	%	*n*	%	*n*	%	*n*	%
Diet (n = 64)	1	2	34	53	22	34	7	11
Imipramine (n = 62)	13	21	28	45	20	32	1	2
Detector (n = 43)	23	54	16	37	4	9	0	0

*From J.B. McKendry, D.A. Stewart, F. Khanna, and C. Netley, Primary enuresis: Relative success of three methods of treatment, *Canadian Medical Association Journal, 113*:953, 1975. Courtesy of the Canadian Medical Association.

The second reason for suggesting that nocturnal enuresis may be allergic in origin is that the same allergens and physical factors that cause bona fide allergies can also cause nocturnal enuresis, as Bray originally showed. We have even encountered children with seasonal enuresis; one child regularly develops nocturnal enuresis at the same time as his father develops hay fever, when the maple is pollenating. An additional child with asthma, when placed on immunotherapy, would on the day following his "shot" regularly wheeze and wet his bed; when the strength of his "shot" was reduced, both his asthma and his nocturnal enuresis subsided. In two instances, cromoglycate, given to one patient by aerosol for asthma and to another orally for gastrointestinal food allergy, has led to a cessation of enuresis, though cromoglycate, in the doses that the author has used it, has not helped appreciably in the management of enuresis. Physical factors that can precipitate asthma, for example exposure to cold, often cause a return of enuresis in the winter months; playing outside in the cold Saskatchewan winters sometimes causes a return of urgency and day dribbling.

A third reason for suggesting an allergic basis for nocturnal enuresis is that the medications most effective in its management —antihistamines, ephedrine, atropine, and Pro-Banthine®—are or have been helpful in the management of other allergies and have antihistaminic and anticholinergic properties, as has imipramine.

There are also reasons for thinking that nocturnal enuresis may not be allergic in origin: first, it is not associated with elevated serum IgE levels. We have measured IgE levels in a normal population of 819, fifty-two of whom were enuretic. The geometric mean IgE levels of the enuretics, adjusted for age, and of the total population as a whole did not differ significantly (Table 7-V).

TABLE 7-V
MEAN SERUM IgE LEVELS IN ENURETICS, NONENURETICS, AND TOTAL POPULATION

	Serum IgE (u/ml)	
	Mean	SD
Enuretics (n = 52)	80	20–324
Nonenuretics (n = 767)	72	22–233
Total population (n-819)	73	22–236

Second, traditional prick skin tests do not usually help in the identification of the supposed offending allergen. The cases reported by Bray were unusual in this respect. However, a negative prick test does not, in our experience, indicate that the patient is free from allergies; it simply means that he is not markedly sensitive to the allergens being tested, or that his allergy is not IgE mediated. Most children sensitive to cow's milk, for example, have negative prick skin tests to cow's milk; cow's milk may, nevertheless, precipitate diarrhea, rhinorrhea, or enuresis, but these are not severe atopic reactions. Were the child to react violently to cow's milk with, for example, an anaphylactic reaction, a drop or two only of milk would precipitate symptoms and the child would have a strongly positive prick test. The lack of strikingly positive skin tests makes the identification of the offending allergens difficult.

When we originally postulated that nocturnal enuresis might be allergic in origin, we compared the frequency of allergic disease in enuretic and control families.[23] We found an increased incidence only of hay fever (allergic rhinitis) in the enuretics. This naturally disappointed us, for we expected to find evidence of an increase in allergic diseases. A later study[9] involving a larger population, however, has shown that it is the specific allergy that tends to run in families. For example, asthma tends to run in families, as do hay fever and eczema; asthmatics do not necessarily have eczema. The prevalence of allergic disorders in the child is closely related to their prevalence in the parent. Enuresis, in this respect, resembles diseases more traditionally called allergic (Table 7-VI), and though it is not an allergic disease in the sense that it is not associated frequently with asthma and eczema, its mode of transmission closely resembles that of allergic diseases in general. This can be seen in the results of the study (Table 7-VI) in which prevalence rates of atopic diseases as well as of enuresis were determined when no parent, one parent, or both parents had the disease in question.

TABLE 7-VI
PERCENTAGE OF CHILDREN WITH ATOPIC DISEASES AND ENURESIS IN 184 FAMILIES WITH 475 CHILDREN

	No parent with disease	*One parent with disease*	*Both parents with disease*
Asthma	3%	24%	—
Hay fever	3%	12%	—
Allergic rhinitis	17%	26%	52%
Allergic bronchitis	11%	38%	—
Eczema	20%	33%	57%
Enuresis	7%	43%	50%

The possible association of nocturnal enuresis with hyperactivity has been of recent concern. With this in view, the prevalence of hyperactivity, as well as of allergic rhinitis and urinary tract infections, was recorded in the last 117 enuretics seen by the author (Table 7-VII).

TABLE 7-VII
THE PREVALENCE RATES OF HYPERACTIVITY, ALLERGIC RHINITIS, AND URINARY TRACT INFECTIONS IN CHILDREN WITH NOCTURNAL ENURESIS

	Boys (n=74)		*Girls (n=43)*	
	Total	*%*	*Total*	*%*
Hyperactivity	25	34	5	12
Allergic rhinitis	16	22	5	12
Urinary tract infections	0	0	8	19

Hyperactivity and allied disturbances of behaviour, but not allergic rhinitis, are appreciably more common in the enuretic than in the local population. Urinary tract infections, as would be expected, are also more common in enuretic girls than in the general population. The frequency with which disturbances in behaviour were associated with nocturnal enuresis was surprising. Breneman,[4] interestingly enough, even before Feingold[7] had made his observation on the relationship between diet and behaviour, had noted that there was often a great improvement in the enuretic's behaviour with diet.

> The surly, hostile, uncooperative enuretic becomes a model child when his malady is corrected. School work, general achievements and ability to solve problems cause parents to ask if the I.Q. has risen. Personality improvements seem to exceed that expected from enuresis control alone. It is so remarkable that it suggests a direct relationship between food allergy and personality traits.

The author too has found that disturbances of behaviour, ranging from overt hyperactivity to moodiness and antisocial behaviour, sometimes accompany nocturnal enuresis, being present in a third of the boys and in 10 percent of the girls. In some instances, as in Breneman's experience, dietary management has led to both continence and a transformation in the child's behaviour. However, the great improvement in the child's disposition is not dependent on the cure of the enuresis, for it has occurred even when the enuresis has persisted. Under such circumstances the parents have kept the child on the restricted diet, even though this has not helped to solve the primary problem, namely the nocturnal enuresis. Imipramine may similarly transform the child's behaviour; it may also do the reverse, making him restless, irritable, and unable to sleep soundly at night. Feingold,[8] studying the hyperactive child, has noted a frequent association with enuresis, and that both are often controlled by a diet free from salicylates and allied products.

In conclusion, the author's approach to the problem of nocturnal enuresis is as follows. The parents are asked to measure volumes of urine passed and to record both days and nights wet, first for one week while on an unrestricted diet and then for two weeks while on a diet free from cow's milk and dairy products, citrus, tomato products, and additives. This is essentially a Feingold diet from which cow's milk and dairy products have been excluded. At the end of three weeks it is possible to assess both the severity of the problem and the response, if any, to dietary management. A five year old, for example, with day dribbling and nocturnal enuresis, with a maximum bladder capacity of 120 ml, is not as likely to respond to any form of treatment as is the five year old whose maximum bladder capacity is 250 ml. Dietary management may increase the bladder capacity appreciably, e.g. from 120 to 240 ml, but the child will probably remain wet at night and become dry during the daytime, a step in the right direction. The addition of imipramine may lead to a further increase in bladder capacity and to both day and night continence. If the child is seven years old and has a minimum bladder capacity of only 150 ml, he is less likely to respond to the use of a wet alarm than is a second seven year old with a maximum bladder capacity of 300 ml.

This approach, though time-consuming to both parents and pediatrician, ensures that the parents take a more understanding view of the child's disorder, and when dietary treatment is successful, the cause of the enuresis is revealed. When the cause is known and can be avoided, the child should never again be troubled unexpectedly by nocturnal enuresis. Although most enuretics grow out of the disorder, many continue to have frequency and a few to have intermittent nocturnal enuresis.[17] In 117 families in which the proband was enuretic, recently analyzed, there were nineteen fathers and nineteen mothers who were enuretic when young; six fathers and fifteen mothers still had to get up at night to pass urine; two parents are enuretic if they have alcohol, a third if he has citrus fruits. If the disability persists in this form, it can prove a handicap, as in the case of a twenty-year-old recovered enuretic, described by Linderholm,[13] who worked as a guide at a fishing camp. He still had urgency and frequency and was handicapped as a guide, for he was unable, as he would have wished, to take women fishing, for when he had the urge to void he never had time to return to the shore. The father of one of the author's own enuretic patients had a similar handicap. He was a construction supervisor and had never been able to work on tall buildings, for he had early learned that if he were to climb the scaffold he would have to descend in a hurry to void.

With regard to medications, imipramine is the drug most likely to ensure dryness and to tide the child over the years until he is prepared to cooperate with the use of a wet alarm. The latter is invaluable in the management of the older child who has a reasonable bladder capacity and who has not responded to other forms of treatment. Whatever the approach, one can confidently say to the parents of all enuretic boys, and of girls who are free from urinary tract infections, that nocturnal enuresis never caused any organic disease, and whatever the treatment, it should not be made more irksome than the disorder it is intended to cure.

With regard to the older patient, if treatment is requested the author uses the combined approach of a detailed allergy history, careful intradermal testing, and dietary management with appropriate immunotherapy.

REFERENCES

1. Bakwin, H.: Enuresis in twins. *Am J Dis Child, 121*:222, 1971.
2. Berg, I., Fielding, D., and Meadow, R.: Psychiatric disturbance, urgency and bacteriuria in children with day and night wetting. *Arch Dis Child, 52*:651, 1977.
3. Bray, G.W.: Enuresis of allergic origin. *Arch Dis Child, 6*:251, 1931.

4. Breneman, J.C.: Allergic cystitis: the cause of nocturnal enuresis. *GP, 20*:85, 1959.
5. Dodge, W.F., West, E.F., Bridgeforth, E.B., and Travis, L.B.: Nocturnal enuresis in 6–10-year-old children: correlation with bacteriuria, proteinuria and dysuria. *Am J Dis Child, 120*:32, 1970.
6. Esperanca, M. and Gerrard, J.W.: Nocturnal enuresis. Comparison of the effect of imipramine and dietary restriction on bladder capacity. *Can Med Assoc J, 101*:721, 1969.
7. Feingold, B.: *Why your child is hyperactive.* New York: Random, 1975.
8. ———: Personal communication.
9. Gerrard, J.W., Ko, C.G., Vickers, P., and Gerrard, C.D.: The familial incidence of allergic disease. *Ann Allergy, 35*:10, 1976.
10. Hallman, N.: On the ability of enuretic children to hold urine. *Acta Paediatr Scand, 39*:87, 1950.
11. Jones, B., Gerrard, J.W., Shokeir, M.H.K., and Houston, C.S.: Recurrent urinary infection in girls: Relation to enuresis. *Can Med Assoc J, 106*:127, 1972.
12. Lapidas, J.: Structure and function of the internal vesical sphincter. *J Urol, 80*:341, 1958.
13. Linderholm, B.E.: The cystometric findings in enuresis. *J Urol 96*: 718, 1966.
14. McKeith, R.: Indications for research. IV: Bladder control and enuresis. In Kolvin, I., McKeith, R.C., and Meadow, S.R. (Eds.): *Clinics in Developmental Medicine,* nos. 48/49. Spastics International Publications, London: Heineman, and Philadelphia: Lippincott, 1973, p. 303.
15. McKendry, J.B., Stewart, D.A., Khanna, F., and Netley, C.: Primary enuresis: Relative success of three methods of treatment. *Can Med Assoc J, 113*:953, 1975.
16. Muellner, S.R.: Development of urinary control in children. *JAMA, 172*:1256, 1960.
17. Oppel, W.C., Harper, P.A., and Rider, R.V.: The age of attaining bladder control. *Pediatrics, 42*:614, 1968.
18. Rutter, M.: Indications for research. III: Bladder control and enuresis. In Kolvin, I., McKeith, R.C., and Meadow, S.R. (Eds.): *Clinics in Developmental Medicine,* nos. 48/49. Spastics International Publications, London: Heineman, and Philadelphia: Lippincott, 1973, p. 292.
19. Starfield, B.: Functional bladder capacity in enuretic and nonenuretic children. *Pediatrics, 70*:777, 1967.
20. Starfield, B. and Mellits, F.D.: Increase in functional bladder capacity and improvement in enuresis. *J Pediatr, 74*:483, 1968.

21. Vulliamy, D.: The day and night output of urine in enuresis. *Arch Dis Child, 31*:439, 1956.

22. Whiteside, C.G. and Arnold, E.P.: Persistent primary enuresis: a urodynamic assessment. *Br Med J, 1*:364, 1975.

23. Zaleski, A., Shokeir, M.H.K., and Gerrard, J.W.: Enuresis: Familial incidence and relationship to allergic disorders. *Can Med Assoc J, 106*:30, 1972.

24. Zaleski, A., Gerrard, J.W., and Shokeir, M.H.K.: Bladder control and enuresis. In Kolvin, I., McKeith, R.C., and Meadow, S.R. (Eds.): *Clinics in Developmental Medicine,* nos. 48/49. Spastics International Publications, London: Heineman, and Philadelphia: Lippincott, 1973.

Chapter 8

HYPERACTIVITY AND THE TENSION-FATIGUE SYNDROME

Doris J. Rapp

Hyperactivity and the tension-fatigue syndrome (TFS) are relatively common pediatric problems that have many features in common. Their prevalence may be on the increase; their etiology is still the subject of debate. This chapter discusses the signs and symptoms of children with hyperactivity and the TFS. Early and recent research in this area will be reviewed. The possible relationship to foods and inhalants will be discussed. Several alternative methods of treatment will be outlined. The potential scope and ramifications of this problem in our society will be mentioned. Easy, practical methods to help physicians determine and eliminate etiologic factors related to hyperactivity so as to obviate the need for drug therapy will be stressed.

Hyperactivity

There is, unfortunately, no unanimity of opinion concerning the exact definition of normal activity versus hyperactivity. Interpretation is often subjective and difficult to quantitate. Parents, teachers, psychologists, and physicians cannot always agree whether a child is or is not hyperactive. One reason for the difference of opinion is that some affected children manifest bursts of hyperactivity, and unless the child is observed during an episode, his actions may be entirely normal. Although the intensity and frequency of hyperactivity vary, most parents complain about their child's purposeless physical activity and inattentive behavior.

Affected children cannot sit through a meal, complete a chore, listen to an entire story, follow directions, or accept discipline. Because of their short attention span and inability to concentrate, learning problems arise. The children generally cannot function at their full potential. An associated delay in speech and impaired motor coordination, as well as perceptual and conceptual problems, contributes to their learning problems. In addition, behavior problems are common. Intermittent or constant irritability, hostility, belligerence, depression, excessive talking, and emotional lability with frequent crying are not uncommon. Varying combinations of hyperactivity, learning, and behavior problems upset family, peer, and school relationships; this in turn has a detrimental effect upon the child's self-image.

Hyperkinesis is defined as impulsiveness, easy distractibility, and inability to concentrate. Common causes include basic personality defects, anxiety, subclinical seizure disorders, sequelae to birth injury or cerebral infection, social or family deprivation or stress, and, possibly, misinterpretation in the eyes of the beholder. At one time it was believed that hyperactive children had minimal brain damage, but as there is no real evidence of organic brain damage, the concept of minimal brain dysfunction (MBD) arose. MBD includes both hyperactivity and learning disability. In 1979 it was recommended that the terms *hyperactivity* and *minimal brain dysfunction* be recalled *attentional deficit disorder* (ADD).[4] Another term, *specific learning disability* (SLD), refers to isolated problems such as dyslexia. Perceptual-cognitive dysfunction and positive "soft" neurological signs also are common.

It is estimated that hyperactivity affects all socioeconomic groups. In the United States alone there are four to five million children with MBD or SLD. The preponderance of hyperactivity and certain learning problems among males has not been explained. As many as 4 percent to 25 percent of children in school have been classified by Feingold as being hyperkinetic.[13] Over 250,000 children use amphetamines or methylphenidate to modify their behavior. Over 250 million methylphenidate tablets are sold annually in the USA.

The Tension-Fatigue Syndrome

Speer, in 1954, initially described the TFS.[52] Crook[9] enlarged on the clinical features. The main symptoms and signs are listed in Table 8-I.

TABLE 8-I

SYMPTOMS AND SIGNS ASSOCIATED WITH THE TFS

	Clinical Features
Behavior	—Wild, maniacal, impulsive, tired, lethargic, lacking energy.
Disposition	—Talkative, restless, inattentive, aggressive, listless, depressed.
Sleep	— Inability to sleep, nightmares, always sleepy.
Symptoms	—Headaches, abdominal pains, leg aches, jittery, restless legs, enuresis, nausea, bloating, abdominal pains, diarrhea and constipation, halitosis, and excessive perspiration.
Signs	—Pallor, circles under eyes, Dennie's sign, nasal stuffiness, aphthous ulcers.

The symptoms encompass a combination of motor and sensory overactivity or fatigue, as well as common behavior problems. Each symptom can range from mild to severe. Some children seem to tire easily; others are too drowsy to function. Some are a little restless; others extremely hyperactive. Many children manifest varying degrees of both fatigue and tension (hyperactivity). Most affected children have evidence of allergy, atopic dermatitis, hay fever, or asthma.

Historical Review

Rowe,[48,49] in 1931 and 1950, described the syndrome of allergic toxemia. His clinical description encompassed the fatigue portions of what we now call the TFS. He noted that fatigue, drowsiness, body aches, depression, irritability, insomnia, fever, chills, and night sweats could be associated with the ingestion of certain foods or exposure to certain pollens and inhalants. Randolph,[39] in 1947, confirmed these findings and differentiated the tired, listless, irritable, and depressed child from the one who is hyperkinetic and hyperexcitable. He noted that affected children or adults often had perennial or seasonal rhinitis, eczema, recurrent headaches, muscle aches, and gastrointestinal complaints. He mentioned problems of discipline, excessive crying, constant talking, and enuresis. He felt that all symptoms might have an allergic basis and that wheat and corn in particular were often to blame.

In 1950, Clarke[5] conducted a survey among allergists to ascertain whether character problems were noted in allergic children. He found that 95/171 responses indicated that personality and learning problems were related to allergy and improved once offending items were eliminated. Many reports described children who had symptoms such as hyperactivity, fatigue, irritability, hostility, depression, insomnia, and learning problems. The elimination of known highly allergenic foods, as well as the removal of dust and pets, and immunotherapy for pollens, appeared to be associated with improvement.

Speer,[52] in 1954, coined the term *allergic tension-fatigue* and gave six examples of this disorder. All children lost their symptoms with the removal of one or more of the following foods from their diets: cow's milk, egg, wheat, corn, and chocolate. Speer emphasized the contrasting features of the syndrome, increase in tension being associated with hyperkinesis and restlessness, and fatigue with emotional instability and lassitude.

Crook,[9] in 1961, studied fifty patients with the TFS. He confirmed that specific foods caused symptoms by 3 withdrawal and challenge periods at 5– to 12-day intervals. He found that 75 percent of the patients had a personal history of nasal, ocular, respiratory, or skin allergy; 66 percent had a strong family history of allergy. The major food offenders he found to be milk, chocolate, and wheat, though some were also sensitive to corn, peanuts, pork, and orange juice. He later added refined sugar to the list. More than half the patients treated by diet had superior to excellent results, while an additional 32 percent (16/50) had a good response. He conducted one double-blind study using milk in capsules to confirm that it caused fatigue, irritability, headache, and stomachache in one child.

In 1970, Kittler and Baldwin[26] emphasized the similarity of symptoms in patients with MBD and the TFS. They randomly placed twenty MBD children with abnormal electroencephalograms and a high incidence of atopy on diets composed either of allergy skin test–positive or –negative foods. Impartial psychological evaluations showed a considerable change in intelligence scores in some children of normal intelligence when on diets that avoided skin test–positive foods. Subjective teacher evaluations of behavior and objective interpretation of electroencephalograms also revealed improvement in some patients who avoided inhalants and probable food offenders. They concluded that a significant percentage of children diagnosed as MBD had allergy as the cause of their problem.

Lockey,[29] in 1971, recognized that food coloring and additives contributed to symptoms in some patients. He devised a sublingual dye test[30] and successfully crusaded for specific food labeling, as well as for the removal of certain harmful FD&C dyes from the market.

In 1978, O'Banion and his associates[36] reported a dietary study on several autistic children. After an appropriate baseline period of observation, each child was fasted for several days. Single foods were then sequentially added to the diet while various parameters, i.e. activity, amount of laughter, and disruptive behavior such as screaming, scratching, biting, and throwing objects, were carefully monitored. Wheat, oats, tomato, sugar, and dairy products were found to be major offending items. Some foods repeatedly altered behavior, others activity. Some were found to cause immediate reactions that lasted a short while; others caused delayed onset reactions that lasted for up to three days.

In 1978, Trites et al.[54] reported that the relationship between hyperactivity and foods was strongest in seventeen out of twenty-two children who also had learning disabilities. Approximately half the hyperactive, learning disabled, or emotionally disturbed children exhibited an allergy to one or more foods by RAST. Although Trites et al. found no statistically significant relationship between hyperactivity and allergy, they found a relationship between hyperactivity, allergy, and the teacher's (Conners[7]) hyperactivity scores.

Buisseret[3] reported the effects of a milk-free diet in seventy-nine children who had eczema, allergic rhinitis, asthma, and intestinal symptoms. He described twenty-seven patients as excessively nervous, timid, high-strung, withdrawn, or prone to nightmares. He found all patients responded favorably to a six-week diet that excluded milk and dairy products.

In summary, the foods that have commonly been found to provoke the TFS include artificial coloring, sugar, milk, wheat, egg, cocoa, corn, citrus, cinnamon, tomato, peanut, and apple. Beef, pork, soy, chicken, yeast, potato, tea, oats, and rice have also been implicated. In addition to foods, inhalants such as house dust, animal danders, feathers, wool, pollens, and mold spores, as well as chemical odors and perfumes, may provoke symptoms in some patients.[8,9,43,44,47,52]

THE RECOGNITION OF HYPERACTIVITY AND TFS

The Patient's History

Symptoms associated with the TFS are often associated with other diseases, but the diagnosis of hyperactivity and the TFS should be suspected under the following circumstances: first, if the hyperactive child has a family and personal history of allergy, an allergic facies, symptoms compatible with the TFS, and specific food-related problems; second, if he had allergic rhinitis and bronchitis when younger; third, if he already has had a negative neurological evaluation, an unsuccessful course of family or psychological counselling, and a poor response to multiple trials of various activity-modifying drugs.

Food likes and dislikes may represent personal preferences, but at times they also indicate definite food problems.[15,39,41,42,45,48] The child who refuses to drink milk, or who dislikes chocolate, or atlernatively who craves them, may have an unsuspected sensitivity. Food sensitivities often affect more than one member of a family and may occur in several generations.[16] If a child was upset by milk as an infant, siblings or parents also may be found to react adversely to cow's milk. Dairy products may cause spells of abdominal pain in one child, enuresis in a second, and hyperactivity in a third.

Physical Examination

The correct diagnosis may be suggested by the child's physical appearance. Table 8-II lists the physical signs and symptoms found in many patients with the TFS and in some with hyperactivity. Table 8-III lists other findings commonly associated with allergy.[31] One physical indicator, the allergic eye wrinkle

TABLE 8-II

SIGNS AND SYMPTOMS ASSOCIATED WITH ALLERGY IN PATIENTS WITH HYPERACTIVITY AND/OR TFS

	Clinical Features
Nose	— Pale, boggy nasal turbinates; watery nasal secretions; an allergic nose wrinkle.
Eyes	— Bilateral erythema; pruritus and tearing; Dennie's sign, extra line fold under each eye (see Fig. 8-1).
Skin	— Antecubital and popliteal eczema.
Lungs	— Expiratory wheezing.

TABLE 8-III

SIGNS OFTEN ASSOCIATED WITH ALLERGY*

- — Allergic shiners (dark eye circles)
- — Puffiness below eyes or puffy upper eyelids
- — Pseudopannus above cornea
- — Marginal upper eyelid eczema
- — Facial pallor in non-anemic patient
- — Swollen vermilion lip edge
- — Cracked corners of mouth
- — Fissured, cracked lips
- — Xerosis of skin with scratch marks
- — Perioral erythema, discoloration or rash
- — Geographic tongue
- — Fissured tongue or buccal mucosa
- — Recurrent aphthous ulcers
- — Red, circular cheek patches
- — Red ear lobes
- — Cracked toe and finger tips

*Adapted from M.B. Marks, *Physical Signs of Allergy in the Respiratory Tract in Children*, 1967.

(Dennie's sign or Morgan's pleat), remains evident for many years in allergic persons (Fig. 8-1). Other symptoms such as puffiness of the eyelids or allergic shiners may wax and wane from day to day. Patients or parents can be taught to observe such flares and may correlate them with exposure to specific foods, inhalants, or contactants.

HYPERACTIVITY AND TFS: CLUES TO PRECIPITATING FACTORS

History

If a child has been hyperactive since infancy, be suspicious of foods ingested prior to the onset of symptoms. Johnstone's studies[23,24] showed that egg, wheat, and milk given prior to nine

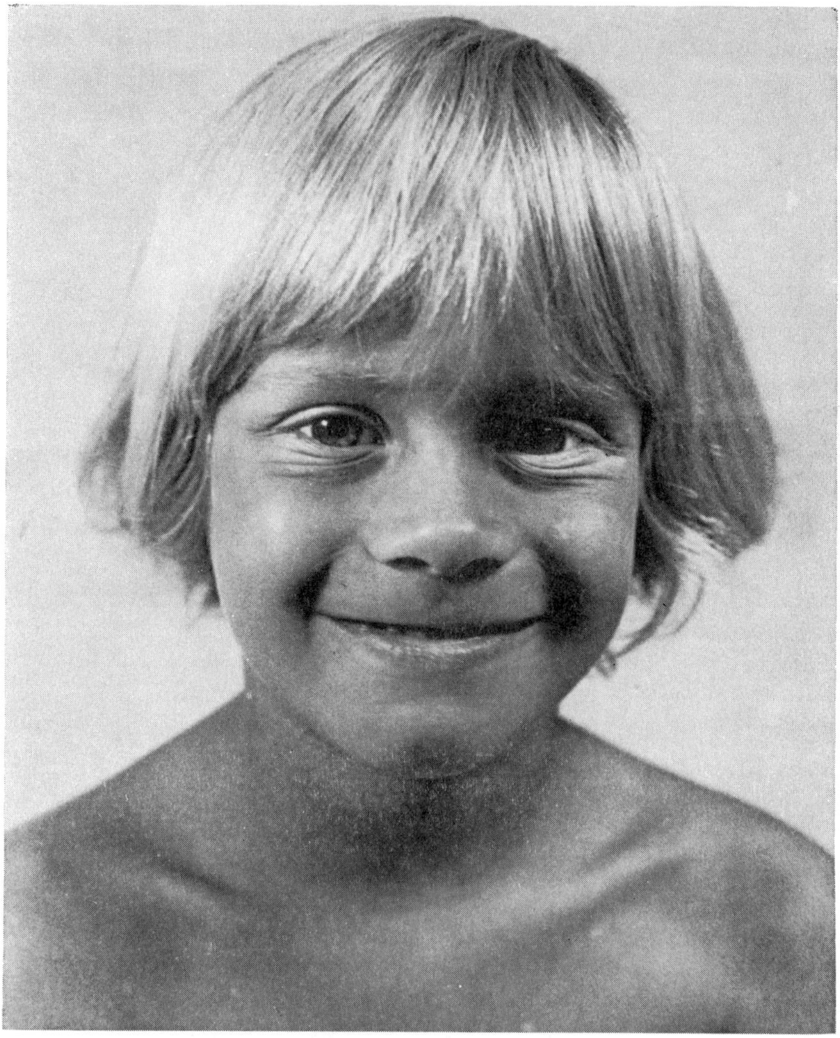

Figure 8-1. Dennie's sign. Courtesy of Bob Sacha.

months of age were associated with an increased incidence of eczema and subsequent perennial rhinitis or asthma in potentially allergic children. Although milk, sugar, corn, wheat, and egg are common precipitating factors in this age group, soya, vitamins, scented baby powder, or paper diapers are also sometimes at fault.[17,40,47]

If hyperactivity is increased during the summer months, pollens or mold spores may be to blame.[5,9,10,43,47,48] Sensitivities to these may be confirmed by appropriate skin tests. Symptoms may respond to appropriate immunotherapy. If hyperactivity during the summer months does not follow a pollen pattern, the ingestion of summer beverages or seasonal fruits should be suspected. If hyperactivity is perennial or noted mainly in the winter months, factors in the patient's home should be suspected. The home is most apt to be at fault if symptoms are noted shortly after a move to a new house, are more severe when the child stays indoors, and are least troublesome when he is camping or on vacation.

If the evidence points to the home, consider pets; dust; furniture; stuffing; carpeting; mattresses; pillows; moldy basement, bathroom or wallpaper; and odors from such diverse items as aerosols, cosmetics, paints, cooking, plastics, tobacco, cleaning solutions, newsprint, or a gas stove or furnace. Note which room seems to cause most symptoms and try to pinpoint exactly what it is in the room that is causing problems. Making the home, particularly the bedroom, more allergy free often helps. If hyperactivity is more conspicuous in school, dust, cleaning solutions, tobacco, perfume, pets, chalk, art supplies, chemically treated paper, and fluorescent lights should be suspected.[1,32,41]

If a patient's problems remain with him regardless of where he goes, and seem to be more severe during the winter months, food may be to blame. No adequate explanation has been given for the observation by Rowe[48] and Rinkel[46] that food sensitivities tend to subside or diminish during the summer months, but this is true. Hyperactivity is thought to lessen during the summer months because children spend more time outside, or are more relaxed on vacation.

Food-related problems should be suspected if a patient's symptoms subside when he does not eat, i.e. when ill or prior to surgery or during religious fasts. If he has an infection, a note should be made if symptoms develop soon after medications have been given. Hyperactivity can be due to ingredients in medications, to dyes, flavors, or sweeteners, or to the drug itself; aspirin and phenobarbitone often aggravate hyperactivity.

Parents should be queried specifically concerning unusual activity patterns associated with holidays such as Easter, Halloween, Christmas, Rosh Hashanah, Yom Kippur, and Chanukah. The ingestion of abnormally large amounts of sugar, chocolate, egg, and artificial coloring at these times may be recalled readily because of repetitive patterns of havoc associated with these celebrations. Details concerning food habits often reveal exact etiologic factors. If a symptom is a daily problem, a frequently eaten food or exposure may be at fault. If hyperactivity occurs sporadically, an infrequent ingestion or exposure is more likely. Parents of hyperactive children should keep daily diet and symptom records for a few weeks to identify the foods and inhalants that may precipitate symptoms. Initially, parents will be able to detect foods that quickly and obviously cause symptoms; later on they may be able to identify those foods which cause delayed symptoms. They should be able to determine the time intervals between the ingestion of foods and the onset of symptoms, and also the duration of the latter. They may, however, err in determining the exact ingredient in the food that is to blame. They may, for example, think that pancakes cause symptoms when the offending food may be corn in the maple syrup.

The relationship between hyperactivity, TFS, and foods is well illustrated by the two following examples.

EXAMPLE 1. Simone was brought up on a proprietary milk formula, and cried constantly from the age of four days. When she was six days old she was placed on an evaporated milk formula and rice, but continued to cry repeatedly. At the age of ten days she developed a diaper rash, and at the age of three weeks vomiting and diarrhea. Symptoms were thought to be due to maternal anxiety, the mother being a nurse and the child her first baby. The mother, however, of her own accord placed her infant on a soya formula without supplementary foods, and within twelve days her baby's dermatitis and the diarrhea and vomiting had subsided, and she began to sleep peacefully. During the next twelve months traces of milk, either alone or in foods, always precipitated a return of her symptoms. When she was two years old she accidentally ingested milk and immediately developed a dermatitis, diarrhea, and hyperactivity.

EXAMPLE 2. Scott was a four-year-old white, adopted child when initially seen. His perennial nasal stuffiness had started at the age of six months and was followed later by a troublesome, persistent cough; he frequently cleared his throat and often vomited mucus daily. He had had, according to his mother, 15 upper respiratory infections a year. He developed urticaria at the age of a year and began to wheeze when he was four. His behavior was intolerable: he hit people, bit his siblings, was violent, aggressive, and destructive, and had at least ten temper tantrums a day. He could not be disciplined. His sleep was interrupted five or six times a night by nightmares. He was sometimes very fatigued and at other times so active that he could only be restrained by being "tied to a piece of furniture." His emotional swings were wide, ranging from elation to extreme depression. He craved milk and cheese. On physical examination he had circles under his eyes, a positive Dennie's sign, and a geographic tongue. He was placed on a strict milk-free diet, and within two weeks he became happy, slept peacefully, and no longer cleared his throat, vomited, or had temper tantrums. His geographic tongue subsided. He played happily and was affectionate. During the subsequent weeks, if he accidentally ingested milk, his previous undesirable symptoms would promptly return. Two years later, at follow-up, his mother stated that he could then drink a glass of milk once a week during the winter, and more frequently in the summer, without experiencing adverse reactions. However, when he ingested more milk, his previous symptoms and geographic tongue returned.

The Relationship Between Foods, Additives and Hyperactivity

Feingold,[13] in 1975, first suggested that artificial food colors and flavors, and foods containing natural salicylates, caused hyperactivity and behavior disorders in some children. He stated that a diet avoiding these factors helped at least 60 percent of hyperkinetic children, and that it enabled 75 percent of these to stop taking activity-modifying drugs. He did not think that allergy was the cause of the TFS and hyperkinesis; he believed that the problem was genetic and nonimmunologic in nature.

Conners,[7] and Harley,[21] both psychologists, subsequently conducted studies similar in design and outcome. After confirmation of hyperactivity and a baseline evaluation, they placed the children under study on a four-week crossover diet. The treatment, a K-P diet,[13] excluded all artificial colors and flavors, nine common fruits that contain natural salicylates, tomato, and commercial candies; it also limited the intake of wheat products. The control diet excluded peanuts, refined sugar, chocolate, and corn products, and also limited the wheat intake. The children's responses were monitored by parents, teachers, and psychologists. The results of their studies were inconclusive and may well have been obscured because both diets excluded a number of foods associated with hyperactivity in children.[10,11,52] A child, for example, who becomes hyperactive after ingesting artificial colors and peanuts would not improve on either diet.

A few children in each group improved when the K-P diet was administered *after* the control diet. Rinkel's observations[45-47] may explain this finding. He found that elimination of some offending foods for more than a two-week period was sometimes followed by a transitory "refractory" period during which symptoms only recurred insidiously. When the K-P diet was administered *before* the control diet, the beneficial effects might have extended into the control period. This effect would not be evident if the K-P diet were given *after* the control diet.

The food industry created the National Advisory Committee on Hyperkinesis and Food Additives in 1975. One of their aims was to evaluate Feingold's claims by the use of chocolate cookies or chocolate bars, each containing 13 mg of food coloring.[21] Placebo cookies and bars were identical in color and taste, but contained no dyes. Subsequent studies might have supported Feingold's hypothesis had the children been sensitive to a 26 mg challenge dose of food coloring. Sensitivities to food colors, as well as to other ingredients in the diet, often are quantitative; for this reason, challenges with an insufficient amount of dye-containing cookies would provide false negative information.[46,47]

Cook and Woodhill[8] found that a Feingold-like K-P diet was helpful in the management of hyperactivity. They found that ten of fifteen children (65%) responded favorably to the K-P diet, and relapsed within three hours of discontinuing it.

Salzman[50] tested thirty-one nonresponsive, hyperactive children with sublingual food coloring. He found that fifteen of thirty-one (50%) had an increase in pulse rate of ten beats per minute, and a falling blood pressure of 15 mmHg or more. When these fifteen patients were placed on the K-P diet, fourteen improved. Accidental ingestion of food coloring was associated with a return of their previous hyperactivity and unacceptable or intolerable behavior.

Williams et al.[57] studied the effect of randomly assigned active or placebo medications in combination with dye-containing or placebo cookies in twenty-six hyperactive children. Double-blind assessments by teachers and parents revealed that stimulant medications controlled hyperactivity more effectively than diet. Seven of the twenty-six children (26%), however, improved on the K-P diet.

Feldman and Tikofsky[14] are presently conducting dye and food studies that attempt to quantitate perceptual motor performance using the Smith Symbol-Digit Modalities Test. They have found that some children become hyperactive and others fatigued with specific sublingual drop or intradermal food challenge.

Swanson[53] has also found that hyperactive children do not react adversely when challenged in a double-blind manner with 26 mg of food colors. Challenges with 100 to 150 mg of dye, however, caused hyperactivity, which interfered with learning.

The author's own interest in hyperactivity began in 1975 when she was asked to see a five-year-old girl with asthma and hay fever; the patient was also extremely hyperactive and appeared to have MBD. Her parents made their home relatively free from inhalant allergens and placed her on a diet free from highly allergenic foods. In less than a week, even though her asthma and hay fever persisted, her behavior became normal. At about the same time, the author was asked to see a second girl, aged nineteen, who had hay fever, extreme fatigue, and daily headaches. Her fatigue and headaches subsided rapidly on a restricted diet. These two patients represented the two extremes of the tension-fatigue syndrome.

Following this, the author studied twenty-four consecutive hyperactive children,[41] 70 percent of whom were atopic. Many had nasal stuffiness, headaches, aching of joints and muscles, spells of abdominal pain, and frequency of micturition or enuresis. Sublingual tests with food colors detected a subgroup of these children who subsequently became repeatedly hyperactive when food colors were ingested. A one-week restricted diet that omitted major allergenic foods was followed by clinical improvement in twelve of the twenty-three patients, and a clearing of most of their chronic TFS symptoms. Single food challenges revealed that the ingestion of the following foods, in order of decreasing importance, was associated with increased activity: food colors, refined sugar, milk, corn, cocoa, wheat, and egg. After the children improved, the parents noted that the following additional foods also were associated with hyperactivity: tomato, apple, orange, grape, peanut, and preservatives. Individualized diets in thirteen of seventeen children resulted in continued improvement over the next six months.

The relationship between foods and additives and hyperactivity in any one child can be demonstrated by first excluding the suspect food (s) or additives from the diet, noting the child's improvement, and then by reintroducing them. To ensure a relapse, it is essential to reintroduce the foods in adequate amounts soon after the child's hyperactivity has subsided, preferably within five to twelve days. If more time is allowed to elapse between recovery and the reintroduction of the foods or colors, or if too little of the challenge food is given, no adverse reactions will be noted. Green[10] also has noted that there may be a refractory period of several days after a food challenge before the food will again cause a reaction.

Adverse reactions to foods also can be demonstrated by double-blind challenge, using encapsulated food extracts. These require special facilities; they are difficult to evaluate stringently in an office setting.

THE TREATMENT OF HYPERACTIVITY

Medications

One method advocated to treat hyperactivity is the use of activity-modifying drugs such as methylphenidate, amphetamines, hydroxyzine, diphenhydramine hydrochloride, thoridiazine hydrochloride, pemoline, chlorpromazine, and imipramine hydrochloride. These drugs are invaluable when the child is unwilling to cooperate or the parent unable to comply with the dietary restrictions. Some parents and physicians, however, find them unacceptable, mainly because of undesirable side effects such as anorexia or dulling of personality. Some children are not helped or are only minimally helped by these medications. A recent addition to the pharmaceutical armamentarium is oral cromolyn, but its role in the management of hyperactivity is yet to be determined.[51] When medications are not helpful, other forms of treatment have to be employed.

Family Guidance

A second common form of adjuvant therapy is family guidance with psychological and social counselling. Most families are grateful for advice and suggestions that enable them to lead a calmer and more normal home life. Therapy of this type often is a helpful, necessary supplement to other forms of treatment, and even when the cause of the hyperactivity is removed, the child and family need help in altering previous maladapted response patterns.

Special Teaching

A third form of therapy includes special education. Children in some communities can be placed in classes with specially trained teachers who help them to cope and learn more effectively. Close, individualized supervision and a paucity of distraction are helpful adjuncts. Many hyperactive children do well in a one-to-one situation, but cannot function well in large groups.

Dietary Management

As has already been indicated, dietary restrictions are often very helpful in controlling hyperactivity. The advantages of dietary treatment are fourfold. First, when foods are the cause of a child's hyperactivity, dietary treatment leads within a week or two to complete recovery. Second, dietary management draws attention to and removes the cause of the child's hyperactivity. Third, it often leads to relief of associated symptoms such as nasal stuffiness, headache, and spells of abdominal pain; the relationship between these symptoms and specific foods is often not recognized by the parents. Fourth, if the entire family is placed on the restricted diet, other members of the family may benefit and may find relief from recurrent unsuspected allergies such as nasal stuffiness and headaches.

Immunotherapy with Food Extracts

An alternative form of treatment, and one that obviates or reduces the need for dietary management, is sublingual or subcutaneous therapy with food extracts. Vaughan and Black[56] described immunotherapy with orally administered or subcutaneous injections of food extracts; they also reviewed a number of previous reports claiming success for this form of treatment. Collins-Williams,[6] in 1955, described oral desensitization to cow's milk. Tuft,[55] in 1955, described successful immunotherapy by injection for a patient with migraine sensitive to wheat. Injection or sublingual therapy with food extracts, however, has not been uniformly successful, and though its value is still debatable, a number of articles have supported its usefulness.[12,20,27,34,38]

Miller,[33] in 1977, conducted a double-blind study on eight patients with diverse medical complaints. One four-year-old boy had marked hyperactivity and behavior problems. The boy's multiple symptoms persisted during the two twenty-day placebo treatment periods, but subsided during both food therapy periods.

O'Shea and Porter[37] conducted a double-blind crossover study in 1978. After titration food testing, children were treated sublingually for two random three-week periods with either a placebo or an extract containing the foods, food coloring, or pollens to which they were sensitive. The extract therapy period was correctly identified by eleven out of fourteen parents and eight out of fourteen teachers.

In 1978, the author[42] reported a single patient who had "hayfever" and the TFS due to cow's milk and food coloring. The patient was able to differentiate, on three occasions because of the prompt recurrence of symptoms, capsules containing cow's milk from those containing sugar, and on two occasions sublingual drops of cow's milk from placebo. All tests were done double-blind.

King and Mandell,[25] in 1978, reported the results of a double-blind study on thirty adults. The patients were tested sublingually with twelve food allergens or chemicals and six placebo solutions. A statistically greater number of nervous symptoms were observed and reported from the allergens than from the placebo challenges.

Levy et al.,[28] in 1978, studied twenty-two hyperactive children to evaluate the effect of yellow dye (FD&C No. 4) challenge during a double-blind crossover dietary trial. They found objective but not subjective confirmation of the diet's efficacy.

In 1979, the second part of the author's original study on hyperactive patients was published.[43] The patients who responded favorably to dietary management were asked to discontinue their diet. They were tested and treated sublingually for the foods to which they were sensitive. They were then allowed to ingest their offending foods in moderation. They continued to do well.

A double-blind evaluation was then completed by eight patients. Each was given two placebos and one food extract solution, all identical in color and taste. Five correctly identified the food extract. The three who did not were asked to resume an entirely normal diet and discontinue all food therapy. Within four weeks, two of these three patients had a recurrence of their hyperactivity. Resumption of the extract therapy caused a prompt remission of symptoms in both patients.

An example of one hyperactive child treated with injections of food extract in a double-blind manner is detailed below. The child had not been helped by sublingual treatment, but was helped by subcutaneous injections of an extract of the foods to which he was sensitive.

Example 3. William, as an infant, was colicky and cried daily until cow's milk was removed from his diet. He first was seen by the author at the age of eleven years. At that time he had been receiving 60 mg of methylphenidate daily for five years to control his hyperactivity; if he missed a dose, his hyperactivity increased. Perennial nasal symptoms had been present since the age of five, and seasonal pollenosis from the age of six. He had received immunotherapy with pollen extract between the ages of eight and eleven. From the age of seven he had complained of weekly spells of abdominal pain associated with headaches, leg cramps at least twice a month, and daily perianal pruritis. He also had diurnal enuresis, flatulence, and halitosis. He was irritable, emotionally labile, and frequently hostile.

When tested sublingually with three drops of equal parts of red, blue and yellow food coloring, he developed nasal congestion and became hyperactive. Three drops of a mixture of equal parts of cocoa, cow's milk, wheat flour, cane sugar, corn syrup, and beaten egg diluted 1:3 with water also caused hyperactivity and "throat clearing." Drops of grape juice and prune juice sublingually produced no symptoms. He then was placed on a diet omitting all food colors, cocoa, milk, wheat, refined sugar, corn, and egg. Within a week his hyperactivity and his other symptoms, except for spells of abdominal pain, had diminished. When the previously omitted foods were returned individually to his diet, the following reactions occurred: milk was followed by headache, abdominal pain, and throat clearing; wheat by belligerence and enuresis; sugar by abdominal pain and muscle aches, giddy behavior, and enuresis; corn by irritability and enuresis; red dyes by irritability and throat clearing, wild behavior, and frequency of micturition; yellow and blue dyes by irritability. Egg and cocoa produced no symptoms. Each offending food was fed at least twice a day, at five-day intervals, to confirm that the foods consistently caused the same symptoms. Prune and grape juice sublingually caused no reactions.

His initial baseline activity score on the parents' Abbot Hyperkinesis Sheet was 22 (normal usually less than 9). After one week on a restricted diet his score fell to 12. During the next five months, while continuing to avoid the foods to which he appeared to be sensitive, William's monthly scores fell gradually to 8. His teacher's Abbott Hyperkinesis Score also fell from 17 to 8 while he was on his limited diet. Sublingual treatment with extracts of the foods to which he had reacted adversely, coupled with relaxation of his diet, did not help to control his symptoms, and his parents' Abbott Hyperkinesis Score rose from 8 to 11. Subcutaneous daily injections of the same extract, however, did help, and he was able to eat in moderation the foods that previously had caused obvious reactions. After two months, injections of food extracts were required only once every forty-eight hours; his parents' Abbott Hyperkinesis Score had fallen to 5. If he ate an excessive amount of one of the foods to which he was sensitive and developed symptoms, an extra injection of food extract led, within twenty minutes, to relief of his symptoms.

To test the efficacy of food injection therapy, three solutions, identical in color, were prepared. In a double-blind manner he was given 0.1 ml of solution A subcutaneously for three days, followed in sequence by solutions B and C, each for three days. His baseline activity score at the onset of the trial was 6. After two days on A he developed a headache, puffiness of the face, irritability, nasal stuffiness, and emotional lability. His activity score rose to 11. After three days on B he cried repeatedly, was unable to concentrate, and became excitable and argumentative. His activity score rose to 16. After three days on C his behavior normalized and his activity score fell to 2. Both he and his family correctly identified C as the food extract.

Treatment with food extract made it possible to gradually reduce the dose of methylphenidate from 60 to 20 mg daily, and later to discontinue it altogether. After 30 months on immunotherapy with food extract he was symptom-free, no longer troubled by nasal stuffiness, headaches, spells of abdominal pain and enuresis, and his behavior was normal.

Hyperactivity: Sequelae and Social Problems

The scope of potential personal, social, and economic problems that may arise from adverse reactions to foods and inhalants is potentially monumental. Battered children,[44] suicides,[45] marital problems, alcoholism,[18] delinquency[2] and possibly crimes of aggression[22,35] and hostility sometimes may be due to, or be sequelae of, abnormal reactions to foods and inhalants. The TFS in the adult may be an unrecognized sequel of hyperactivity in childhood. It may lead to antisocial behavior. For example, of eight children seen by the author who participated in an evaluation of sublingual food therapy,[41,43] three began to steal during placebo treatment. The parents stated that stealing subsided when the children were on restricted diets, and later on unrestricted diets while receiving sublingual therapy with food extracts. An example of this type of behavior follows.

Example 4. Sean, an eleven-year-old, white male, had a long history of perennial nasal stuffiness, abdominal pain, and leg cramps. He was irritable, clumsy, restless, hostile, and fought with family and friends. Stealing was a serious problem. Prick skin tests were negative. Within a week of being placed on a diet that excluded major allergenic foods, his abdominal pain and leg cramps subsided and his hyperactivity diminished. He was fighting only once a day, and for the first time in his life was able to play happily with the other children. As foods were re-added to his diet it was found that mainly food colors and sugar caused irritability, hostility, and violent behavior. After he had been on a diet excluding the major offending food items for several months, he was skin tested and began sublingual food therapy. On this treatment he continued to do well, while ingesting sugar and food coloring in moderation.

At a later date, all food therapy was discontinued and he was asked to ingest an entirely normal diet. Within three weeks, for the first time in eight months, he began to steal at home, in stores, and at school. His teachers noted a dramatic recurrence of his former behavior and activity problems. Reinstitution of food therapy was associated with a remission of his symptoms within a few days. Three years later he continues to be moderately improved in activity and behavior.

In conclusion, there is no doubt that many children respond well to activity-modifying drugs and counselling. After variable periods of time, drugs and psychosocial therapy may be discontinued. Many such children become normal, productive adults; some, however, do not respond to medications or guidance. They are unable to realize their full potential, develop innate talents, or manifest their true personalities until their problems have been recognized and treated, preferably before going to school. The longer these children are allowed to remain maladjusted the more likely they are to become antisocial or chronically ill adults. The methods outlined here indicate the various approaches to the management of hyperactivity in children. Appropriate dietary management can often quickly lessen a patient's hyperactivity and lead to relief of associated allergies. Adequate dietary control in our society is difficult, and the addition of appropriate sublingual or subcutaneous injections often make it possible for patients to eat offending foods in moderation, thus enabling them to live a more normal life.

REFERENCES

1. Blume, K.A.: *Air Pollution in the Schools.* Chicago: The Human Ecology Research Foundation, 1968.
2. Borcal, A. and Rabkin, L.Y.: A precursor of delinquency. The hyperkinetic disorder of childhood. *Psychiatric Quarterly, 48*:387, 1974.
3. Buissert, P.D.: Common manifestation of cow's milk allergy in children. *Lancet, 1*:304, 1978.
4. Cantwell, D.P.: The hyperactive child. *Hosp Pract, 14(1)*:65, 1979.
5. Clarke, T.W.: The relation of allergy to character problems in children: A survey. *Psychiatric Quarterly, 24*:21, 1950.
6. Collins-Williams, C.: Acute allergic reactions to cow's milk. *Ann Allergy, 13*:415, 1955.
7. Conners, C.K., Goyete, C.H., Southwich, D.A., Lees, J.M. and Adrulonis, P. A.: Food additives and hyperkinesis: A controlled double-blind experiment. *Pediatrics, 58*:154, 1976.
8. Cook, P.S. and Woodhill, J.M.: The Feingold dietary treatment of the hyperkinetic syndrome. *Med J Aust, 2*:85, 1976.
9. Crook, W.G.: *Can Your Child Read? Is He Hyperactive?* Jackson: Professional Books, 1977.
10. Crook, W.G., Harrison, W.W., Crawford, S.E. and Emerson, B.S.: Systemic manifestations due to allergy. *Pediatrics, 27*:790, 1961.
11. Davison, H.M.: Cerebral allergy. *South Med J, 42*:712, 1949.
12. Dickey, L.D.: Sublingual antigen testing and therapy for inhalants, foods and petrochemicals. In Dickey, L.D. (Ed.): *Clinical Ecology.* Springfield: Thomas, 1976, pp. 544-555.
13. Feingold, B.F.: *Why Your Child is Hyperactive.* New York: Random House, 1975.
14. Feldman, H.T. and Tikofsky, R.S.: In press (personal communication).
15. Gerrard, J.W., Heiner, D.C., Ives, E.J., and Hardy, L.W.: Milk allergy: Recognition, natural history and management. *Clin Pediatr, 2*:634, 1963.
16. Gerrard, J.W.: Allergy in infancy. *Ped Annals, 3*:9, 1974.
17. Glaser, J. and Johnstone, D.E.: Prophylaxis of allergic disease in children. *N Engl J Med, 274*:715, 1966.
18. Goodwin, D.W., Schulsinger, F., and Hermansen, I.: Alcoholism and the hyperactive child syndrome. *J Nerv Ment Dis, 160*:349, 1975.
19. Green, M.: Sublingual provocation testing for foods and FD&C dyes. *Ann Allergy, 33*:374, 1974.
20. Hansel, F.K.: Sublingual testing and therapy. *Trans Amer Soc Ophthalmol Otolaryngol Allergy, 11*:93, 1970.
21. Harley, J.P., Ray, R.S., Tomasi, L., Eichman, P.L., Matthews, C.G.,

Chun, R., Cleeland, C.S., and Traisman, E.: Hyperkinesis and food additives: testing the Feingold hypothesis. *Pediatrics, 61*:818, 1978.
22. Hippchen, L.J.: Biochemical approaches to offender rehabilitation. *Offender Rehabilitation, 1*:115, 1976.
23. Johnstone, D.E. and Dutton, A.: Dietary prophylaxis of allergic disease in children. *N Engl J Med, 274*:715, 1966.
24. Johnstone, D.E.: The natural history of allergic disease in children. *Ann Allergy, 38*:387, 1977.
25. King, D.S. and Mandell, M.: M.: A double-blind study of allergic cerebral-viscero-somatic malfunctions evoked by provocative sublingual challenges with allergenic extracts: Statistical confirmation of the induction of psychological (mental) and somatic symptoms by provocative testing. Presented at the 12th Advanced Seminar in Clinical Ecology, Key Biscayne, Florida, 1978.
26. Kittler, F.J. and Baldwin, D.G.: The role of allergic factors in the child with minimal brain dysfunction. *Ann Allergy, 28*:203, 1970.
27. Lee, C.H., Williams, R.L., and Binkley, E.L.: Provocative testing and treatment for foods. *Arch Otolaryngol, 90*:113, 1969.
28. Levy, F., Dumbrell, S., Hobbes, G., Ryan, M., Wilton, N., and Woodhill, J.M.: Hyperkinesis and diet: A double-blind crossover trial with a tartrazine challenge. *Med J Aust, 1*:61, 1978.
29. Lockey, S.D.: Reactions to hidden agents in foods, beverages and drugs. *Ann Allergy, 29*:461, 1971.
30. ———: Hypersensitivity to tartrazine (FD&C yellow #5) and other dyes and additives present in foods and pharmaceutical products. *Ann Allergy, 38*:206, 1977.
31. Marks, M.B.: *Physical Signs of Allergy of the Respiratory Tract in Children.* Kalamazoo. Upjohn Company, 1967.
32. Mayron, L.W., Ott, J., Nations, R., and Mayron, E.L.: Light, radiation and academic behavior. *Academic Therapy, 10*:33, 1974.
33. Miller, J.B.: A double-blind study of food extract injection therapy: A preliminary report. *Ann Allergy, 38*:185, 1977.
34. Morris, D.L.: Use of sublingual antigen in diagnosis and treatment of food allergy. *Ann Allergy, 27*:289, 1969.
35. Moyer, K.E.: *The Psychology of Aggression.* New York: Har-Row, 1976, pp. 69-73.
36. O'Banion, D., Armstrong, B., and Cummings, R.H.: Disruptive Behavior: A dietary approach. *J Autism and Child Schizophr, 8*:325, 1978.
37. O'Shea, J.A. and Porter, S.F.: A double-blind study of children with hyperkinetic syndrome treated with multi-allergen extract sublingually. Presented at the 12th Advanced Seminar in Clinical Ecology, Key Biscayne, Florida, 1978.
38. Pfeiffer, G.O.: Sublingual diagnosis and treatment. *Trans Amer Soc*

Ophthalmol Otolaryngol Allergy, 15:109, 1975.
39. Randolph, T.G.: Allergy as a causative factor of fatigue, irritability and behavior problems in children. *J Pediatr, 31*:560, 1947.
40. Rapp, D.J.: *Questions and Answers About Allergies and Your Child.* New York: Drake Pub, 1974, pp. 236-242.
41. ———: Does diet affect hyperactivity. *J Learning Disabilities, 11*:383, 1978.
42. ———: Double-blind confirmation and treatment of milk sensitivity. *Med J Austr, 1*:571, 1978.
43. ———: Food allergy treatment for hyperkinesis. *J Learning Disabilities 12*:608 1979.
44. ———: *Allergies and the Hyperactive Child.* New York: S & S, 1979.
45. Rinkel, H.J., Randolph, T.G., and Zeller, M.: *Food Allergy.* Springfield: Thomas, 1951.
46. Rinkel, H.J.: Food allergy: The role of food allergy in internal medicine. *Ann Allergy, 2*:115, 1944.
47. Rinkel, H.J., Lee, C.H., Brown, D.W., Willoughby, J.W., and Williams, J.M.: The diagnosis of food allergy. *Arch Otolaryngol, 79*:78, 1964.
48. Rowe, A.H.: *Food Allergy.* Philadelphia: Lea & Febiger, 1931.
49. ———: Allergic toxemia and fatigue. *Ann Allergy, 8*:72, 1950.
50. Salzman, L.K.: Allergy testing, psychological assessment and dietary treatment of the hyperactive child syndrome. *Med J Austr, 2*:248, 1976.
51. Simeon, J., O'Malley, M., Tryphonas, H., Graham, D., Mastronardi, M., Simeon, S., and Griffin, J.: Cromolyn DSG effects in hyperkinetic and psychotic children with allergies. Paper presented at the Second International Symposium on Food Allergy, Oct. 16-20, 1978, Mexico City.
52. Speer, F.: Allergic tension-fatigue in children. *Ann Allergy, 12*:168, 1954.
53. Swanson, J.: Behavioral responses to artificial color. Paper presented at the Second International Symposium on Food Allergy, American College of Allergy, 1978, Mexico City.
54. Trites, R., Tryphonas, H., and Ferguson, B.: Treatment of Hyperactivity in a Child with Allergies to Foods. In Fine, M. (Ed.): *Case Studies in Hyperactivity.* Springfield: Thomas, in press.
55. Tuft, L.: *Allergy Management in Clinical Practice.* St. Louis: C.V. Mosby Company, 1973, p. 311.
56. Vaughan, W.T. and Black, J.H.: *Practice of Allergy,* 3rd ed. St. Louis: C.V. Mosby Company, 1954, pp. 321-323.
57. Williams, J.L., Cram, D.G., Tausig, E.T., and Webster, E.: Relative effects of drugs and diet on hyperkinesis behavior: An experimental study. *Pediatrics, 61*:811, 1978.

Chapter 9

THE PREVENTION OF FOOD ALLERGY

JOHN W. GERRARD

ALLERGIC REACTIONS can occur only to allergens to which the child has been exposed, and though they may occur on what seems to be the first exposure, this must have been preceded by previous single or repeated exposures. Children take several seasons to develop hay fever, and adults, on moving to a new district, may take several years to acquire new inhalant sensitivities. The same relationship probably applies to foods, but it is less clear-cut. The child may have been sensitized *in utero* to foods taken by the mother, or subsequently to traces of foods, egg for example, in foods such as custard. The child may, under these circumstances, react to his first overt encounter with a food. Systemic reactions to foods will occur only if food antigens are absorbed.

Gastrointestinal Permeability to Food Antigens

It is generally thought that foods are thoroughly digested in the gastrointestinal tract and that they are absorbed only in the form of their constituent amino acids, hexoses, pentoses, and fatty acids. This is not the case, for trace amounts of ingested foods are absorbed in antigenic form. This was first clearly demonstrated by Walzer,[35] using the P-K test and sera from individuals very sensitive to egg and fish. He injected the sera intradermally into individuals who were at the time avoiding the food to be tested. Twenty-four hours or more later he gave them the food to eat, and in nearly every instance the injected site became red, itchy, and swollen, indicating that some of the food had been absorbed in antigenic form. Reactions were most obvious when the food was taken raw or after a fast; under these circumstances reactions were also rapid, the shortest reaction time being only two minutes. Eighty-three percent of the positive reactions occurred within thirty minutes. Negative reactions occurred only if the subject on whom the test was being carried out was himself very atopic, presumably because receptor sites on mast cells in his skin were already fully saturated with his own IgE. Walzer concluded that the absorption of some food in antigenic form was a natural phenomenon. That this is so can easily be demonstrated by any investigator using serum from a patient very sensitive to a food, injecting the serum into his own skin, and twenty-four hours later ingesting the food in question by mouth. That foods are absorbed in this form is also demonstrated by patients with food-induced urticaria; they differ from the normal, not in absorbing food antigens, but in mounting an IgE response. Although this, the absorption of food antigens, is a natural phenomenon, it occurs more readily in babies during the first few days of life,[14] and in infants after gastroenteritis;[26] under the latter circumstances food proteins may even be detected in the urine. The greater absorption of food antigens in early infancy may be due to the immunological immaturity and the low levels of secretory IgA in the gut at this time, for the immune system plays an important role in holding at bay and limiting the absorption of macromolecules.[32-34]

Antenatal Sensitization

If *in utero* sensitization is to occur, the foods eaten by the mother must not only enter her own circulation but also cross the placenta to stimulate antibody production in the fetus. Immunoglobulin E does not cross the placenta; IgE-mediated allergies are therefore not passively transferred. IgE antibodies can, however, be made *in utero*, for fetal lung and liver are capable of synthesizing IgE as early as eleven weeks.[23] IgE antibodies have also been detected in amniotic fluid at thirteen weeks.[29] Matsumura et al.[20] have studied ten totally breast-fed babies who developed eczema due to egg. The eczema cleared completely when the mothers avoided egg. As the maternal amniotic fluid in each instance contained hemagglutinating antibody to egg, Matsumura postulated antenatal sensitization. He did not demonstrate that IgE sensitization had actually occurred, but that it may do so is suggested by Lyon's[19] observation that breast-fed babies tend to be sensitive and prick test–positive to foods that the mother has taken in abundance during the pregnancy. Lyon gave as an example the case of a baby on the breast developing extensive angioedema to corn and white navy beans. This baby's mother was penniless, and throughout her pregnancy had lived for the most part on corn and white navy beans. It was suggested that it was for this reason the baby had become sensitive to these two foods. Ratner,[25] a few years later, made very similar observations, and went on to suggest that foods taken in abundance during pregnancy might well sensitize the baby. It was probably on account of these observations that when formula feeding became fashionable and cow's milk allergy more widespread, Glaser and Johnstone[11] and Johnstone and Dutton[16] suggested that prevention of allergic disease was best insured by keeping the mother on a diet free from cow's milk and dairy products and egg, and by bringing the baby up on a soya formula.

As antenatal sensitization is possible, and as foods taken in great abundance by the mother are most likely to sensitize her baby *in utero,* it would seem wise for the expectant mother with a strong family history of food allergy to avoid eating too much of any one food and to enjoy a mixed diet, possibly rotating her foods.

Breast Feeding and the Prophylaxis of Food Allergy

If food antigens are as readily absorbed as appears to be the case, and particularly if they are absorbed more readily in infancy than in later childhood, the prophylaxis of food allergy will entail bringing up the baby on the breast[21]—the breast milk contains a minimum of foreign protein—and delaying the introduction of foods, particularly those which are highly allergenic, for as long as is compatible with sound nutrition and normal growth and development. Breast milk, unfortunately, is not by itself free from hazards. Though one would not expect babies, on a priori grounds, to be allergic to breast milk as such, it may exceptionally be the case. There is, in the literature, one very suggestive case report,[18] that of a breast-fed baby who vomited repeatedly and who, when given cow's milk at the age of five days, tolerated it. When discharged home at the age of nine days she was given one more breast feed, at the mother's request, and died of anaphylaxis. There are many more case reports of babies being sensitive to foods ingested by the mother and presumably transmitted to the baby in her milk. A characteristic example was published by Talbot[31] sixty years ago: the baby developed eczema whenever the mother ate chocolate. Commenting on this problem, Shannon,[27] three years later, noted, "Our forefathers believe that foods ingested by the nursing mother might affect the child through the breast milk. We, however, have discarded that belief almost universally and have relegated it to the shelves of superstition simply because we have not proved it to be true." O'Keefe,[24] the year previously, reported a series of breast-fed babies with eczema precipitated by foods (cow's milk, egg, oats and codfish) that the baby had never been given, but that the mother was eating. The eczema cleared in each instance when the mother herself avoided the food in question. Sensitivities to the foods were frequently associated with positive prick tests. Shannon[27] himself had under his care a partially breast-fed baby with widespread urticaria associated with definite or doubtful positive prick tests to a number of foods. The baby in question was taken off all foods, apart from the breast, but the urticaria persisted until the mother was also taken off the same foods. Shannon felt certain that foods taken by the mother must have entered her own milk and must have caused her baby's symptoms. He then set out to demonstrate, using egg as the antigen, that egg eaten by a mother could be detected in her milk. He first sensitized guinea pigs to breast milk obtained from mothers both avoiding and ingesting egg, and then injected the guinea pigs with egg. If the injections were made intrathecally the guinea pigs sensitized by breast milk from mothers eating egg developed anaphylaxis; those sensitized by breast milk from mothers avoiding egg did not. He repeated the experiments, but on the second occasion sensitized the guinea pigs with egg and then injected them with breast milk; only if the mothers were eating egg did the guinea pigs then develop anaphylaxis. Schloss and Worthen[26] tried unsuccessfully to repeat these experiments, throwing doubt on Shannon's conclusions. A few years later Donnally,[6] using the newly introduced P-K test, not only demonstrated that foods taken by the mother entered her milk but also, by comparing the sizes of the wheals produced by breast milk from mothers eating egg and by varying dilutions of egg in breast milk whey, estimated that egg protein was present in breast milk of mothers eating egg in concentrations between 10^{-6} and 10^{-9}.

The Avoidance of Sensitization in Breast-Fed Babies

These observations suggest that breast-fed babies can be sensitized to foods eaten by the mother. Kaplan and Solli's[17] recent experience confirmed this. They noted, when comparing 18 age-matched, breast– and formula-fed babies from highly atopic families, that the breast-fed group (primarily breast-fed for 6 months) were more likely to develop IgE antibodies to cow's milk protein and urticaria, wheezing, and severe diarrhea after ingesting cow's milk than were those brought up on cow's milk. The differences were statistically significant ($P < .03$). Björkstén and Saarinen[2] confirmed these findings, noting that breast-fed babies, when compared with bottle-fed babies from similar atopic backgrounds, were more likely during the first six months of life to develop IgE antibodies to cow's milk, often confirmed by RAST tests, than were babies brought up on formula. The observation that babies brought up on breast milk were more likely to develop IgE antibodies to cow's milk than were babies brought up on cow's milk is so contrary to current dogma that breast is best, that Kaplan had difficulty in getting her observations published. They are, nevertheless, in keeping with the earlier observations of Ratner[25] and Shannon[27] that allergies to cow's milk and to other foods in breast-fed babies are often associated with positive prick tests, and are often severe. Clinical observations that colic in breast-fed babies often subsides when the mother herself avoids cow's milk[15] confirm the effect of diet on breast milk and on the behaviour of the baby. Breast-feeding does not, therefore, guarantee freedom from so-called food allergies. This is also in keeping with the author's own experience.[9] Eighteen instances have been encountered in which breast-fed babies were sensitive to foods being ingested by the mother. The symptoms produced in the baby included diarrhea, vomiting, eczema, colic, rhinorrhea, and bronchitis. The food to which the babies were most commonly sensitized was cow's milk, but sensitization also occurred to oranges, egg, chocolate, tomato, apple, banana, coffee, and strawberry.

It is important that the physician be aware that breast-fed babies can be sensitized to foods ingested by the mother, for he may be tempted, particularly if the baby presents with diarrhea, to suggest that breast-feeding be discontinued and a formula substituted. If the baby is sensitive to cow's milk this will almost certainly compound the baby's problems.

For optimal protection against the development of food allergies, prolonged breast-feeding is recommended for the baby, and a varied diet for the mother. The vagaries of food allergy are such that no comprehensive plan can be offered all babies at special risk, but if specific food allergies are present in the family, such foods are probably best avoided by the mother or eaten only infrequently. When the baby himself is offered foods, he should be offered them singly so that any adverse reactions can be identified and the food avoided.

Formula Feeding

If a baby cannot be breast-fed, and there is a strong family history of cow's milk allergy, some would recommend placing the baby on a soya formula or on a hypoallergenic formula such as Nutramigen®. Reactions to soya are, however, so common, occurring in 20 percent of those allergic to cow's milk, that it would seem wise to approach each case individually. Safer formulas, to which reactions are less likely to occur, are, in our experience, Nutramigen and Pregestimil.® These are also less likely than cow's milk or soya to stimulate antibody production.[7] If the child is to be given a formula derived from cow's milk, we would recommend a modern "humanized" formula; such formulas meet the baby's nutritional needs and provide him with a food that is less allergenic than unprocessed cow's milk. If this is tolerated he should remain on it until he is at least a year old. The introduction of new foods should be delayed for as long as is compatible with good nutrition; foods that are liked and tolerated should, if possible, be given once every four to five days; those which are not tolerated should be avoided.

We cannot ensure that babies brought up either on breast milk or on formulas remain free from allergies, but we can at least recognize allergic reactions when they arise and do our best to minimize their effects. As already indicated, adverse reactions to the same food in breast– and in formula-fed babies tend to differ. The reactions in the breast-fed baby are commonly due to trace amounts of food present in the mother's milk, and are often associated with positive prick and RAST tests. Reactions in the formula-fed baby are usually due to relatively large amounts of the food in question and in such instances are commonly associated with negative prick and RAST tests. This is in keeping with the experience of most pediatricians, for it is unusual to encounter a baby brought up on formula who has such a violent reaction to his formula, whether it be vomiting, diarrhea, or collapse, that the inference that he is allergic to cow's milk is unavoidable. More commonly, his symptoms are less clearly cow's milk–related, and his nasal stuffiness and rhinorrhea may be thought to be due to an infection; their relationship to cow's milk may not even be suspected.

The varying published prevalence rates of cow's milk allergy[1,4,10,13] are probably due to how widely the cow's milk allergy net is spread, what symptoms are included, and how carefully cases are screened. Colic, for example, is considered by some to be a manifestation of allergy,[30] and by others not. The feature that has militated against the recognition of so-called cow's milk allergy has been the unavailability of tests, whether prick, intradermal, or laboratory, that might at least point clinicians in the right direction. Because such tests are lacking, there has been a need to repeatedly demonstrate adverse reactions to cow's milk by withdrawal and challenge. In Goldman's well-known study,[12] three such challenges were required. If all patients who had reacted adversely to cow's milk had had positive prick tests, and had there been a clear-cut relationship between the degree of clinical sensitivity and the size of the response to the prick tests, no such repeated challenges would have been necessary. More recently, considerable light has been shed by May[3,4,22] and his colleagues, using double-blind food challenge, on the relationship between a history of adverse reaction to foods and positive prick tests. In extreme forms of type I hypersensitivity states, reactions to foods are so dramatic and the response to prick tests so obvious, with large wheal and flare responses, that even a single challenge is avoided; if a challenge is suggested by the physician it is often refused by the parent or the patient. This frequent lack of laboratory corroboration of the allergic response to cow's milk, combined with the need of the modern scientific investigator for objective evidence of a reaction, has spurred some clinicians[28] to suggest that mucosal changes in response to milk challenge are much more valid than a succession of watery stools.

If babies with cow's milk allergy are to be helped optimally the relationship between their formula and their symptoms must first be recognized. The recurrent rhinorrhea, bronchitis, and/or diarrhea must not be ascribed to a series of infections—some proved and others not. Its postulated relationship to a food should be recognized, and the food identified. In this context, it should be noted that Frick[8] has observed that viral infections in infancy are often associated with a rising IgE level and the development of clinical allergy. These observations are in keeping with the postulate that if IgE is involved in the primary immune response, cross-reactivity between viral and food antigens might well trigger new allergies. We have also observed that measles, perhaps through nonspecific inhibition of T-helper cells (tuberculin-positive individuals often become temporarily tuberculin-negative following measles), and immunizations may both precipitate the development of new allergies to antigens, e.g. cow's milk, previously tolerated.

It is generally taught that food allergy is relatively common in infants and young children, but rare in the adult, for those with food allergies tend to grow out of their sensitivities. This generalization is too all-embracing to be accepted without reservations. Some people with type I hypersensitivity to foods seem to retain their sensitivities almost indefinitely, so much so that such sensitivities are often referred to as fixed. To those with prick test–negative hypersensitivity, the common form of cow's milk allergy, three possibilities may arise. First, the child, when later given cow's milk, may refuse it and will therefore remain symptom-free on this account; in Saskatchewan, 5 percent of men and 20 percent of women dislike and avoid cow's milk as such. Second, when later offered cow's milk, he may drink it and remain symptom-free, or third, he may drink it and, particularly if he drinks large quantities of it, may once more develop clinical symptoms that may not be identical to the ones previously caused by the offending food. These symptoms, as in the child, are varied and include nasal stuffiness, recurrent rhinorrhea, bronchitis, indigestion, heartburn, diarrhea, headaches, lassitude, or polyarthritis. Deamer[5] has drawn attention to the insidious manner in which symptoms tend to return. Their relationship to milk ingestion is far from obvious, and is usually not suspected by the patient. It can be demonstrated by a cessation of symptoms when milk is avoided, and their return when it is reintroduced. To ensure relative freedom from illness, the mothers of babies with food sensitivities should be advised to avoid giving their children the foods to which they are sensitive, on a relatively permanent basis. I have yet to see a child come to any harm through avoiding foods, ranging from cow's milk to citrus fruits, to which he was sensitive in infancy. I have seen many become ill because they were given them repeatedly. Who, by analogy, having found that a feather pillow caused nasal stuffiness and wheezing, would repeatedly suggest that the child later be asked to sleep on this same pillow, but this is the sort of advice, with reference to milk, that many well-meaning relatives and some physicians still give. If the child dislikes the food when offered it, there is no good reason for making him take it. If he likes the food, he may be allowed it, preferably on a rotary basis, and not more frequently than once every five to seven days, provided it does not precipitate a return of his symptoms. Children who develop sensitivities to cow's milk seem prone to develop sensitivities to other foods, particularly highly allergenic ones, if they are given frequently and in large amounts. Foods are best given in moderation, and on a rotary basis. Cow's milk is the most common food allergen, not because it is particularly allergenic, but simply because it is consumed by so many people in such large quantities.

It is all too easy to become so concerned or immersed in the problem of overt or potential reactions to foods that nonallergic diseases and the contribution of inhalants to the child's symptomatology are overlooked. House dust and animal danders are still important allergens,[21] though they are being replaced in many homes by cigarette smoke, sometimes an irritant but also on occasion an allergen, deodorants, perfumes, hair sprays, natural gas, propane, and emanations from plastic materials. I do not think that we can, by prophylactic measures, prevent the development of allergies, but we can certainly reduce their prevalence and, by identifying them early and instituting suitable treatment, minimize their effects on our patients.

In conclusion, although most people do not suffer from allergic reactions, or experience only the occasional trivial one, a sizeable segment of the population is handicapped by allergies that make them sufficiently ill to require medical attention. Some are resigned to learning to live with their medical problems. The majority of these subjects come from allergic families. There is no way in which to ensure that they will not develop allergies, but the prevalence and severity of food allergies can at least be minimized by bringing up children as suggested here, and by identifying and providing appropriate treatment for allergies as and when they arise.

REFERENCES

1. Bachman, K.D. and Dees, S.C.: Milk allergy. 1. Observations on incidence and symptoms in "well" babies. *Pediatrics, 20:*393, 1957.
2. Björkstén, F. and Saarinen, U.M.: IgE antibodies to cow's milk in infants fed breast milk and milk formulae. *Lancet, 2:*439, 1978.
3. Bock, S.A., Buckley, J., Holst, A., and May, C.D.: Proper use of skin tests with food in diagnosis of hypersensitivity to food in children. *Clin Allergy, 7:*375, 1977.
4. Clein, N.W.: Cow's milk allergy in infants. *Ann Allergy, 9:*195, 1951.
5. Deamer, W.C., Gerrard, J.W., Speer, F.: In press.
6. Donnally, H.H.: The question of the elimination of foreign protein (egg white) in woman's milk. *J Immunol, 19:*15, 1930.
7. Eastham, E.J., Lichauco, T., Grady, M.I., and Walker, W.A.: Antigenicity of infant formulas: Role of immature intestine on protein permeability. *J Pediatr, 93:*561, 1978.
8. Frick, O.L., German, D.F., and Mills, J.: Development of allergy in

children. I. Association with virus infections. *J Allergy Clin Immunol, 63*:228, 1979.

9. Gerrard, J.W.: Allergy in breast fed babies to ingredients in breast milk. *Ann Allergy, 42*:69, 1979.
10. Gerrard, J.W., MacKenzie, J.W.A., Goluboff, N., Garson, J.Z., and Maningas, C.S.: Cow's milk allergy: Prevalence and manifestations in an unselected series of newborns. *Acta Paediatr Scand (Suppl), 234:* 1973.
11. Glaser, J. and Johnstone, D.E.: Prophylaxis of allergic disease in the newborn. *JAMA, 153*:620, 1953.
12. Goldman, A.S., Anderson, D.W., Sellers, W.A., Saperstein, S., Kniker, W.T., and Halpern, S.R.: Milk allergy. 1 Oral challenge with milk and isolated milk proteins in allergic children. *Pediatrics, 32*:425, 1963.
13. Halpern, S.R., Sellars, W.A., Johnson, R.B., Anderson, D.W., Saperstein, S., and Reisch, J.S.: Development of childhood allergy in infants fed breast, soy, or cow's milk. *J Allergy Clin Immunol, 51*:139, 1973.
14. Heiner, D.C.: Absorption of immunologically active wheat protein in man. *In Macromolecular Aspects of Protein Absorption and Excretion in the Mammalian Intestine*. Report of the 15th Ross Conference in Pediatric Research. Ross Laboratories, Columbus, Ohio, 1964, p. 106.
15. Jakobsson, I. and Lindberg, T.: Cow's milk as a cause of infantile colic in breast-fed infants. *Lancet, 2*:437, 1978.
16. Johnstone, D.E. and Dutton, A.M.: Dietary prophylaxis of allergic disease in children. *N Engl Med J 274*:715, 1966.
17. Kaplan, M.S. and Solli, N.J.: IgE to cow's milk protein (CMP) in breast-fed atopics. *J Allergy Clin Immunol*. In press.
18. Leveuf, J. and Vignes, H.: *Centre bl d ges Heilk, 28*:12, 389, 1934. Quoted by Wergelund, H.: Three fatal cases of probable familial allergy to human milk. *Acta Paediatr (Suppl I), 35*:321, 1948.
19. Lyon, G.M.: Allergy in an infant of three weeks. *Am J Dis Child, 36:* 1012, 1928.
20. Matsumura, T., Kuroume, T., Oguri, M., Iwasaki, I., Kanbe, Y., Yamada, T., Kawabe, S., and Negishi, K.: Egg sensitivity and eczematous manifestations in breast-fed newborns with particular reference to extra-uterine sensitisation. *Ann Allergy, 35*:221, 1975.
21. Matthew, D.J., Taylor, B., Norman, A.P., Turner, M.W., and Soothill, J.E.: Prevention of eczema. *Lancet 1*:321, 1977.
22. May, C.D.: Objective clinical and laboratory studies of immediate hypersensitivity reactions to foods in asthmatic children. *J Allergy Clin Immunol 58*:500, 1976.
23. Miller, D.L., Hirvonen, T., and Gitlin, D.: Synthesis of IgE by the human conceptus. *J Allergy Clin Immunol, 52*:182, 1973.
24. O'Keefe, E.S.: The relation of food to infantile eczema. *Boston Med Surg J, 183*:569, 1920.

25. Ratner, B.: A possible causal factor of food allergy in certain infants. *Am J Dis Child, 35*:277, 1936.
26. Schloss, O.M. and Worthen, R.W.: The permeability of the gastro-enteric tract of infants to undigested protein. *Am J Dis Child, 11*:342, 1916.
27. Shannon, W.R.: Demonstration of food proteins in human breast milk by anaphylactic experiments on guinea pigs. *Am J Dis Child, 22*:223, 1921.
28. Shiner, M., Ballard, J., Brook, C.G.D., and Herman, S.: Intestinal biopsy in the diagnosis of cow's milk protein intolerance without acute symptoms. *Lancet, 2*:1060, 1975.
29. Singer, A.D., Hobel, C.J., and Heiner, D.C.: Evidence for secretory IgA and IgE in utero. *J Allergy Clin Immunol, 53*:94, 1974.
30. Speer, F.: Colic and allergy. *Arch Pediatr, 75*:271, 1958.
31. Talbot, F.B.: Eczema in childhood. *Med Clin North Am, 1*:985, 1918.
32. Walker, W.A., Isselbacher, K.J., and Bloch, K.J.: Intestinal uptake of macromolecules: Effect of oral immunisation. *Science, 177*:608, 1972.
33. Walker, W.A., Wu, M., Isselbacher, K.J. and Bloch, K.J.: Intestinal uptake of macromolecules. III. Studies of the mechanism by which immunisation interferes with antigen uptake. *J. Immunol, 115*:854, 1975.
34. Walker, W.A.: Host defence mechanisms in the gastrointestinal tract. *Pediatrics, 57*:901, 1976.
35. Walzer, M.: Studies in absorption of undigested protein in human beings. *J Immunol, 14*:143, 1927.

Chapter 10

THE MANAGEMENT OF FOOD ALLERGY

Joseph B. Miller

Reactions to foods fall into two clinical types, immediate and delayed. Immediate reactions often occur within minutes after taking the food in question, whereas delayed reactions may occur many hours later.

IMMEDIATE REACTIONS

Immediate reactions tend to cause anaphylaxis, angioedema, urticaria, asthma, vomiting, and acute diarrhea. These are easily recognized as allergic reactions, not only because of their sudden appearance, but also because they usually are precipitated by infrequently eaten foods taken just before the reaction occurs. These foods are relatively easy to identify and include nuts, eggs, strawberries, mushrooms, fish, shellfish, and some legume and seeds such as peanut, soy, cottonseed, mustard, and buckwheat. The foods need only be taken in small amounts to produce obvious reactions. On each re-exposure, an immediate reaction tends to recur, so that even after the lapse of many years, if the food is taken again, the same reaction occurs. These reactions are often associated with positive prick tests and can often be confirmed, as Bock et al have shown[6-8] by double-blind challenge. IgE levels often are elevated and radioallergosorbent tests (RAST) often are positive.[9,10]

DELAYED REACTIONS

Delayed reactions to foods also involve the gastrointestinal tract, but often with vague symptoms such as indigestion, flatulence, abdominal pain, discomfort, and aphthous stomatitis; they may also involve the respiratory system with recurrent moderate laryngeal edema, rhinitis, and asthma; the nervous system with headache, mental torpor, depression, hyperactivity, and sleeplessness; the skeletal system with arthralgias and myalgias; and the skin with pruritus, eczema, chronic urticaria, and adult acne. Symptoms are not often considered to be due to food sensitivity because they do not usually occur immediately after meals and the foods that usually precipitate them are those which are eaten daily and in relatively large amounts. The foods commonly incriminated include cow's milk, chocolate, wheat, corn, egg, coffee, citrus fruits, beef, pork, chicken, and other such regularly consumed dietary staples. The foods that cause delayed reactions can also cause immediate reactions, and vice versa, but it usually requires only a small amount of the food to cause an immediate reaction, and a larger amount to cause a delayed reaction.

Delayed, unlike immediate, sensitivity may not be permanent, and symptoms usually do not recur after each response. For example, if the food is avoided for fourteen days or longer, a degree of tolerance begins to build up and the food may no longer precipitate symptoms. If it is once more regularly taken in large amounts, the original symptoms will almost certainly return; if taken at intervals of four or more days, they may not. If the food is first avoided for four to fourteen days, i.e. for a sufficiently long time for symptoms to subside, but not long enough for tolerance to occur, and if it is then taken in normal amounts by itself, the original symptoms usually will return, often in an exaggerated form. It is as though the regular ingestion of a food causes symptoms to be partially obscured or masked, but when the food is taken after four to fourteen day's abstinence, symptoms are enhanced and tend to occur soon after ingestion so that the relationship between the food and the symptoms become abundantly clear.[68] A food, for example egg, taken daily may cause only cyclic or intermittent headaches; when egg products are avoided, headaches will subside. If, however, egg is taken again after a week's avoidance, the headache will return and may be unusually abrupt, severe, and prolonged; it may even cause additional symptoms such as vomiting or vertigo.

Another unusual feature of the delayed type of food sensitivity is that although avoidance of a frequently eaten, symptom-producing food may in the long run lead to tolerance and relief of symptoms, the first omission of the food may lead to so-called withdrawal symptoms.[69] A patient, for example, who had been in the habit of ingesting corn products several times each day developed severe headache, disorientation, and inability to concentrate or think clearly for three days when she suddenly stopped eating corn. Similar severe or bizarre symptoms can follow the sudden avoidance of any food to which the patient has become habituated or addicted. This delayed type of food sensitivity is usually associated with negative prick tests, low IgE levels, and negative RAST.

Difficulty in Recognizing Delayed Food Reactions

Features that make the delayed type of food allergy difficult to recognize include first, the long latent period that elapses between the ingestion of the food and the manifestation of symptoms; second, the variability of the response; third, the bizarre nature of many of the symptoms; and fourth, that symptoms may at times be caused by hidden ingredients or additives rather than by the food itself.

With regard to the *long latent period,* a patient with migraine due to wheat may eat spaghetti at noon one day and awake early the next morning with a severe headache; it is unlikely that the headache will be ascribed to a food, let alone to wheat. A second patient may eat pork at dinner one day and develop vertigo after lunch on the following day; he may not only fail to correlate pork with the vertigo, but may tentatively attribute the vertigo to foods eaten at lunch.

The classic example of the long latent period and the unexpected discovery and inadvertent confirmation of a food sensitivity is that described by Walter Alvarez[3] concerning his own reaction to chicken. He used to suffer from "dumb Mondays," i.e. inability to think clearly and work productively on Mondays. By keeping a diet diary, he finally detected the relationship between eating chicken and chicken gravy on Sundays and his "dumb Mondays." He then eliminated his "dumb Mondays" by avoiding chicken and chicken gravy on Sundays. Later, he developed an overwhelming craving for chicken while on a camping trip where chicken was not available. When he returned from the trip, he compulsively ate an entire chicken at his first meal and suffered a severe reaction, including hallucinations and four days of severe depression.

If a patient eats a food in moderate quantities at least two or three times a week, he may experience only insidious delayed symptoms and will not suspect the food in question. If he eats the food occasionally in a more rapidly absorbed form (such as chicken gravy), he may have more intense symptoms of the delayed type and he will not correlate them with the food unless he is a very accurate observer and uses a diet diary or deliberate challenge feedings. If, by chance, he avoids the food for four to fourteen days, his next exposure to it will tend to produce more obvious immediate symptoms, particularly if the quantity ingested is large or if he eats it in two closely spaced meals. Even so, he may still deny any correlation between the food and symptoms because, as he says, he has often eaten the food in the past and it has never bothered him before. When he again resumes eating it frequently, symptoms will usually immediately revert to the insidious delayed type and will not obviously be related to the food; he may, therefore, become even more certain that he is not sensitive to it.

A second factor that makes the identification of the delayed type of food sensitivity difficult is the *variability of symptoms produced.* Symptoms may be negligible if the amount of the food taken is very small, but may be severe or unusual if the amount taken is large, particularly if taken in two consecutive meals after four to fourteen days of abstinence. Some patients have a single symptom caused by many different foods; one patient may develop asthma from ingesting any one of five different foods, and another migraine from any one of ten different foods. Other patients may experience symptoms referable to several different systems, developing nasal stuffiness, nausea and mental dullness from each of several different foods. Still others have different symptoms from different foods, such as nasal stuffiness after ingesting beef, asthma after egg, headache after yeast, and insomnia with night sweats after rice. As described, different responses can be caused at different times in the same patient by varying the amount of the food, the frequency of its ingestion, and the form in which it is ingested. For example, corn in the form of corn syrup or corn alcohol may cause a more obvious or severe reaction than corn on the cob.

A third factor that militates against making a diagnosis of food allergy is that many patients have *bizarre symptoms*. They may not have classical asthma, hay fever, urticaria, or eczema, and for this reason their symptoms are thought to be functional in origin. This is not surprising, for their symptoms—bloating, crampy abdominal pain, diarrhea, flushing, chills, limb and joint pains, unexplained profuse perspiration, headaches, tiredness and depression—have not yet been correlated with any laboratory evidence of organic disease.[70] The natural, almost inevitable conclusion is that the symptoms are functional and that the patient is a hypochondriac. This conclusion often is enhanced by discovering that the patient has compulsive feeding habits, such as drinking endless cups of coffee or, in one of Finn's patients,[16] eating raw potato. Many such patients also seek help from vitamins, nutritional supplements, tranquilizers, and other medications; sensitivity to such products may in fact perpetuate their symptoms.

These patients are not basically neurotic, but they are less able to cope with daily problems because their allergic symptoms distract and bewilder them. They shop for relief from physician to physician, their self-esteem diminishes, and their anxieties increase when they are told repeatedly that their symptoms are "only due to nerves." They receive symptomatic and supportive care rather than specific treatment. Many who are not primarily depressed by specific cerebral allergic reactions become secondarily depressed from the feeling of being hopelessly trapped. They may end by receiving multiple medications, surgical procedures, electroshock therapy, or prolonged psychotherapy.

To the allergist who deals primarily with immediate hypersensitivity, the list of symptoms discussed here will seem strange and unfamiliar. They are, nevertheless, precipitated by both foods and inhalants. That this is so has been attested to by many observant allergists, some of whom were themselves sensitive to foods and suffered many of the symptoms and syndromes just described.[18,70,75,78]

The fourth factor that makes a diagnosis of delayed food sensitivity unlikely is that it may not be the food itself that causes symptoms, but *hidden additives and chemicals* added to the food either before or after processing. Grapes sprayed with insecticides or wheat with herbicides may cause symptoms in highly sensitive patients, while the same foods free from chemicals may not. Salmon in resin-lined cans may provoke symptoms, but freshly caught may not. Cow's milk passed through homogenizing eqiupment and delivered in waxed cartons containing cornstarch or in bottles washed with detergents may cause symptoms, but raw cow's milk may not. Steaks broiled in a gas oven or fried in a Teflon®-lined pan may cause symptoms, but steaks broiled in an electric oven may not. In the above instances, there may not be a consistent reaction to the same food because the reaction is really to a hidden agent, and the postulated relationship between ingestion and symptoms may therefore be dismissed.

A final factor that sometimes clouds the issue is that patients and physicians may ascribe these reactions to nonspecific factors such as spiciness, greasiness, roughness, acidity, natural salicylates, tyramine content, or enzyme deficiencies. Most physicians simply do not think in terms of delayed reactions or hidden ingredients and have no diagnostic tools in their armamentarium for delineating these factors.

DIAGNOSIS

The preceding paragraphs have outlined the main features of the two common types of food sensitivity, as well as the factors that make it difficult to correlate foods with symptoms in patients with the delayed type of food sensitivity. There are, however, aids to diagnosis. These are the history, skin tests, laboratory aids, dietary challenge, and elimination diets.

The History

In the immediate type of food allergy, the history often provides invaluable information since, as already indicated, patients often know which foods precipitate symptoms and which symptoms are precipitated by each food. Further investigations may do no more than confirm what the patient already suspects.

The history is not as helpful in the delayed type of food sensitivity. The patient may not suspect that foods, much less which specific foods, are precipitating the symptoms. In fact, many of the foods eventually incriminated will often be those which the patient is sure are best tolerated. Therefore, as Bock et al.[6] state, the physician must be aware of the syndromes likely to be precipitated by foods. As discussed, these include disorders often thought to be functional: headaches, insomnia, hyperactivity, lassitude, aphthous stomatitis, abdominal discomfort, flatulence, diarrhea, myalgias, and arthralgias; as well as those which are generally considered to have an allergic component, including recurrent laryngeal edema, rhinitis, asthma, eczema, and chronic urticaria.

The clinician can often deduce useful information from his patients through knowledge of the cyclic nature of food sensitivity, and the roles of masking, craving, addiction, tolerance, withdrawal symptoms, and exaggerated reactions that might have occurred in the past when the food was omitted and reingested. Familiarity with hidden food ingredients, chemical additives, and food labelling practices is also helpful, and will be discussed below in detail.

Skin Tests

In immediate type of food allergy, using fourteen common foods in concentrates of 1:20 w/v, Bock et al.[6] showed that prick tests that produced a 3mm or greater wheal helped to identify those who could be shown by double-blind challenge to have clinical hypersensitivity. But not all those with positive prick tests reacted to the double-blind challenge. Some were categorized as having subclinical hypersensitivity, since their symptoms were not precipitated by a single feeding of a small amount (4 to 8 grams) of the food. Symptom production from the use of two or more such foods taken simultaneously was not studied. The best correlation of prick tests with reactions to foods, in their experience,[7] was with egg; 53 percent (10 of 19 with positive prick tests) had symptoms on double-blind challenge. By contrast, only 20 percent (2 of 10 with positive prick tests) had symptoms from soy on double-blind challenge. Thus, subclinical hypersensitivity is very common. No corn reactions were reported, but this may have been at least partly because corn products were allowed in the basic diet (corn oil margarine, white vinegar, etc.), and also because the placebo capsules contained corn sugar (dextrose).

In the delayed type of food sensitivity, prick tests are usually negative, and if positive are only weakly so.[12,14,78,84] Such tests, therefore, are of little or no help. Intradermal tests, by contrast, are often very useful in identifying the foods precipitating symptoms. Not only do they often produce local wheals, but it is often found that when a single food extract is injected intradermally, the patient experiences the same symptoms as those produced by ingestion of the food.[56] In some instances, such symptoms may be produced in the absence of a positive wheal; such symptom induction is of great diagnostic value in skin-test negative patients. Intradermal testing is also of great value in determining the concentration of the extract to be used in immunotherapy. This technique for testing requires meticulous attention to detail; the reward for this effort is in the ability to protect the patient from his symptom-producing foods by using food extract injection therapy employing doses determined by these tests. Since this procedure plays an essential role in the treatment of many patients with delayed type of food sensitivity, a special section is devoted to it at the end of this chapter.

Laboratory Aids

A number of investigators have recently studied the comparative value of history, RAST, prick tests, and oral challenge in immediate food allergy.[2,5,9,10,34] Chua[9] and colleagues found that prick tests correlated with clinical history in 72 percent of cases of immediate type of food allergy, and RAST in 54 percent. The

RAST is thus less reliable than the prick test, and neither is as reliable as history, challenge, and, in my experience, intradermal tests appropriately performed and interpreted. There seems to be a general consensus that RAST fairly commonly identifies anaphylactic sensitivities, particularly due to peanut, egg, and fish, but that it usually does not identify clinical sensitivities to other foods such as cow's milk, wheat, and soy. Björkstén et al.[5] found, when studying patients sensitive to wheat, that there was a good correlation between positive wheat RAST and baker's asthma due to inhaled wheat flour. However, this was not the case in patients exhibiting clinical hypersensitivity to ingested wheat. The latter patients may have had the delayed type of food sensitivity.

Dietary Challenge

Dietary challenge is probably the tool most commonly employed for detection of food sensitivity. It is simple in concept but deceptively difficult to implement. Dietary challenge is usually not very informative unless the patient first avoids all traces of the specific food to be challenged for at least four days, preferably for seven, and then eats a large quantity of that specific food in simple form. A single feeding may produce no symptoms; in these cases, a second feeding should be taken in two or three hours to insure an adequate challenge. Then, if no immediate reaction occurs, and there are good reasons for suspecting the food in question, it should be taken three times a day for at least three consecutive days while checking carefully for onset of delayed symptoms. If the food is avoided for two weeks or longer before being reintroduced, a degree of tolerance may develop and the subsequent challenge may be negative.

Ambulatory patients eating self-chosen meals often find it difficult or impossible to carry out these required dietary restrictions or to properly note and record subtle symptoms occurring at work, at school, or in the midst of other activities. Challenge is most reliable in severe anaphylactic types of allergies, but is not safe to use in these situations.

Elimination Diets

Omitting dietary challenge entirely and placing the patient directly on an elimination diet has been employed successfully by many.[11,71,78] Restricted diets usually contain only a limited number of "less allergenic" foods. Some patients respond well and can later identify the foods to which they are sensitive when they reintroduce them into the diet. Others do not respond, since they are allergic to some of the allowed foods, or while on the elimination diet, they quickly become sensitive to them through repetitive ingestion. Many drop out because they are unable or unwilling to follow severe dietary restrictions.

Randolph,[63] Rea,[73] and others have successfully managed patients with very complex food and chemical sensitivities by first hospitalizing them and then, under carefully controlled conditions, fasting them for four to five days to clear symptoms. Then, under close observation to detect food sensitivities, they have given them individual, natural, less chemically contaminated foods. After sensitivity to foods has been established, they finally have switched patients onto ordinary, commercially available foods to detect chemical sensitivities.[38,50,62] This is far more accurate and reliable than the ambulatory challenge procedures commonly employed. If these patients are sensitive to a great many foods that are difficult to avoid, they can usually be helped a great deal by food extract immunotherapy.

TREATMENT

Dietary Management

Some fortunate patients can readily be helped by fairly simple diets because their symptoms are precipitated by only a few foods. Others are sensitive to so many foods that dietary management is difficult or impossible. A surprisingly large number of these patients seem to be sensitive to nearly all the foods they eat very frequently. In such cases, dietary management alone is usually unsuccessful, and immunotherapy with food extracts is usually needed. In what follows, an outline is given of diets designed for patients with narrow, intermediate, and broad food sensitivities. The first avoids currently or previously suspected foods plus cow's milk products and chocolate. The second avoids these same foods in addition to wheat and corn. The third excludes all these foods and also all other cereals, all beverages (except water and unsweetened fruit juices), beet and cane sugar, commercially prepared foods containing artificial colors, artificial flavors, preservatives, and other chemical additives, and all other complex processed foods ("factory foods") that contain multiple or unknown ingredients.

Diet #1. This is a milk– and chocolate-free diet. Some patients, particularly infants and children, can achieve excellent relief by completely avoiding any foods to which they are suspected to be sensitive, as well as milk products and the chocolate family. The chocolate family, or Sterculiaceae, includes the cocoa bean, cola nut, and karaya gum derived from *Sterculia* trees of East India. Milk and other avoidance lists are available from allergy laboratories. Cow's milk and chocolate are two of the most commonly allergenic foods in the Western diet; cow's milk also may be responsible for other problems such as lactose malabsorption.

If Diet #1 relieves symptoms adequately within one to three weeks, each of the avoided foods can be re-introduced individually by the challenge method described earlier, if deemed safe and desirable. Challenge-negative foods may be taken regularly; challenge-positive foods should be avoided completely for at least three to six months. If they are then tolerated, they may be rotated into the diet no more frequently than at one meal every four days to maintain tolerance.

Diet #2. This diet can be instituted at the start if a more restricted diet is indicated and if the patient is cooperative. Diet #2 avoids the same foods as does Diet #1, with the addition of wheat and corn. It is intermediate between the simplest of diets and the more comprehensive diet used for patients with multiple sensitivities.

Milk, chocolate, wheat, and corn are ingredients of a great many processed foods. When placed on Diet #2, some patients exclaim that there is nothing left for them to eat. They can be reassured by pointing out that this is a temporary baseline diet, and that they are still allowed all meats, fowl, seafoods, eggs, vegetables, fruits, salads, oils, corn– and wheat-free starches, sweets, juices, nuts, berries, and other foods, as long as they are obtained in unprocessed form and are known not to be contaminated with milk, chocolate, wheat, or corn. They must avoid only four of more than 400 individual simple available foods (Table 10-I).

TABLE 10-I
Individual Simple Foods*

	MEATS
80	Beef
80	Goat
99	Hare
80	Lamb
123	Pork
99	Rabbit
116	Squirrel
128	Venison, European red
133	Venison, white tailed
	FOWL
110	Chicken
77	Duck
77	Goose
104	Guinea fowl
110	Peafowl
110	Pheasant
110	Quail
102	Turkey
110	Egg (chicken, duck, etc.)
	SCALEFISH
82	Amberjack
91	Anchovy
119	Bass, Oriental spotted
119	Bass, white
75	Beluga
84	Black bass, largemouth
84	Black bass, smallmouth
84	Black bass, spotted
113	Bluefish
84	Bluegill
117	Bonita
83	Buffalofish
122	Butterfish
89	Carp
98	Catfish
98	Catfish, Mississippi
83	Chub
93	Cod
115	Croaker
90	Dolphin, common
88	Dolphin fish
115	Drum, freshwater
78	Eel, common
79	Flounder, left-eyed
111	Flounder, right-eyed
79	Flounder, southern
79	Flounder, summer
111	Flounder, winter
119	Grouper
94	Grunt, common
94	Grunt, gray
94	Grunt, yellow
93	Haddock
83	Hagfish
111	Halibut, Atlantic
79	Halibut, California
111	Halibut, Pacific
85	Herring
83	Lumpfish
117	Mackerel, Atlantic
117	Mackerel, frigate
82	Mackerel, jack
117	Mackerel, king
117	Mackerel, Spanish
85	Menhaden
103	Mullet, gray
103	Mullet, striped
103	Mullet, white
92	Muskellunge
112	Paddlefish, North American
118	Perch, ocean
119	Perch, white
109	Perch, yellow
92	Pickerel
92	Pike, northern
109	Pike, walleye
85	Pilchard (sardine)
111	Plaice
93	Pollock
82	Pompano
121	Porgy
84	Pumpkinseed
115	Redfish
101	Red snapper
119	Rockfish
118	Rosefish
114	Salmon, Atlantic
114	Salmon, coho
114	Salmon, pink
119	Sea bass, black
85	Shad
93	Silver hake
103	Silversides
106	Smelt, common
120	Sole
115	Squeteague
75	Sturgeon
83	Sucker
83	Sucker, white
84	Sunfish
84	Sunfish, longeared
114	Trout, brook
114	Trout, brownlake
114	Trout, rainbow

*The number preceding each food refers to the numerical location of the food family in Table 10-III.

TABLE 10-I (continued)

117	Tuna, bluefin
117	Tuna, skipjack
111	Turbot
115	Weakfish
87	Whitefish
115	Whiting, king
82	Yellow jack
	CRUSTACEANS
81	Crab
97	Crayfish
97	Lobster
97	Prawn
108	Shrimp
	MOLLUSKS
95	Abalone
125	Clam
107	Oyster
105	Scallop
96	Snail, edible
100	Squid, North American
	VEGETABLES
36	Artichoke, Chinese
19	Artichoke, globe
36	Artichoke, Japanese
19	Artichoke, Jerusalem
40	Asparagus
32-G	Bamboo shoots
32-G	Bamboo sprouts
39	Beans
	acaia
	adsuki
	alfalfa
	asparagus
	black
	broad
	bush
	butterbean, calico
	butterbean, white
	carob
	fava
	fenugreek
	frijole
	guar gum
	gum arabic
	jack
	kidney, red
	kidney, white
	lablab
	licorice
	lima
	navy
	pinto
	pole
	snapbean
	soybean
	stringbean
	tamarind
	tepary
	tonka
	tragacanth
	wax
	yambean
18	Beets
22	Broccoli
22	Brussels sprouts
19	Burdock root
22	Cabbage, Chinese
22	Cabbage, common
22	Cabbage, savoy
8	Cabbage palm
39	Carob
71	Carrot
22	Cauliflower
71	Celeriac
71	Celery
19	Celtuce
18	Chard, Swiss
71	Chervil
19	Chicory
40	Chives
22	Collards
11	Comfrey
32-D	Corn
19	Dandelion
65	Eggplant
19	Endive, common
19	Endive, French (escarole)
71	Fennel, sweet
22	Horseradish
22	Kale
22	Kohlrabi
19	Lettuce
2	Mushroom
41	Okra
71	Parsnip
39	Peanut
39	Peas
	blackeye
	butterpeas
	chick (garbanzo)
	cowpea
	creme
	crowder
	English
	field
	green split
	lady finger
	lentil
	pigeon pea, common
	purplehull
	snow
	Spanish
	yellow eye
	yellow split
32-D	Popcorn
21	Potato, sweet
65	Potato, white
22	Radish
22	Rape
54	Rhubarb
22	Rutabaga
19	Salsify
3	Seaweed
18	Spinach
23	Squash
65	Tomato
65	Tomato, strawberry
65	Tomato, tree
2	Truffle
22	Turnip
22	Watercress
22	Wintercress
27	Yam, American
27	Yam, Chinese
27	Yam, Indian
19	Yarrow
40	Yucca

TABLE 10-I (continued)

FRUITS & BERRIES

58	Apple
59	Apricot
45	Banana
57	Blackberry
28	Blueberry
57	Boysenberry
44	Breadfruit
23	Cantaloupe
15	Caper
23	Chayote
65	Cherry, ground
41	Cherry, Surinam
59	Cherry, sweet
59	Cherry, wild
61	Citron
58	Crabapple
28	Cranberry
64	Currant
8	Dates
57	Dewberry
16	Elderberry
44	Fig
43	Gooseberry, American
65	Gooseberry, cape
64	Gooseberry, English
73	Grape, American
73	Grape, European
61	Grapefruit
47	Guava
60	Guava, black
44	Hops
28	Huckleberry, black
47	Jambolan
20	Juniper
61	Kumquat
61	Lemon
61	Lime
28	Lingonberry
57	Loganberry
58	Loquat
48	Lotus, Chinese
5	Mango
23	Melon, casaba
23	Melon, honeydew
23	Melon, Persian
44	Mulberry
13	Muscadine
23	Muskmelon
59	Nectarine
61	Orange, common
61	Orange, mandarin
61	Orange, sour
17	Papaya
6	Pawpaw, American
59	Peach
58	Pear
65	Pear, melon
26	Persimmon, American
26	Persimmon, Oriental
12	Pineapple
45	Plantain
59	Plum, American
59	Plum, beach
59	Plum, common
59	Plum, Damson
59	Plum, Oriental
59	Plum, Pacific
56	Pomegranate
13	Prickly pear
59	Prune
23	Pumpkin
58	Quince
73	Raisin
57	Raspberry, black
57	Raspberry, red
58	Redhaw
47	Roseapple
58	Rose hips
73	Scuppernong
54	Sea grape
59	Sloe
57	Strawberry, beach
57	Strawberry, cultivated
57	Strawberry, meadow
39	Tamarind
61	Tangelo
61	Tangerine
23	Watermelon
28	Wintergreen (berry)

MEALS, STARCHES & CEREALS

74	Arrowroot, East Indian
67	Arrowroot, Fiji
24	Arrowroot, Florida
14	Arrowroot, Queensland
42	Arrowroot, West Indian
32-A	Barley
54	Buckwheat
39	Flour, carob
39	Flour, lima bean
39	Flour, soybean
9	Malanga
42	Maranta
30	Meal, cassava
32-D	Meal, corn
41	Meal, cottonseed
23	Meal, pumpkin
19	Meal, sunflower
32-E	Millet
32-C	Oats
9	Poi
32-B	Rice
32-B	Rice, wild
32-A	Rye
32-D	Starch, corn
8	Starch, Sago
30	Tapioca
9	Taro
32-A	Wheat
2	Yeast (in bread)
30	Yuca
40	Yucca

SALADS

19	Artichoke, Jerusalem
37	Avocado
65	Bell pepper
19	Burdock, leaves
22	Cabbage, Chinese
22	Cabbage, common
22	Cabbage, savoy
71	Carrot
22	Cauliflower
71	Celeriac
71	Celery
19	Celtuce

TABLE 10-I (continued)

71	Chervil
19	Chicory
40	Chives
23	Cucumber
19	Dandelion leaves
19	Endive, French (escarole)
54	Garden sorrel
23	Gherkin, Indian
40	Leek
19	Lettuce
2	Mushroom
49	Olive
40	Onion
71	Parsley
65	Pepper, garden varieties
22	Radish
40	Shallot
18	Spinach
65	Tomato (all varieties)
70	Water chestnut
22	Watercress
22	Wintercress

OILS

8	Coconut
32-D	Corn
41	Cottonseed
49	Olive
8	Palm
39	Peanut
19	Safflower
52	Sesame seed
39	Soybean
19	Sunflower seed

VINEGAR

58,2	Apple
32,2	Grain
32A,2	Malt
73,2	Wine

SPICES, FLAVORINGS & SEASONINGS

47	Allspice
71	Angelica
71	Anise
36	Balm
36	Basil
37	Bay leaf
36	Bergamot
57	Burnet
71	Caraway
74	Cardamom
36	Catnip
19	Chamomile
65	Chili (paprika)
71	Cicily, sweet
37	Cinnamon
36	Clary
47	Clove
29	Coca leaf
66	Cola
71	Coriander
71	Cumin, black
71	Cumin, common
71	Dill
71	Fennel
71	Fennel, sweet
39	Fenugreek
40	Garlic
74	Ginger
36	Hoarhound
36	Hyssop
36	Lavender oil
40	Leek
39	Licorice
71	Lovage
46	Mace
36	Marjoram
36	Mint
22	Mustard, black
22	Mustard, Indian
22	Mustard, white
46	Nutmeg
10	Oil of birch (wintergreen)
40	Onion
40	Onion, Welsh
36	Oregano
34	Orris root
71	Parsley
36	Pennyroyal
53	Pepper, black
65	Pepper, cayenne
65	Pepper, chili (paprika)
65	Pepper, garden
53	Pepper, white
36	Peppermint
51	Poppyseed
36	Rosemary
34	Saffron
36	Sage
40	Sarsaparilla
37	Sassafras
36	Savory
52	Sesame seed
40	Shallot
36	Spearmint
19	Tansy
19	Tarragon
36	Thyme
39	Tonka bean
74	Turmeric
50	Vanilla bean
60	Woodruff

NUTS & SEEDS

59	Almond
31	Beechnut
38	Brazil nut
35	Butternut
5	Cashew
31	Chestnut, American
31	Chestnut, Chinese
31	Chestnut, Spanish
31	Cinquapin
25	Chufa (ground nut)
8	Coconut
10	Filbert
10	Hazelnut
35	Hickory nut
62	Litchi nut
55	Macadamia nut
38	Paradise nut
39	Peanut
35	Pecan
20	Pine nut (pinon)

TABLE 10-I (continued)

5	Pistachio	1	Sugar, maple	68	Tea
52	Sesame seed	32-F	Syrup, cane	39	Tea, alfalfa
19	Sunflower seed	32-D	Syrup, corn	11	Tea, comfrey
39	Tepary	1	Syrup, maple	19	Tea, kaffir
35	Walnut, black			72	Tea, lemon verbena
35	Walnut, English		*BEVERAGES*	69	Tea, linden lime
35	Walnut, white	4	Agave		(flower)
70	Water chestnut	69	Basswood fruit		
25	Water chestnut,	66	Chocolate		*GUMS*
	Chinese	66	Cocoa	39	Acacia
		8	Coconut milk	3	Carrageen
	SWEETS	60	Coffee	63	Chicle
76	Honey	7	Ginseng, American	39	Guar
32-F	Sorghum	7	Ginseng, Asian	39	Gum arabic
18	Sugar, beet	33	Mate' (Yerba)	66	Karaya
32-F	Sugar cane	80	Milk: cow, goat, etc.	3	Kelp
32-D	Sugar, corn	58	Rose hips	39	Tragacanth
8	Sugar, date	39	Soybean milk		

If this diet adequately relieves symptoms within one to three weeks, each omitted food can be challenged individually and then allowed, avoided, or rotated on a trial basis as described in Diet #1. If symptoms are still not adequately relieved and the patient is unable to undertake a comprehensive regime such as Diet #3, the omission-challenge procedure can be continued for additional frequently eaten foods in the patient's diet, such as egg, orange, peanut, beef, chicken, etc.

Diet #3. If a stringent diet is indicated from the beginning, or if Diet #2 does not provide adequate symptom relief, Diet #3 can be instituted. This diet avoids suspected foods, milk products, the chocolate family, and all cereal grains including wheat, corn, rice, rye, oats, barley, and millet. It also avoids cane and beet sugar, all beverages (except water and unsweetened fruit juices), all commercially prepared foods containing artificial flavors, preservatives, and other chemical additives, and all other complex processed and factory-mixed foods with multiple and unknown ingredients.

As will be noted, this diet combines the outstanding features of the cereal-free elimination diet of Rowe,[80] the multiple exclusion diet of Speer,[83] and the chemical avoidance diet of Randolph.[67] Below is a list of some examples of the forbidden, complex, factory-made, chemicalized "foods":

Canned soups	Potted meats	Bottle drinks
Soup mixes	Cured ham	Colored beverages
Dips	Bacon	Colored gelatin desserts
Catsup	Bologna	Packaged custards
Sauces	Mixed cereals	Packaged puddings
Salad dressings	Sugared cereals	Sherbets
Mayonnaise	Diet breads	Ice cream
Barbecue sauce	Snack crackers	Frozen pies
Sausages	Candies	Meat extenders
Lunch meats	Canned "drinks"	"Convenience" foods
Wieners	Powdered drinks	"Instant" anything

This diet includes, for the most part, those foods on which man depended for his daily diet before the agricultural revolution 10,000 years ago. At that time, mankind survived on relatively simple, natural foods such as meat, fowl, fish, eggs, vegetables, fruits, berries, nuts, and honey. Although this diet is not easy to follow in this age of restaurant eating, travel, and manufactured foods, it is nourishing and sustaining. Many nutrition-conscious people use it by choice.

The patient on a natural diet eats simple foods from natural sources of known origin. For example, raw pork may be bought and cooked at home with onions or other known tolerated ingredients, but ham, bacon, sausage, or other processed pork products should not be eaten; fresh beef may be used, but corned beef, canned beef stew, etc., should be avoided. Fresh or frozen vegetables are usually tolerated, although they often contain minute amounts of pesticides and herbicides, which may cause reactions in the very sensitive patient. If this is the case, it may be necessary to purchase organic foods, as will be discussed in a later section.

Not only is it difficult to keep track of the changing contents of processed foods, but the labels on such products are often incomplete and confusing. In the case of "standardized" foods, the labels offer no ingredient information whatsoever. A standardized food is one, e.g. ice cream or beer, for which the FDA has prescribed a broad general list of allowed ingredients. The specific ingredients in such foods need not be listed on the labels except ingredients not included in the FDA list. It is for such reasons that complete avoidance of factory-processed foods is advised. Even certain unprocessed foods should not be eaten initially by patients on this diet because they may cause confusing pharmacologic effects, e.g. caffeine-containing foods, or may be difficult to obtain in unprocessed form, or simply complicate the diet. Some may be introduced carefully later. Foods to be omitted are underlined in the Rotary Diet Charts (Table 10-II).

THE ROTARY DIET (Table 10-II). Patients with food sensitivities should try to eat as varied a diet as possible and should not ingest the same food too frequently. A patient placed on Diet #1 (omitting known allergenic foods plus milk, chocolate, cola drinks, and karaya gum) may substitute orange juice or other products too frequently and may develop new sensitivities to these previously tolerated beverages and foods. The patient may then have to avoid these foods to which new sensitivities have developed and, in doing so, will probably eat some of the remaining foods more frequently; as a result, he may develop still more sensitivities. In this way, the patient may rapidly become sensitive to most of the foods in his normal diet.

Since the development of new food sensitivities is much less common when foods are eaten infrequently, a patient can usually preserve most of his remaining food tolerances by following a diet that includes ingestion of any one food only once every four days.[77] The four-day rotation can be combined with each of the three diets previously discussed.

A patient on Diet #1 may thus be instructed to avoid all suspected foods, milk, and the chocolate family, and to rotate all other foods. A patient on Diet #2 may be instructed to avoid suspected foods, milk, the chocolate family, wheat, and corn, and to rotate all other foods. A patient on Diet #3 may be instructed to avoid suspected foods and the forbidden foods listed, and to rotate the remainder.

Rotating foods serve three purposes. First, it reduces or eliminates symptoms from foods that the patient eats frequently.

Second it helps in the identification of specific food allergies, since it breaks the masking that accompanies repetitive eating. Third, it enables the patient to continue tolerating the currently safe foods presently in his diet, since people with food allergies tend to become sensitive to foods ingested too frequently.

In the rotary diet, if beef is eaten at dinner on Monday, it should not be eaten again in any form (as hamburger, roast, steak, gravy, or soup) until dinner on Friday. If chicken is eaten at dinner on Tuesday, it should not be eaten again in any form (such as soup or in salad) until dinner on Saturday. If pork is eaten at dinner on Wednesday, it too should not be eaten again in any form, e.g. ham, bacon, sausage, nonvegetable shortening, Jell-O® and other pork-containing products until dinner on Sunday. Turkey can be eaten on Thursday, and not repeated until Monday. The home freezer is a great aid to those on rotary diets, since large amounts of foods can be prepared and the leftovers stored frozen in small portions, one of which can be thawed and reheated every four days.

Rotary diets cannot be followed casually. They must be committed to paper. Meals must be planned, written out, and shopped for in advance. Three meals a day for four days means twelve menus to be constructed. The same twelve meals can again be used the following four days, with minor planned variations. These variations are designed to omit a newly suspected food or to add a new, hopefully tolerated, food from time to time for the final "fine-tuning" of the diet. This can be done successfully, but requires constant label reading, careful shopping and cooking, a minimum of eating in restaurants, and regular note keeping. Fortunately, a rotary diet is necessary only with the occasional patient who has multiple severe sensitivities.

Although the rotary natural diet represents an unusual pattern of eating for these times, it is highly nutritious and much safer than the usual American diet with its heavy emphasis on sweets, salts, spices, starches, and chemicalized foods. It emphasizes the better foods and omits the poorer ones. Meats are available every day in the form of beef, pork, chicken, or turkey. Other meats and fowl can be used, for example, lamb, venison, duck, dove,

TABLE 10-II
ROTARY DIET DAY 1

BREAKFAST	LUNCH	DINNER
111. Atlantic halibut Pacific halibut plaice right eye flounder turbot winter flounder	77. duck goose	110. chicken egg peafowl pheasant quail
32-C. oat	107. oyster	109. walleye pike yellow perch
73. American grapes European grapes muscadines raisins	105. scallop	88. dolphin fish
8. cabbage palm coconut (meal, oil, nut) date date sugar Sago starch	125. clam	90. common dolphin; 76. honey
60. black guava coffee woodruff	115. croaker freshwater drum King whiting redfish squeteague weakfish	22. broccoli Brussels sprouts cabbage cauliflower Chinese cabbage collard horseradish kale kohlrabi mustard radish rape rutabaga turnip watercress wintercress
	121. porgy	2. mushroom truffle yeast
	100. North American squid	30. cassava meal (yuca) tapioca
	65. bell pepper cape gooseberry cayenne pepper chili (paprika) eggplant ground cherry melon pear potato (white, Irish) strawberry tomato tomato tree tomato	32-A. barley rye wheat
	15. caper	49. olive (ripe, black), (oil)
	43. American gooseberry	62. litchi nut
	44. breadfruit fig hops mulberry	10. filberts hazelnuts oil of birch (wintergreen flavor)
	52. sesame seed, oil	58. apple (vinegar) crabapple loquat pear quince redhaw rosehips
	51. poppyseed	

page 1

DAY 1

BREAKFAST	LUNCH	DINNER
Broiled flounder Fresh grapes Coffee with date sugar	Potato soup, chili pepper seasoning with oysters Redfish or croaker dipped in potato flour, fried in sesame oil Baked potato with pepper and salt Eggplant strips dipped in potato flour fried in sesame oil Sliced tomato Tomato juice or water	Chinese cabbage, radish, apple wedges, cauliflower salad with apple vinegar and olive oil Baked or broiled chicken Mushroom gravy thickened with tapioca Homemade bread with wheat, honey, yeast, and water Broccoli Rutabaga Tapioca and apple dessert with honey or deep dish apple pie with honey Apple juice or water
Fried flounder (dipped in coconut meal, fried in coconut oil) Oatmeal with raisins and date sugar Coffee with date sugar	Roast duck Bell pepper stuffed with eggplant seasoned with cayenne pepper Layers of sliced potato and tomato, sesame seed and oil as casserole Tomato juice or water Figs	Cabbage slaw, radish, watercress, olives, hardboiled eggs with olive oil and cider vinegar Chicken dipped in cassava meal or wheat flour and fried in olive oil Turnips or rutabaga Baked apple with honey and filberts
Oatmeal with chopped dates Fresh coconut wedges Coconut milk or coffee	Oysters dipped in potato flour, fried in sesame oil French fried potatoes in sesame oil Sliced tomato and bell peppers Tomato juice or water Figs	Fried yellow perch using cassava meal or wheat flour and olive oil Cauliflower Collards or mustard Radishes and olives Pear

ROTARY DIET DAY 2

BREAKFAST

- 114. salmon, trout
- 79. California halibut, left eyed flounder, southern flounder, summer flounder
- 32-D. corn (grits, starch, vegetable, oil, meal syrup) popcorn
- 61. citron, grapefruit, kumquat, lemon, lime, orange, tangelo, tangerine
- 64. currant, English gooseberry
- 6. American pawpaw
- 55. macadamia nut

LUNCH

- 99. hare, rabbit
- 95. abalone
- 117. mackerel, tuna, bonita
- 120. sole
- 91. anchovy
- 75. beluga, sturgeon
- 96. edible snail
- 41. cottonseed (meal, oil), okra
- 71. angelica, anise, caraway, carrot, celeriac, celery, chervil, coriander, cumin, dill, fennel, lovage, parsley, parsnips, sweet cicily, sweet fennel
- 45. banana, plantain
- 26. persimmon
- 9. malanga, poi, taro
- 11. comfrey (vegetable, tea)
- 69. basswood, linden (tea)
- 31. beechnut, chestnut, chinquapin
- 70. water chestnut

DINNER

- 80. beef
- 104. guinea fowl
- 87. whitefish
- 106. common smelt
- 82. amberjack, jack mackerel, pompano, yellow jack
- 21. sweet potato (vine tuber)
- 40. asparagus, chives, garlic, leek, onion, sarsaparilla, shallot, Welsh onion, yucca
- 24. Florida arrowroot
- 32-B. rice, wild rice
- 50. vanilla bean
- 12. pineapple
- 38. Brazil nut, paradise nut
- 20. juniper, pine nut

page 3

DAY 2

BREAKFAST	LUNCH	DINNER
Trout (mealed)/fried in corn oil Grapefruit and orange sections/ corn syrup Hot lemonade/corn syrup	Tuna/water chestnuts Okra (fry in cottonseed meal & oil) Carrot sticks/celery Banana	Roast beef/garlic Wild rice (plain gravy) Boiled small onions Asparagus Baked sweet potato
Tangerine/orange sections/corn syrup Corn meal pancakes/corn syrup Grapefruit or orange juice	Baked mackerel Parsnips Boiled okra Carrot/celery Baked banana	Steak/sliced onions Rice/steak gravy Asparagus Brazil nuts/sweet potato/ pineapple Pineapple juice
Grits Salmon/lemon juice Half grapefruit/corn syrup Juice	Rabbit (cottonseed meal and fried in cottonseed oil) Okra (boiled or fried) Baked plantain Carrots Persimmon	Casserole ground beef, onion slices, chives, rice Asparagus Sliced pineapple Sweet potato custard with pure vanilla

page 4

ROTARY DIET DAY 3

BREAKFAST

- 118. ocean perch, rosefish
- 103. mullet, silversides
- 113. North American paddlefish
- 54. buckwheat, garden sorrel, rhubarb, sea grapes
- 57. black raspberry, boysenberry, burnet, dewberry, loganberry, red raspberry, strawberry
- 32-F. sorghum, sugar cane
- 68. tea

LUNCH

- 80. goat
- 102. turkey
- 83. buffalofish, chub, hag, lumpfish, sucker, white sucker
- 85. herring, menhaden, pilchard (sardine), shad
- 32-G. bamboo shoots, sprouts
- 23. cantaloupe, casaba melon, chayote, cucumber, gherkin, honeydew melon, muskmelon, Persian melon, pumpkin (seed, meal, vegetable), squash (all kinds), watermelon
- 67. Fiji arrowroot
- 74. cardamom, East Indian arrowroot, ginger, tumeric
- 46. mace, nutmeg
- 16. elderberry
- 1. black walnut, butternut, English walnut, hickory nut, pecan

DINNER

- 80. lamb
- 116. squirrel
- 101. red snapper
- 94. grunt (common, gray and yellow)
- 92. muskellunge, northern pike, pickerel
- 27. American yam (plant tuber, not vine), Chinese potato, Indian yam
- 14. Queensland arrowroot
- 19. burdock root, camomile, celtuce, chicory, dandelion, endive, escarole, French endive, globe artichoke, Jerusalem artichoke, kaffir (tea), lettuce, safflower (oil), sunflower (seed, meal, oil), tansy, tarragon, yarrow, salsify
- 36. artichoke-Chinese and Japanese, balm, basil, bergamot, catnip, clary, horehound, hyssop, lavender, marjoram, mint: common, horse, round leaf, curled, oregano, pennyroyal, peppermint, rosemary, sage, savory, spearmint, thyme

page 5

DAY 3

BREAKFAST	LUNCH	DINNER
Broiled mullet Rhubarb sauce/cane sugar Black raspberries/cane sugar Raspberry juice or water Hot tea	Sardines or other allowed fish Bamboo sprouts Baked chayote Cucumbers Cantaloupe Arrowroot custard/maple syrup, nutmeg and pecans	Baked red snapper or other allowed fish Globe artichokes/herbed safflower oil Baked American yams Salad of lettuce, endives, escarole/safflower oil and oregano, thyme and savory Kaffir tea or water Dandelion tea
Buckwheat pancakes/sorghum syrup Strawberries/cane sugar Pan-broiled ocean perch Hot tea/cane sugar	Baked turkey Stewed zucchini squash with turmeric Baked pumpkin with nutmeg, maple syrup and pecans Cucumber slices Watermelon or honeydew melon	Lamb/mint Heart of lettuce/herbed sunflower oil Fried American yam slices Globe artichokes/safflower oil and herbs Camomile tea or water
Buckwheat groats/sorghum syrup Raspberries/cane sugar Mullet or ocean perch Hot tea	Baked turkey with gravy of natural juices Acorn squash with nutmeg, walnuts and maple sugar Bamboo shoots Cantaloupe	Squirrel (boiled) with oregano American yams/peppermint Chopped lettuce, sunflower seed, Jerusalem artichoke slices, escarole, dandelion leaves with safflower oil and herbs Globe artichokes Yarrow tea or water Dandelion tea

ROTARY DIET DAY 4

BREAKFAST

- 122. butterfish
- 93. cod, haddock, pollock, silver hake
- 32-E. millet
- 59. almond, apricot, cherry (fresh), nectarine, peach, plum, prunes, sloes, wild cherry
- 72. lemon verbena (tea)
- 33. mate' (yerba mate')

LUNCH

- 81. crab
- 97. crayfish, lobster, prawn
- 108. shrimp
- 98. catfish, Mississippi catfish
- 113. bluefish
- 78. common eel
- 39. acacia gum, adsuki bean, alfalfa, asparagus bean, carob, English pea, fava bean, fenugreek, garbanzo bean, guar, jack bean, kidney bean, lablab bean, lentil, licorice, lima bean, navy bean, peanut (nut, oil), peas (all kinds), pinto bean, snapbean, soybean (flour, nut, oil, milk), stringbean, tamarind (fruit), tepary, tonka bean (imitation vanilla), tragacanth gum, yambean
- 17. papaya
- 56. pomegranate
- 13. prickly pear
- 3. carrageenan, kelp (seaweed)

DINNER

- 123. pork
- 84. black bass (largemouth, smallmouth, spotted), blue gill, longeared sunfish, sunfish, pumpkinseed
- 119. grouper, rockfish, white bass, white perch
- 37. avocado, bay leaf, cinnamon, sassafras
- 42. West Indian arrowroot (maranta starch)
- 47. allspice, cloves, guava, jambolan, roseapple, Surinam cherry
- 53. black and white pepper
- 34. saffron, orris root
- 28. black huckleberry, blueberry, cranberry, lingonberry, wintergree berries
- 18. beet, beet sugar, spinach, Swiss chard
- 4. agave
- 7. ginseng
- 25. Chinese water chestnut, chufa (groundnut)
- 5. cashew, mango, pistachio

page 7

DAY 4

BREAKFAST	LUNCH	DINNER
Millet cereal Prunes Broiled peaches Lemon verbena tea or mate' Allowed fruit juice	Crab claws or lobster English peas Peanut butter (pure) Papaya Carob	Pork chops with black pepper Sliced beets with bay leaf Avocado Spinach
Codfish Allowed fresh fruit (apricots, peach, cherries) Juice of fruit Millet bread (cook millet, allow to get cold and slice)	Catfish fried with soy flour and oil Lentil soup with shrimp Salad of navy, pinto, kidney, stringbeans with soy oil Pomegranate Fenugreek tea	Fresh pork ham with cloves and beet sugar Swiss chard Avocado and cashews Cranberry sauce and beet sugar Cranberry juice
Allowed fish, baked or broiled Prunes Millet cakes (pancakes) Fresh fruit (nectarines, plums, peach, etc.) Hot fruit juice	Boiled shrimp Stringbeans Soy crackers with peanut butter (pure) Prickly pear Carob	Allowed fish, broiled or baked with saffron Chinese water chestnuts Beets Spinach Blueberries with beet sugar Sassafras tea, beet sugar

quail, pheasant, partridge, rabbit, and squirrel. Fish also is an excellent source of protein and may be eaten daily or twice daily, as long as fish from any one family is not eaten more frequently than once every four days. A list of the foods and the families to which they belong is presented with the rotary diet in Table 10-II and 10-III. Many of these and other uncommonly eaten foods can be obtained from specialty food shippers (Table 10-IV).

TABLE 10-III
FOOD FAMILY CLASSIFICATION

Plant Family Classification
1. Acaraceae (maple): maple sugar and syrup
2. Agaricaceae (fungi): mushroom, truffle, yeast
3. Algae (algae): carrageen, kelp or seaweed
4. Amaryllis (amaryllis): agave
5. Anacardiaceae (cashew): cashew, mango, pistachio
6. Annonaceae (buttercup): American pawpaw
7. Araliaceae (ginseng): ginseng
8. Arecaceae (palm): cabbage palm (oil), coconut (meal, milk, oil), date (date sugar), Sago starch
9. Araceae (Arum): malanga, poi, taro
10. Betulaceae (birch): filbert, hazel nut, oil of birch (wintergreen flavoring)
11. Boraginaceae (borage): comfrey
12. Bromeliaceae (pineapple): pineapple
13. Cactaceae (cactus): prickly pear
14. Cannaceae (canna): Queensland arrowroot
15. Capparidaceae (caper): caper
16. Caprifoliacea (honeysuckle): elderberry
17. Caricaceae (papaya): papaya
18. Chenopodiacea (goosefoot): beet (beet sugar), spinach, Swiss chard

*Adapted from: A.H. Corwin, The rotating diet and taxonomy, in L.D. Dickey (Ed), *Clinical Ecology,* 1976. Courtesy of Charles C Thomas, Publisher, Springfield, Illinois.
F. Speer and R.J. Dockhorn, *Allergy and Immunology in Childhood,* 1973. Courtesy of Charles C Thomas, Publisher, Springfield, Illinois.
Manual for Those Sensitive to Foods, Drugs and Chemicals, 3rd ed., 1969. Courtesy of the Environmental Health Association of Greater Washington.

TABLE 10-III (continued)

19.	Compositae (sunflower): burdock leaves, burdock root, celtuce, chamomile, chicory, dandelion, endive, escarole (French endive), globe artichoke, Jerusalem artichoke, kaffir, lettuce, safflower (oil), salsify, sunflower (meal, oil, seed), tansy, tarragon, yarrow
20.	Coniferae (conifer): juniper, pine nut or pinon
21.	Convoluculaceae (sweet potato): sweet potato (vine tuber, Ipomoea batatas species)
22.	Cruciferae (mustard): broccoli, Brussels sprouts, cabbage (Chinese, common, savoy), cauliflower, collards, horseradish, kale, kohlrabi, mustard, radish, rape, rutabaga, turnip, watercress, wintercress
23.	Cucurbitateae (gourd): cantaloupe, casaba melon, chayote, cucumber, gherkin (Indian), honeydew melon, muskmelon, Persian melon, pumpkin (meal, seed), squash (all kinds), watermelon
24.	Cycadaceae (cycad): Florida arrowroot (Zamia)
25.	Cyperaceae (sedge): Chinese water chestnuts, chufa or groundnut
26.	Ebenaceae (ebony): American persimmon, Oriental persimmon
27.	Dioscoreaceae (yam): American yam, Chinese potato, Indian yam
28.	Ericaceae (heath): black huckleberry, blueberry, cranberry, lingonberry, wintergreen berry
29.	Erythrosylaceae (coca): coca leaf (flavor, Coca Cola)
30.	Euphoribaceae (spurge): cassava, tapioca, yuca
31.	Fagaceae (beech): beechnut (American, European), chestnut (American, Chinese, Spanish), chinquapin
32-A.	Graminneae, Hordeae (grass): barley, rye, wheat
32-B.	Graminneae, Oryzeae (grass): rice, wild rice
32-C.	Graminneae, Aceneae (grass): oats
32-D.	Graminneae, Haydeae (grass): corn (grain, oil, starch, sugar, syrup, vegetable), popcorn
32-E.	Graminneae, Paniceae (grass): millet (browntop, common, ditch, finger, foxtail, Japanese, pearl)
32-F.	Garminneae, Andropogoneae (grass): can syrup, sorghum, sugar cane
32-G.	Graminneae, Bambuseae (grass): bamboo (shoots and sprouts)
33.	Iliacaceae (holly): mate' (Yerba mate')
34.	Iridaceae (iris): orris root, saffron (flavors)
35.	Juglandaceae (walnut): black walnut, butternut, English walnut, hickory nut, pecan, white walnut

TABLE 10-III (continued)

36.	Labiatae (mint): balm, basil, bergamot, catnip, Chinese artichoke, clary, common mint, curled mint, hoarhound, horse mint, hyssop, Japanese artichoke, lavender, marjoram, oregano, pennyroyal, peppermint, rosemary, roundleafed mint, sage, savory, spearmint, spike lavender, thyme, water mint
37.	Lauraceae (laurel): avocado, bay leaf, cinnamon, sassafras
38.	Lecythiadaceae (sapucaya): Brazil nut, paradise nut
39.	Leguminosae (legume): acacia gum, adsuki bean, alfalfa (tea), asparagus bean, beans (all varieties), carob bean, fava bean, fenugreek, garbanzo pea, guar, gu marabic, jack bean, lablab bean, lintil, licorice, peanut, peas (all varieties), soybean, tamarind, tepary bean, tonka bean, tragacanth, yambean
40.	Liliaceae (lily): asparagus, chives, garlic, leek, onion, sarsaparilla, shallot, Welsh onion, yucca
41.	Malvaceae (mallow): cottonseed (meal, oil), okra
42.	Marantaceae (arrowroot): West Indian arrowroot (Maranta starch)
43.	Melostomadaceae (melostomad): American gooseberry
44.	Moraceae (mulberry): breadfruit, fig, hops, mulberry
45.	Musaceae (banana): banana, dwarf banana, plantain
46.	Myristiceae (nutmeg): mace, nutmeg
47.	Myrtaceae (myrtle): allspice, clove, guava, jambolan, roseapple, Surinam cherry
48.	Nymphaeaceae (water lily): Chinese lotus
49.	Oleaceae (olive): olive (oil)
50.	Orchidaceae (orchid): vanilla bean
51.	Papaveraceae (poppy): poppyseed
52.	Pedaliaceae (pedalium): sesame seed and oil
53.	Piperaceae (pepper): black and white pepper
54.	Polygonaceae (buckwheat): buckwheat, garden sorrel, rhubarb, sea grape
55.	Proteaceae (protea): macadamia nut
56.	Punicaceae (pomegranate): pomegranate
57.	Rosaceae, Rosoideae (berries): blackberry, black raspberry, boysenberry, burnet, dewberry, loganberry, red raspberry, strawberry
58.	Rosaceae, Pomoideae (pomes): apple, crabapple, loquat, pear, quince, redhaw, rose hips
59.	Rosaceae, Prunoideae (stone fruits): almond, apricot, nectarine, peach, plum, prune, sloe, sweetcherry, wild cherry
60.	Rubiaceae (madder): black guava, coffee, woodruff

TABLE 10-III (continued)

61.	Rutaceae (citrus): citron, grapefruit, kumpquat, lemon, lime, orange, tangelo, tangerine
62.	Sapindaceae (soapberry): litchi nut
63.	Sapotaceae (sapodilla): chicle
64.	Saxifragaceae (saxifrage): currant, English gooseberry
65.	Solanaceae (nightshade): bell pepper, cape gooseberry, cayenne pepper, chili (paprika), eggplant, garden peppers, ground cherry, melon pear, potato (white), strawberry tomato, tomato, tree tomato
66.	Sterculiaceae (cola nut): chocolate, cocoa, cola, karaya gum
67.	Taccaceae (tacca): Fiji arrowroot (Tacca)
68.	Theaceae (tea): tea
69.	Tiliaceae (linden): basswood, lime or linden (for tea)
70.	Trapaceae (water chestnut): water chestnut
71.	Umbelliferae (parsley): angelica, anise, black cumin, caraway seed, carrot, celeriac, celery, chervil, coriander, cumin, dill, fennel, lovage, parsley, parsnip, sweet cicily, sweet fennel
72.	Verbenaceae (verbena): lemon verbena (tea)
73.	Vitaceae (grape): American grape, European grape, muscadines, raisins, scuppernongs
74.	Zingiberaceae (ginger): cardamom, East Indian arrowroot, ginger, turmeric
	Crustaceans, Mollusks, Fish, Birds, Mammals
75.	Acipenseridae: beluga, sturgeon
76.	Apidea (bee): honey
77.	Anatidae: duck, goose
78.	Anguillidae: common eel
79.	Bothidae: California halibut, left-eyed flounder, southern flounder, summer flounder
80.	Bovidae: African buffalo, American bison, Brahman, cattle (cow's milk), goat, sheep
81.	Cancridae: crab
82.	Canrangidae (jack): amberjack, jack mackerel, pompano, yellow jack
83.	Catostomidae (sucker): buffalofish, chub, hag, lumpfish, sucker, white sucker
84.	Centrarchidae (sunfish): bluegill, largemouth black bass, longeared sunfish, pumpkinseed, smallmouth black bass, spotted black bass, sunfish
85.	Clupeidae: herring, menhaden, pilchard (sardine), shad
86.	Columbidae: pigeon
87.	Coregonidae: lake whitefish
88.	Coryphaenidae: dolphin fish

TABLE 10-III (continued)

89.	Cyprinidae: carp
90.	Delphinidae: common dolphin
91.	Engraulidae: anchovy
92.	Esocidae (pike): muskellunge, northern pike, pickerel
93.	Gadidae: cod, haddock, pollock, silver hake, tomcod
94.	Haemulidae: common grunt, gray grunt, yellow grunt
95.	Haliotidae: red, pink and green abalone
96.	Helicidae: edible snail
97.	Homaridae: crayfish, lobster, prawn
98.	Ictaluridae: catfish, Mississippi catfish, yellow bullhead
99.	Leporidae: Belgian hare, cottontail, domestic rabbit, jackrabbit, snowshoe rabbit
100.	Loliginidae: North American squid
101.	Lutjanidae: red snapper
102.	Meliagridae: turkey
103.	Mugilidae: mullet, silversides, white bait
104.	Numididae: guinea fowl
105.	Pectenidae: scallops
106.	Os:meridae: common smelt
107.	Ostreidae: oyster
108.	Peneidae: shrimp
109.	Percidae: walleye pike, yellow perch
110.	Phasianidae: chicken (egg), domestic pheasant, Indian pheasant, peafowl, quail
111.	Plueronectidae: Atlantic halibut, Pacific halibut, plaice, right-eyed flounder, turbot, winter flounder
112.	Polydonitdae: North American paddlefish
113.	Pomatomidae (bluefish): bluefish
114.	Salmonidae: salmon, trout
115.	Sciendidae: croaker, freshwater drum, king whiting, redfish, squeteague, weakfish
116.	Sciuridae: prairie dog, squirrel, woodchuck
117.	Scombridae: albacore, Atlantic mackrel, bluefin tuna, bonita, king mackerel, skipjack tuna, Spanish mackerel
118.	Scorpaenidae: ocean perch, rosefish
119.	Serranidae: black sea bass, brown grouper, Oriental spotted bass, red grouper, rockfish, speckled hind, white bass, white perch

TABLE 10-III (continued)

120.	Soleidae: common sole, European sole
121.	Sparidae: porgy
122.	Stromateidae: butterfish
123.	Suidae: pig
124.	Tetraonidae: prairie chicken, ruffled grouse (partridge)
125.	Veneridae: clams
	Uncommon Animal Food
126.	Antilocapridae: pronghorn antelope
127.	Castoroidae: beaver
128.	Cervinae: American elk, European red deer
129.	Chelidridae: snapping turtle
130.	Didelphidae: opossum
131.	Equidae: horse
132.	Musticeiti: blue whale, fin whale, Greenland whale, humpback whale, North Atlantic whale, Pacific gray whale, sperm whale, white whale
133.	Odocoileinae: caribou, moose, reindeer, white tailed deer
134.	Phocidae: common seal
135.	Procyoninae: raccoon
136.	Ranidae: American bullfrog, European edible bullfrog
137.	Ursidae: black bear, brown bear, grizzly bear

Commercial vitamin and mineral preparations are usually unnecessary and are often better avoided because of the substances from which they are made, the chemical residues of processing, and the excipients and fillers in the finished products. Simple, wholesome foods contain plenty of vitamins and minerals. An adequate vitamin-mineral intake usually can be ensured by eating only the foods in the natural diet, by eating some fruits and salads in the raw state, and by cooking with a minimum of water for a minimum amount of time and using the cooking water for soups and sauces. The recently popularized slow-cooking, low temperature, minimum water–requiring utensils and steaming racks are convenient tools for achieving these ends. Inexpensive food grinders allow small amounts of ordinary cooked foods to be pureed, so that many of the foods prepared for the entire family can be ground and fed to the allergic infant.

The need for calcium supplementation after the age of three in most patients on milk avoidance probably is unnecessary, but if the diet is deficient in calcium, extra calcium should be provided. It may be necessary to avoid colored capsules, tablets containing cornstarch, and liquid calcium preparations containing sugar or corn syrup.

Charts showing four days of menus for the rotary diet, in which entire food families are rotated, are outlined in Table 10-II. Each patient, however, must sit down with a pencil and paper and draw upon these four days of over 400 listed foods to construct his own meals, including only those tolerated and to which there is no known sensitivity.

The Diet Diary

After beginning a diet, it is essential to keep an accurate diary of all foods eaten, preferably in blue ink, and a record, on the same diary, of symptoms and their time of occurrence in red ink (Fig. 10-1). Errors in choice of foods and in frequency of ingestion of allowed foods will show up automatically.

In addition, the patient with complex problems should record activities such as exposures to inhalants, including dusts, molds, feathers, fur-bearing animals, cooking odors, and chemical odors such as perfumes. The patient should be made aware of the problem of "outgassing" or volatilization of vapors from things such as new cars, new carpets, and other home furnishings and structural materials. He should also record chilling, undue fatigue, poor sleep, or other special stresses. Women should note correlations of symptoms with menstrual cycles. The weather and season are important also, since symptoms may occur more readily in some patients with rapid drops in environmental temperature, cool nights, humid or foggy mornings, rain, changes in wind velocity and direction, and pollen seasons. Some patients develop symptoms when they are too warm or overdressed, or when the heat of a thermostatically controlled, forced-air heating system automatically turns on. Some are susceptible to both

NAME:________________ 14 DAY DIET DIARY DATE:______________

1st DAY	2nd DAY	3rd DAY	4th DAY	5th DAY	6th DAY	7th DAY
SYMPTOMS						
MEDICATION						
BREAKFAST						
SYMPTOMS						
MEDICATON						
LUNCHEON						
SYMPTOMS						
MEDICATION						
DINNER						
SYMPTOMS						
MEDICATION						
8TH DAY	9th DAY	10th DAY	11th DAY	12 DAY	13th DAY	14th DAY
SYMPTOMS						
MEDICATION						
BREAKFAST						
SYMPTOMS						
MEDICATION						
LUNCHEON						
SYMPTOMS						
MEDICATION						
DINNER						
SYMPTOMS						
MEDICATION						

RECORD FOODS AND MEDICATION IN BLUE AND SYMPTOMS IN RED

Figure 10-1. The Diet Diary.

chilling and overheating.

As described, symptoms from an allergenic food may not occur immediately after eating it but may occur later that day, during the night, or even on the following day. In some patients, symptoms from a single exacerbation are prone to occur on two or three consecutive nights, with relative freedom from symptoms during the intervening daytime hours. Total stress loads, not just total allergic loads, and long-delayed reactions have to be taken into consideration to pinpoint causative foods in some complex patients. Detailed notes on the diet diary are a most valuable aid in making these correlations.

The Food Ledger

It is also important to set up and maintain a food ledger consisting of a single sheet of paper with four columns (Fig. 10-2). The first column should list all the foods that are tolerated, i.e. those which do not cause any symptoms. The second column should list all foods that questionably produce symptoms of mild or moderate degree. These eventually must be tried again and moved either to the first or third column.

The third column should contain all foods that cause definite mild symptoms. These ordinarily should be avoided, but some can occasionally be eaten if the list of tolerated foods remains very limited. The fourth column should list all foods that cause severe symptoms. These foods should be totally eliminated for at least three months, after which foods causing less severe reactions may cautiously be tried again in small quantities. Tolerance to some foods changes, and it may be necessary to move a food from one column to another from time to time.

Prompt Relief of Food Reactions

If a patient has an adverse reaction to a food, he may obtain relief by taking one heaping teaspoonful of bicarbonate of soda in a glass of ice water, followed by a second glass of water. Intravenous bicarbonate has been reported to be useful in the management of acute, severe reactions.[65]

The elimination of food can be accelerated by the induction

FOOD LEDGER

TOLERATED (Live on These)	POSSIBLE MILD SYMPTOMS (Try Again)	DEFINITE MILD SYMPTOMS (Avoid if Possible)	POSSIBLE OR DEFINITE SEVERE SYMPTOMS (Avoid!)

Figure 10-2. The Food Ledger.

of vomiting, the administration of a laxative, or both. In general, the mildest and safest laxative is unflavored liquid magnesium hydroxide (milk of magnesia), but certain unflavored saline laxatives, e.g. Epsom salt or Fleet Phospho-Soda®, are faster and more reliable. Laxative pills, chewing gums, or flavored preparations should be avoided, for they themselves can produce allergic reactions. In some instances, a laxative combined with a therapeutic fast for a day or two may be used to relieve acute symptoms. During the fast, adequate amounts of a suitable water should be taken. The fast should be broken only with known tolerated foods, preferably taken one at a time. Additional foods should then be added one by one so that if reactions occur the offending food can be identified.

Starting the Diet

It often takes several days, sometimes one to two weeks, after starting a diet for the body to eliminate offending foods already present in the gastrointestinal tract, bloodstream, and tissues. It also takes time for some patients to become completely focused on the fine points of their diets. They tend to make many dietary mistakes at first. Because of these factors, one may continue to experience symptoms during the first days or weeks of a rotary diet. If symptoms finally clear and later recur, this recurrence should be noted in red in the proper place on the diet diary, and the food causing the recurrence should then be sought.

At first, it is best to keep the diet simple, eating as few foods with each meal as possible, to more readily detect reactions from individual foods. The ideal initial diet for the patient with many food sensitivities includes only one food per meal for the first four days, no more than two foods per meal for the second four days (repeating the first food, if tolerated, and adding one new food), no more than three foods per meal for the third four-day period, etc. Not all patients have the self-discipline to achieve the ideal, and it is not intended that all should be forced to follow this pattern. Reasonable compromises must be made when indicated.

To avoid excessive hunger and weight loss, the patient should be instructed that the quantity of each food is not limited. Eventually, for a particular meal, he may choose as many tolerated foods as are wanted. There may well be some weight loss during the first weeks of the diet, partly due to fluid elimination and partly due to the avoidance of sweet, spicy, salty, and high calorie foods. This may be useful in patients who are obese because of food addiction, and the addiction may be broken by the rotary diet. If weight loss is excessive or undesirable, food extract injection therapy can be instituted and the patient can then usually tolerate the formerly nontolerated foods without rotation.

A few examples of menus and ways in which the allowed foods can be prepared for given meals are included with the charts. The tastes and culinary ingenuity of the individual may suggest many additional methods of food combination and preparation. Many special cookbooks and other publications are available for additional ideas.

The rotary diet charts (Table 10-II) are like a supermarket with the entire stock on the shelves. It is not necessary to eat every food in stock, but rather to choose carefully from those that are available. The specific foods chosen for each meal must be recorded in the diet diary. Those which cause symptoms when inadvertently eaten too frequently should be tried again on a four-day rotation. Those which cause symptoms, even when rotated, must be noted in the diet diary and should be avoided.

Food Families

Some knowledge of food families (Table 10-II) is helpful in the management of food allergy. A patient who is sensitive to one member of a food family may be sensitive to another, although this is by no means always true. Cross-reactivity often does exist within the grass family (Graminneae), which includes cereals, sugar cane, sorghum, bamboo sprouts and shoots, and Chinese water chestnuts. Patients sensitive to an edible member of a food family, such as wheat, may also be sensitive to wheat flour or a related food in inhaled particulate form, as in baker's asthma; they may also be sensitive to inhaled cooking odors of this and related foods (osmyls), and to related grass pollens. Patients with cereal sensitivity may have grass hayfever and increased symptoms from grain ingestion during grass season.

It is for this reason that it is sometimes necessary to rotate an entire food family so that only one member of the family is taken every four days. The rotation of entire families is not always necessary, and it is often possible to eat one member of a food family every two days, or even daily so long as no specific food is eaten more often than once every four days. This should be attempted in stages after the patient becomes relatively symptom-free.

Every food family containing foods considered to be acceptable, nutritious, and obtainable has been listed in the rotary diet charts (Table 10-II). Each food family has been enclosed in a box in the charts. The underlined foods are those to be omitted in the stricter natural food diet #3. Each box in the four-day rotary diet contains the common edible members of one family; no family is repeated in the entire four-day diet. Milk and chocolate have been excluded from all four days of the rotary diet.

Plant family classifications (Table 10-III) have been listed alphabetically and enumerated with the numbers corresponding to the family boxes on the rotary diet charts (Table 10-II) and to the individual simple food listings (Table 10-I), which will allow the patient to easily identify the family name of any given food. However, it is not necessary to memorize the names of the food families to follow the rotary diet charts.

Rare Foods

The number of foods to which a patient may be sensitive is highly variable. A patient may obtain adequate results simply by avoiding one or two foods, or may have such widespread sensitivities that he may have to devote a great deal of time and thought toward planning proper nourishment. It is very important to maintain good nutrition and relative absence from incapacitating symptoms, but it is also important to try not to become faddist, compulsive, or sympathy seeking. Life should not be restricted any more than necessary, and all conversations should not revolve around personal food problems.

Foods that were never or rarely eaten by a given individual may be tolerated better than those which were past dietary staples. Some excellent foods not often found in the average Western diet are available. These foods may be obtained from diet or gourmet sections in the local supermarkets, from health food stores, from home gardens and farms, from sport fishermen and hunters, and from specialized food shippers. Examples of such foods are mangos, papayas, venison, rabbit, squirrel, bluefish, ling, crayfish, Alaskan king crab, South African lobster tails, macadamia nuts, American yams (not sweet potatoes), Chinese cabbage, leaks, shallots, and flours made from a variety of substances such as sunflower seed meal, pumpkin seed meal, lima bean flour, cassava meal, and poi.

It is also well to remember that some people who are exquisitely sensitive to traces of chemicals in their foods often feel better on organic diets. Organically grown foods may be more expensive and may or may not be more nutritious than non-organically grown foods, but by reducing specific chemical exposures and total chemical loads, they are of great value to the chemically sensitive patient.

The Patient's Role

The successful management of food allergies is largely dependent on the attitude and cooperation of the patient. Dietary instructions must be followed meticulously. Restaurant meals may have to be avoided, at least for a while, since restaurant flavorings, additives, oils, or other materials cannot always be identified. If restaurant meals cannot be avoided, selections must be simple, such as a plain broiled steak (no butter, seasonings, or tenderizer), a dry baked potato with natural gravy from the broiled steak, head lettuce or sliced tomato salad, and melon or other fruit for dessert. Complex salad dressings must be avoided; olive oil with lemon wedges or wine vinegar (grape and yeast) can be used if tolerated. Fresh or dried fruits and nuts are nourishing and convenient "fillers," although care should be taken to avoid dried fruits treated with additives, if these are a problem.

Many patients ask what to do about food at parties. Parties themselves should not be avoided, but it is best to satisfy hunger at home and then eat only safe, known foods at the party. The patient should avoid diet deviation, but if deviation is inevitable, a careful diet diary should be kept so that when symptoms occur, the causative foods may be pinpointed.

The Manufacturer's Role: Food Labelling

Most processed, packaged, and canned foods contain hidden ingredients of both natural and synthetic origin. Labelling is often incomplete and misleading.

Sugars, starches, oils, protein fragments, alcohols, and other derivatives of natural foods usually carry the allergenicity of the specific food source. For example, the allergenicity of corn may be carried by corn alcohol, corn sugar, cornstarch, corn oil, and corn oil margarines. Such derivatives often contain deliberate chemical additives and may accidentally be contaminated with minute residual amounts of the chemicals used in processing. These additives and chemicals may be of natural or synthetic origin, the synthetic ones usually being derived from petroleum, coal tar, and cellulose from plant or wood pulp.

Hidden Natural Ingredients

Among the natural foods commonly incorporated into other foods as labelled or unlabelled ingredients are egg, milk, soy, cottonseed, pork, beef, yeast, corn, wheat, and peanut. However, this is not always easy for the consumer to determine because of unfamiliar labelling used by food technologists. For example, all of the following ingredients are egg derivatives: vitellin, ovovitellin, livetin, ovomucin, ovomucoid, and albumin.[18,72]

Milk

Milk avoidance must include avoidance of all foods made from milk or milk derivatives. Casein, caseinate, lactose, and whey may not be recognized as milk but are, in fact, milk derivatives. Most "nondairy" creamers surprisingly contain milk products (sodium or calcium caseinate or lactose), and all of them contain ingredients from other unexpected sources such as corn, soy, animal and vegetable fats, and petroleum.[20,41] Powdered artificial sweeteners usually contain lactose (milk) or dextrose (corn) as well as saccharin (derived from coal tar).[43] Disodium cromoglycate inhalant powder for asthma contains lactose. Milk is absent from kosher bread (challah) and from some French, Italian, Syrian, and other special breads, as can usually be determined from their labels.

Milk powder is used as a filler in frankfurters, sausages, sauces, gravies, and many other such products. Milk derivatives are found in most margarines (including some labelled as 100% corn oil margarines), butter, cheese, cottage cheese, ice cream, sherbet, junket, yogurt, creamed soups, puddings, waffles, and candies (including, chocolate). Coffee Rich® and Mocha Mix® do not contain milk derivatives. Gerber's Meat Base® formula, Cho-Free®, and soybean formulas are free of milk, but some milk-sensitive infants are also sensitive to the beef, soy, corn, and other ingredients used as milk replacements. Margarines and cheeses are further complicated with various dyes, flavors, and preservatives introduced at the factory to produce uniform products with prolonged shelf lives.[30] A list of milk-containing products should be furnished to the milk-sensitive patient.

Chocolate

When chocolate is to be avoided, cola drinks and karaya gum (often listed on labels as a "vegetable gum") should also be omitted. For simplicity in instructing patients, this family often is referred to as the chocolate family. Cola drinks not only contain derivatives of the cola nut but also many other ingredients, including an extract of the coca leaf (Erythroxylaceae).

Egg

Egg derivatives are commonly found as labelled and unlabelled ingredients in baking powder, cakes, pancakes, packaged cake and pancake mixes, cookies, doughnuts, pastries, waffles, pretzels, French toast, pies, muffins, meringues, hollandaise sauce, tartar sauce, some salad dressings, icings, marshmallows, many candies and candy bars, and some sausages and lunch meats. Egg is often used in the production of root beer foam, and may be used to clarify wines and coffee.[19,75]

Soy

Soy is another common hidden ingredient in foods. Lecithin, food "extenders" and factory-made, low cholesterol food substitutes (such as certain Morningstar Farms® products) are derived largely from soy and also contain many spices and chemicals.[40,42] Soybean flour is used in some breads, cakes, rolls, pastries, doughnuts, and crackers. Soy is used in cereals, as a nut (roasted soybeans), and in sauces, e.g. soy sauce, teriyaki sauce, La Choy Sauce®, etc.[21] Tuna, sardines, and other foods are often packed in soy oil. Popcorn, potato chips, processed fried fish, and other substances are often fried in soy oil. Soy oil is also used as the base for many salad dressings and mayonnaises that are simply labelled as containing vegetable oil. It is added to sausages, lunch meats, hard candies, chocolate, caramels, and margarines, as well as being the base for many milk-free infant formulas.

Cottonseed

Cottonseed oil is used almost interchangeably with soy oil. Cottonseed flour is also used in some bakery products such as Fig Newtons®. Cottonseed flour or meal is sometimes used to make gin and xylose,[22] a sugar substitute used in soft drinks. There are innumerable additional uses for cottonseed and other oils in industry. Cottonseed allergy is uncommon but is often severe in degree.[81]

Vegetable Oils and Their Derivatives

Liquid shortenings usually contain oil from only one source, the source being printed on the label. Solid white vegetable shortenings contain unlabelled mixtures whose ingredients vary from time to time, depending chiefly on the current market prices of individual oils from which they are made.[54] Liquid Crisco Oil® is pure soy oil with BHA and BHT (butylated hydroxy anisole and butylated hydroxy toluene).[54] Louanna® is labelled as containing cottonseed oil, with no preservatives.[39] Wesson Oil® used to be only cottonseed oil, but now contains soy oil as well.[44] A wide variety of oils usually containing preservatives can be found in supermarkets, including soy, cottonseed, coconut, peanut, olive, almond, safflower, palm, and sesame oils. Oils without preservatives can be obtained from some health food stores and specialized food shippers (Table 10-IV).

Pork, Beef, Lamb

Shortening not labelled as of vegetable origin is usually derived from pork (lard), beef, or lamb. Almost all gelatin desserts such as Jell-O are now made from both pork and beef,[86] except Knox® gelatin, which is made only from beef.[46] However, some chemically sensitive patients are unable to tolerate beef-derived gelatin. This apparently is due to the residual amounts of chem-

TABLE 10-IV
SOME ORGANIC FOOD SHIPPERS*

1. Vita Green Farms P. O. Box 878 1525 W. Vista Way Vista, California 92083 Phone (211) 714-2163	Fresh fruits and vegetables
2. Max Kozek Produce 651 S. Kohler Street Los Angeles, California 90021 Phone (213) 622-6093	Fresh fruits and vegetables, year round
3. Shiloh Farms Sulphur Springs, Arkansas 72768 Phone (501) 298-3297	Bottled water, fruits, and juices, vegetables, baked goods, dairy products, nuts, grains, honey, flours, meats and seafoods
4. Erewhon Trading Company, Inc. 342 Newbury Street Boston, Massachusetts 02115 Phone (617) 262-3420	Brown rice, dried beans, sea vegetables, soybean products, condiments, oils, noodles, beverages, etc.
5. Breads for Life 1727 E. Division P. O. Box 3484 Springfield, Missouri 65804 Phone (417) 865-7350	Breads, baked goods, and cereals
6. Kennedy Natural Food Store 1051 W. Broad Street Falls Church, Virginia 22046 Phone (703) 533-8484	A variety of natural foods
7. Caledonia Packing Company Caledonia, Minnesota 55921	Strawberries, raspberries, corn, asparagus and peas
8. Al Mueller 233 Dade Avenue Ferguson, Missouri 63135	Sweet potatoes
9. Briggs Way Company Ugashik, Alaska 99683	Glass-canned natural Alaskan salmon with no seasonings or preservatives
10. Lee Anderson Coachella, California 92236 Cobalds Date Company	Dates (unfumigated) and date sugar

*This is not an endorsement of any shippers or any product.

TABLE 10-IV (continued)

SOME SOURCES OF UNUSUAL MEATS AND FISH	
(Not Necessarily Organic)	
1. Czimer Food, Inc. Route 1, Box 285 Lockport, Illinois 60441 Phone (312) 925-7800	Organic foods and exotic meats such as game and game birds of the United States and a few foreign animals
2. Burhop's 545 N. State Street Chicago, Illinois 60605	Fresh seafood

SOME SOURCES OF INFORMATION	
1. Natural Foods and Farming P. O. Box 210 Atlanta, Texas 75551	Can provide lists of organic growers directly or through magazine *Natural Foods and Farming*. Can provide names of secretaries of state chapters of Natural Foods Associates who may provide names of growers
2. *Organic Gardening Magazine* 33 Minor Street Emmaus, Pennsylvania 18049	Can provide lists of organic farms in each state

icals remaining from processing techniques, since many of these patients can tolerate fresh, nonprocessed beef.

Yeast

Yeast is found primarily in baked goods, alcoholic beverages, B vitamins, and products that contain vinegar, e.g. catsup, mayonnaise, and barbecue sauce. Those products which are labelled as "enriched" usually contain yeast-derived vitamins of the vitamin B complex series. This includes packaged cold cereals and macaroni, consumer products which one would not expect to contain yeast. Black tea is yeast fermented and is another unlikely source of this food.[37] Torula, listed on the labels of some processed and smoked foods, is a yeast. Some commercial citric acid and some monosodium glutamates are also yeast fermented.

Wheat

Wheat includes everything made from the wheat grain, including wheat flour, wheat germ, bran, etc. Of course, this includes all bakery products such as bread (even most rye breads and pumpernickel contain wheat), crackers, cookies, pies, doughnuts, matzos, and pretzels. It also includes spaghetti, macaroni, noodles, dumplings, alphabet soups, wheat batters on fried foods, and wheat cereals such as Wheaties®, Cream of Wheat®, Grape Nuts®, and farina; also all frankfurters and sausage in which wheat flour is used as a filler and most products labelled as containing gluten. Special wheat-free breads and crackers (such as rice crackers, 100% rye bread, and Ry-Krisp®) may be used by some patients. Recipes for wheat-free, corn-free, and milk-free breads are published in special cookbooks for allergic and celiac patients.[35,47,79,82]

Corn

Corn products are found in a great number of foods both as known and hidden ingredients. Examples are foods that contain cornmeal, cornstarch, corn oil, corn sugar, corn syrup, corn sweetener, dextrose, glucose, dexin, dextrin, dextrimaltose, and corn alcohol (beer, bourbon, Scotch, blended whiskeys, vodka, gin, some wines, and many liqueurs). Commercial fructose is now also made from corn. Malt is generally yeast-fermented from corn and wheat as well as barley.

Almost all factory-processed foods contain corn derivatives such as corn sugar, corn sweetener, citric acid, or monosodium glutamate. These include candies, cakes, cookies, pastries, ice cream, cake icings, powdered sugar, gelatin desserts, canned fruits and juices, powdered fruit drinks such as Kool-Aid®, powdered sugar, jams, jellies, syrups, peanut butter, catsups, chili, barbecue sauce, mayonnaise, salad dressing, chewing gum, tacos, enchiladas, tortillas, Fritos®, and Chee-Wees®. As mentioned, commercial table salts contain dextrose.

Most infant formulas also contain corn derivatives. There are, however, some corn-free formulas: Gerber's Meat Base,® Mull-Soy®, Neo-Mull-Soy, Cho-Free®, and Soyalac®. Many medications contain corn derivatives, e.g. cough syrups, cough drops, lozenges, pills, tablets, suppositories, and baby powders.

Cornmeal is often used as a dry lubricant on the floors of bakery ovens and becomes cooked into the undersurfaces of bread loaves. Cornmeal and cornstarch are used in some paper milk cartons, in baking powders, and in the glue on stamps, envelopes, and adhesive tape.

Vinegars

White grain vinegar, which is the vinegar most commonly used in the United States, carries the allergenicity of wheat, corn, and other grains and sugars, as well as yeast. The primary vinegar in Great Britain is malt,[25] made from barley, but sometimes with adjuncts of other grains such as corn and rice.[24] Wine or grape vinegar is the one most commonly used on the European continent.[25] Plain wine vinegar and apple cider vinegar are free from corn and wheat. Olives canned in ferrous gluconate and water are free from corn and wheat. The citric acid employed commercially usually is made from molasses, fermented by *Aspergillus niger*. It is also derived from lemon or yeast-fermented, pineapple canning wastes.[26]

Starches

Wheat flour and cornstarch can be replaced in diets by tapioca, arrowroot starch, rice flour, potato flour, lima bean flour, soy flour, and other flours commonly found in supermarkets and health food stores. Foods that might ordinarily be fried in wheat or corn batter also can be placed in Pyrex® dishes and baked in their own juices, thus eliminating the need for batter and a frying oil or butter. Most table salts contain corn sugar (dextrose) as well as sodium silicoaluminate and iodide, and these are unsuitable for some highly corn sensitive, chemically sensitive, or iodide sensitive patients. If salt is to be added, plain sea salt can be obtained from most health food stores.

Careful label reading is required; the presence of "food starch" or "modified food starch" on a label might indicate a starch of wheat, corn, sorghum, arrowroot, cassava (tapioca), or potato origin. To avoid inadvertent ingestion of wheat or corn, foods labelled as containing food starch should not be used in this diet. Arrowroot starch and tapioca are much less frequently allergenic than are wheat and corn, and manufacturers should be encouraged to use these in their products and designate on the label the type of starch used.

Alcohols

As mentioned, alcoholic extracts of foods are absorbed very rapidly, cause more immediate reactions, and therefore can be used to pinpoint sensitivities not otherwise so apparent. Most beers contain corn products, though Michelob® is made with rice and is corn free. Rums are made primarily from cane sugar and many are corn free. Bacardi Rum® contains grape but is free of corn. Jamaican rums must be free of all noncane alcohol by law.

Alcoholic beverages are derived from foods and carry the allergenicity of their food origin.[76] Most American beers are made with corn grits, but they also contain other ingredients such as barley, malt, hops, and yeast.

Whiskeys, including "straight corn whiskey," contain a vast array of ingredients. One popular brand is advertised as "containing 94 ingredients for your taste pleasure." Gin is equally complicated. Many people believe that vodka is made from potatoes, but this is not usually true.[23] American vodka is as complex as blended whiskeys and gin. However, aquavit is made from potatoes. Tequila is made from cactus.

In making wine and brandy, the fermentation of the grapes and other fruits does not naturally proceed beyond a concentration of about 14 percent alcohol; any patient who is able to partake of yeast and grapes, or whatever fruit the product is made from, usually can tolerate wine and brandy. However, any product listed on the label as containing greater than 14 percent alcohol contains additional distilled alcohol from other sources, often from corn. Exceptions are wines and brandies that are themselves distilled to greater than 14 percent alcohol content. Cognac has no additives, but many brandies contain grain alcohol and synthetic colors and flavors. Cordials and liqueurs often contain added sugar, spices, and aromatics. Caramel color is usually from heat-processed sugars, and the sugar itself is filtered through lime.[45]

This explains why a patient can often tolerate one alcoholic beverage better than another. For example, a patient who gets symptoms from most beers, whiskeys and fortified wines, but not from Michelob, Bacardi Rum or unfortified wines, is almost certainly corn sensitive. One who gets symptoms from Michelob but not from other beers is probably rice sensitive. A patient who exhibits symptoms from all liquor may be sensitive to yeast or to several foods such as corn, rice, and grapes.

The more rapid absorption of alcohols and sugars also explains why some patients have no detectable symptoms when challenged with whole corn, cornstarch or corn oil but exhibit definite symptoms when challenged with corn alcohol or corn sugars. Headache, vertigo, diarrhea, and other symptoms of corn sensitivity are common from the glucose-loading dose used for the glucose tolerance test, but their significance usually is missed by both the patient and the physician.

Artificial Colors and Flavors

Artificial colors and flavors have been incriminated as causative agents in hyperactivity, behavior problems, and learning disorders in children.[15] In addition, clinical experience also implicates many other chemical food additives such as preservatives, thickeners, gums, suspending agents, emulsifiers, surface active agents, chelating agents, sequestrants, buffers, acidulants, texture modifiers, antioxidants, freshness preservers, antibacterials, antibiotics, mold retarders, humectants, organic solvents, enzymes, vitamins, minerals, alcohol (e.g. glycerol, sorbitol, and mannitol) , non-nutritive sweeteners, and flavor potentiators, e.g. sugar, salt, monosodium glutamate, citric acid, eugenol, nucleotides, and maltol.

Medications

Medications often contain hidden food and chemical ingredients.[49] A particular capsule or tablet may contain starch as a filler, usually derived from corn, but sometimes from wheat, potato, sorghum, arrowroot, cassava (tapioca) or other sources.[27] Medications also may contain a binder such as zinc, calcium, or magnesium stearate, made from the stearic acid of pork, beef, or lamb fat.[49] Color usually is derived from coal tar and synthetic compounds[36,51,85] and flavoring from aromatic hydrocarbons that are, in turn, usually derived from petroleum.[28,53] A final coating or glaze on hard tablets may contain either corn syrup or plastic films of petrochemical origin.

Liquid medications also contain many artificial colors and flavors and may also contain synthetic alcohol, usually derived from petroleum. If the medication is thick, it often contains natural gums (karaya, acacia, tragacanth, arabic, guar, or carob bean gum), methylcellulose (derived from wood or plant pulp), carrageenan (derived from Irish moss, a dried seaweed) or other suspending and emulsifying agents.[60]

Chemicals in Fruits, Vegetables and Meats

Patients with multiple food and chemical sensitivities usually do better to avoid all foods that have passed through a factory on the way to the supermarket. However, this does not guarantee freedom from inadvertent exposures, particularly to chemicals.

Fresh fruits and vegetables that would ordinarily appear to be very good choices may present enormous problems to the chemically sensitive patient because of unexpected processing procedures. Nearly all produce available from commercial grocers has been treated in the fields with insecticides. Peaches, apples, and cherries are the most seriously affected, often being sprayed or treated with insecticides ten to fifteen times per season.[66] In addition, fruits are sometimes sprayed at the market counters to prevent fruit fly and other insect infestation. Although the fruits and vegetables may be washed or even peeled, the chemicals have often penetrated the pulp.[66]

Cosmetic alterations of foods also may cause difficulties. The appealing shine on many fruits and vegetables is often due to coating with vegetable or mineral oils or petrochemically derived waxes.[31,67] Since these chemicals are not water soluble, washing is not an effective method of removal. Among the types of produce that may be treated in this manner are rutabagas, cucumbers, green peppers, apples, parsnips, and squash. Peeling can reduce chemical exposures but does not entirely eliminate them and some foods, e.g. green peppers, do not lend themselves to peeling.

All commercially dried fruits are treated with sulfur dioxide unless otherwise stated on the package.[67] This is also a cosmetic modification, serving to prevent some discoloration of the products. All dates crossing state lines are fumigated with methyl bromide[66] in accordance with federal regulations.

Bananas, which are picked green, are usually exposed to a petroleum-derived gas, ethylene, which destroys the green chlorophyll and hastens apparent ripening.[88] Such bananas may not be tolerated by the petrochemically sensitive patient. Some patients say that they can distinguish these bananas from nongassed ones because gassed bananas develop large brown spots as they ripen and have a "green" taste, whereas nongassed bananas or less gassed bananas ripen with small, stippled brown spots and have a sweeter taste.[65] Apples, pears, oranges, and tomatoes are also often exposed to ethylene.[67] Oranges are often also dyed with artificial colors.[52,67]

Eggs may be dipped in penicillin solutions to retard spoilage. The penicillin penetrates the shell and contaminates the contents. Chicken can also be a problem. Antibiotics, coccidiostats, hormones, growth stimulants, and other chemicals are often added to their feed.[89] Killed, plucked, eviscerated chickens are sometimes placed in an ice slush bath containing antibiotics to retard bacterial growth.[32] The patient who is exquisitely sensitive to chemicals may be bothered by the traces of these materials remaining in the poultry products.

Chemicals in Canned and Packaged Foods

Certain foods in cans cannot be tolerated by some patients who can tolerate the same foods in glass jars. A major cause of this is the plastic or phenolic resin liner of the can.[64]

Some methods of storing and preparing foods may also cause symptoms in hypersensitive patients. The soft plastic wrappers (such as Handi-Wrap®) used to cover foods have been reported to produce reactions in certain patients.[64] Some patients who have an apparent allergy to coffee discover that they tolerate coffee roasted with electric heat but not coffee roasted with a gas flame.[64]

Chemicals in Frozen Foods

Frozen fish is often dipped in antibiotics before freezing to retard spoilage.[33] Frozen potatoes are often treated with chemicals such as sodium acid pyrophosphate and sodium EDTA to prevent discoloration.[29] They are also often coated with methylcellulose to harden when subjected to frying, so as to produce a crisp outer shell with a tender, moist interior.[13] Coatings or batters on frozen fried chicken, fried shrimp, etc., often contain not only wheat flour and cornmeal, but sometimes egg, seasonings, monosodium glutamate, texture modifiers, and preservatives.[42]

Water

Water is also a problem for an increasing number of people. In an effort to provide water that is as safe from bacteriological and chemical contamination as possible, most water reaching the consumer via municipal systems has undergone a great deal of processing. Some patients are very sensitive to the chemicals used.[59] Evaporation of chlorine can be achieved by boiling the water for thirty minutes, or by drawing it into a glass pitcher and leave it uncovered overnight.

The use of distilled water may also prove helpful, although distilled water in soft plastic containers can cause symptoms due to the leaching of the plastic solvents into the water. In this case, it may be necessary to buy distilled water in glass bottles. Unfortunately, the filters through which the water is distilled may be made from resins and the bottle caps may be lined with plastic. There are many brands of glass-bottled water, and a tolerated one may be determined for each patient by trials.

There are rare patients who find that only water drawn directly from a well or spring can be tolerated. This water would then preferably be stored in glass bottles with natural cork stoppers.

Unintentional Chemical Contaminants

It is inevitable that some chemicals used to control bacteria, mold, insects, and rodents in food factories should accidentally enter the consumer products. This is also true of detergents, organic solvents used to clean food vats, and lubricating agents used for the equipment. There are strict guidelines set by the Food and Drug Administration with regards to the quantities of such indirect contaminants in food. Unfortunately, although the levels of these chemicals may not be high enough to cause a toxic reaction in the general population, they can cause reactions in some hypersensitive patients.

The Producer-Consumer Interface

Life is a hazardous obstacle course for many broadly sensitive patients. They literally must pick their way through a jungle of chemicals and allergens in the supermarket. Manufacturers should use minimum concentration of less toxic and less sensitizing additives, use natural rather than synthetic ingredients whenever possible, and omit chemicals such as artificial colors that add nothing to the nutritional value of the product. Food processors who do not label their products completely place an unacceptable health burden on a rapidly growing segment of the public they serve. It may well be that industrial processing of foods is causing some of the increase in chemical sensitivities noted in the population in recent years.

INTRADERMAL TESTING AND IMMUNOTHERAPY WITH FOOD EXTRACTS

Both prick and intradermal tests are more useful in food sensitivity diagnosis than most allergists realize. Of course, no *in vivo* tests should be used for a specific food in a patient with a history of anaphylaxis to the food. Patients with marked IgE-mediated food allergy of subanaphylactic degree often show positive prick tests to the etiologic foods, as demonstrated by the studies of Bock et al.[6-8] Patients with moderate IgE-mediated, and those with non–IgE-mediated (delayed), sensitivites are usually prick test–negative. Many patients with negative prick tests have positive intradermal tests.[55-57] Others with definite food sensitivities have negative intradermal whealing responses but develop mild transient symptoms when tested intradermally to each specific allergenic food; induction of such symptoms is even more valuable diagnostically than a positive wheal.

An added advantage of intradermal testing is that weaker or stronger dilutions can be chosen so that precise and controlled amounts of a specific extract can be delivered into the skin, making it possible to safely test patients with varying degrees of sensitivity. At the same time, it enables one to measure the degree of sensitivity to each food in each patient by a multiple dilution bioassay of each food extract. Those who are more sensitive to the antigen tend to have a positive reaction to a more dilute dose, and conversely.

This method of assaying an individual's sensitivity to inhalant antigens has been compared by many workers with the results of RAST and histamine release, the only other objective methods of measuring specific sensitivities.[1,4,17,48,58,61] Reisman,[74] summarizing his own findings and those of others, has concluded that multiple dilution skin tests correlate well with the patient's sensitivities and with RAST and histamine release but are usually more reliable. Multiple dilution testing has the additional advantage that the results of testing are immediately available. Intradermal testing, using multiple serial dilutions, in my experience, has the same advantages in determining the degree of the patient's immediate and delayed sensitivity to food antigens.

I learned this food testing technique from its originator, Carleton Lee. When he began carrying out intradermal tests on the above lines, he very quickly became aware that dilutions of the antigen that were associated with positive wheals frequently precipitated symptoms. These symptoms often correlated closely with those previously or subsequently produced by ingestion challenge. For example, a patient who wheezed after ingestion of beef also wheezed after the intradermal injection of beef extract in sufficient strength to cause positive whealing. When Lee injected weaker dilutions, each dilution being one-fifth the strength of the previous dilution, he often found that the injection of the strongest dilution that produced a negative wheal was associated with prompt relief of the patient's symptoms. He called this relieving phenomenon *neutralization.* His next step was to give regular injections of the relieving dose and to follow this with oral challenge of the food in question in an amount that previously caused wheezing. When this was done, it was often found that the injection was protective and that ingestion of the food no longer precipitated symptoms.

My observations have been identical with Lee's. I have been following his precepts with remarkable success for fifteen years, and have outlined the details of technique and response in a book[56] and a double-blind study.[55] These phenomena can be verified by any practicing allergist. Mechanisms have not yet been delineated, but Walker's[87] finding that intraperitoneal injections of protein antigens in the rat are associated with a significant decrease in the absorption of those same antigens when given by mouth may reflect a similar phenomenon in humans.

Methods and Concepts

If this approach is to be useful in the management of food and other allergies, it is essential to *standardize* the equipment (syringes, needles, and even rules for wheal measurements), the technique of the intradermal injection, the site of the injection (this author uses the lateral aspect of the upper arm), and the serial dilutions (1:5). I always inject 0.05 ml unless I expect the patient to be sensitive, when 0.01 ml is injected as a preliminary screening dose. The 0.01 ml volume is defined operationally as the volume required to produce a 4 mm wheal.

The *interpretation of the wheal* is crucial to this method. Wheals associated with this form of food allergy do not resemble the tremendous wheals with pseudopodia encountered in testing individuals highly sensitive to pollens. The two important features of the wheal are, first, its growth, and second, its physical characteristics. The wheal that grows 2 mm in diameter (the mean of the largest and smallest diameters) in ten minutes usually is a positive wheal. Such wheals retain or increase their initial characteristics, i.e. they are blanched, hard, raised, and discoid with sharply demarcated elevated edges. A wheal that grows less than 2 mm in diameter in ten minutes and that becomes soft and flesh-colored and melts into the surrounding skin is negative. Erythema may be associated with both positive and negative wheals in some patients; its presence therefore is not taken into consideration. The clinical significance of a positive wheal is that it represents a stronger dilution than the treatment dilution.

The Treatment Dose

The treatment dose is usually 0.05 ml of the strongest dilution of the extract that produces a negative wheal; this amount usually clears symptoms produced by stronger or weaker dilutions. To give an example, if Dilution #4 is the treatment dilution, it produces a negative wheal and all weaker dilutions usually also produce negative wheals. Stronger dilutions usually produce progressively larger wheals. The strongest negative wheal dilution, #4 in this example, will relieve symptoms in about 75 percent of tests. In 15 percent of tests, even though Dilution #4 produces a negative wheal, symptoms are not relieved until the next weaker dilution, #5 in this example, is given; and in 5 percent, the third negative wheal dilution (#6 in this example), etc. In brief, the treatment dilution is the strongest dilution that can be given intradermally without inducing a positive wheal or provoking symptoms, and that relieves symptoms produced by previously administered dilutions. It is the maximum tolerated intradermal dilution.

This dilution can be determined in several ways, as illustrated in the following examples. If the first test injection produces a positive wheal, with or without symptoms, one should move consecutively to weaker dilutions; provided no symptoms have been induced, the first dilution with a negative wheal is the treatment dilution (Fig. 10-3a). If symptoms are induced and the first negative wheal dilution does not clear them completely, consecutively weaker dilutions should be administered until symptoms are relieved (Fig. 10-3b). If the treatment dilution is passed while proceeding weaker on negative wheal dilutions, the symptoms may increase in severity ("underdose" symptoms), but this can be corrected by again administering consecutively stronger dilutions until symptoms clear. This still should be associated with a negative wheal (Fig. 10-3c).

If the first test injection produces a negative wheal and induces symptoms, consecutively stronger dilutions should be given until clearing occurs (Fig. 10-3d). If too strong a dilution is given, a positive wheal usually will be produced, signalling the necessity to again administer the next weaker dilution (Fig. 10-3e). Relief of symptoms usually is more clear-cut when the treatment dose is administered the second time. In some cases, symptoms become more severe with stronger dilutions even though no positive wheal is formed ("overdose" symptoms). In such instances, weaker dilutions must be given to relieve symptoms (Fig. 10-3f,g). When given weaker dilutions, a patient may feel better but not completely symptom-free on one dilution, and worse on a still weaker dilution. Complete relief of symptoms usually will be obtained by readministering either the strongest dilution with a negative wheal or the dilution on which the patient previously reported that he was better but not quite symptom-free (Fig. 3-10h). Waiting an additional five to ten minutes may occasionally be necessary to provide time for improving symptoms to clear. An occasional slow-reacting patient requires twenty to thirty minutes between most or all test doses. In infants, wheals are often evanescent and must be evaluated at five minutes, although ten minutes are still usually required for symptom clearing.

Having determined the treatment dose for each antigen to which the patient is sensitive by the procedures summarized in Fig. 10-4, these antigens are combined in one extract using dilutions that testing revealed relieved symptoms. This extract, given subcutaneously twice weekly, leads within a few weeks to a diminution and sometimes to complete relief of symptoms.

Although testing usually is simple, logical, and straightforward, the following situations may be encountered:

Bound Wheals. Sometimes a certain concentration will be associated with both a positive wheal and with clearing of symptoms. When this happens, it is thought that only a small portion

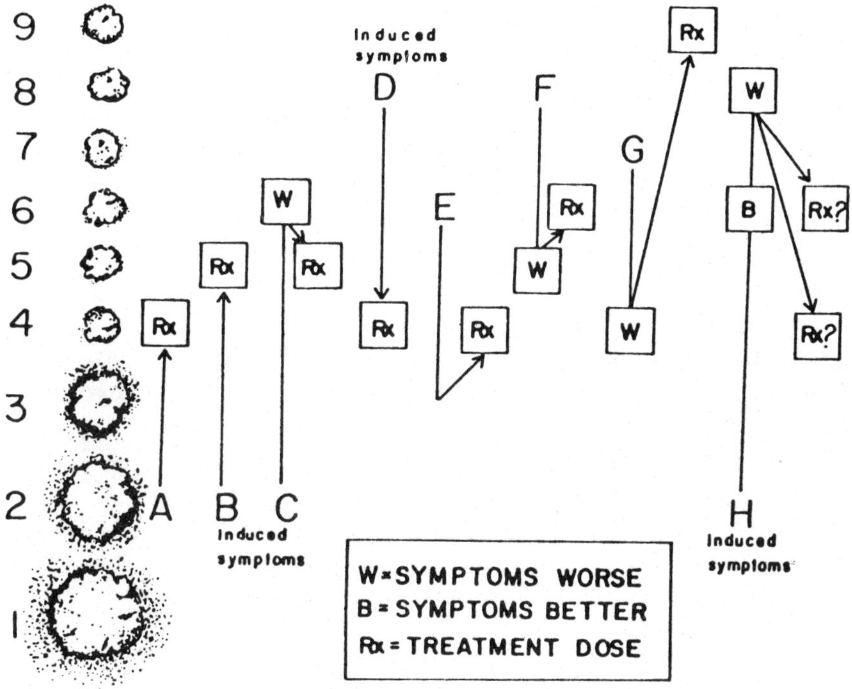

Figure 10-3. Wheal and symptoms guidelines to treatment dilutions.

of the injected antigen is immediately absorbed, and this relieves symptoms; most of the antigen, however, remains bound in the firm, discoid wheal, only to be released later, causing delayed reactions. Dilutions that cause positive wheals, even though they

Begin with 0.05/#2

- → Positive wheal. Use 0.05/#3, 0.05/#4, etc.
- → Negative wheal, induces persistent symptoms. Use 0.05/#3, 0.05/#4, etc.
- → Negative wheal, induces transient symptoms. This is the treatment dilution.
- → Negative wheal, relieves pre-existing symptoms. This is the treatment dilution.
- → Negative wheal, no symptoms. Not sensitive, or this is the treatment dilution. Review history; challenge; relieve symptoms induced by challenge; therapeutic trial.

Figure 10-4. The basic method of neutralizing testing.

appear at first to relieve symptoms, should not be used as treatment doses.

Positive Wheal But No Symptoms. Sometimes an injected food extract will cause a positive wheal but will not precipitate symptoms. If there is clinical suspicion by history or oral challenge that the food under study contributes to the patient's symptomatology, the food should be included in the extract, the treatment dilution being the strongest dilution with a negative wheal.

Symptoms But No Positive Wheal. Sometimes the extract does not cause positive whealing but does precipitate symptoms. Again, if there is any evidence that the food being studied contributes to the patient's symptomatology, it should be used in therapeutic trial, and the strength of the extract to be included should be the strongest dilution that relieves symptoms.

The Very Sensitive or Brittle Patient. Patients who might experience severe reactions to test doses because they have a history of anaphylaxis, laryngeal edema or severe asthma, or because they have severe concomitant disease such as angina or emphysema, are included under this heading. Food testing should begin with those foods eaten daily which the patient thinks do not contribute to his symptomatology. Foods known to have caused a severe reaction should be avoided. Testing should proceed cautiously with weak dilutions and with small volumes, i.e. with 0.01 ml (Figs. 10-5 and 10-6). When the presumptive treat-

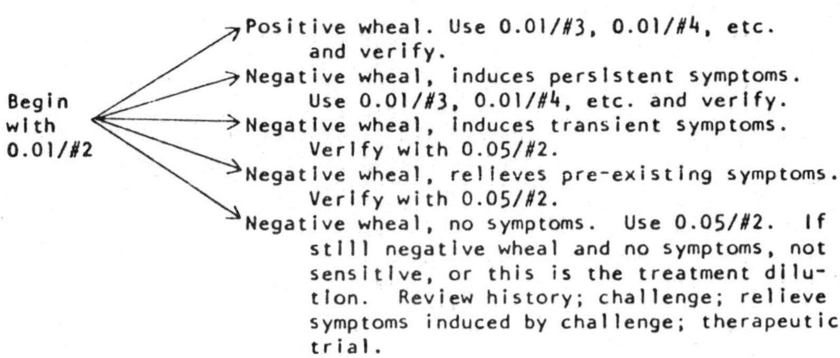

Figure 10-5. Testing the first foods—new nonbrittle patients.

Begin with 0.01/#4, 0.01/#8, etc.

→ Positive wheal: Screen consecutively weaker to strongest negative wheal dilution on which no induced symptoms persist, and verify.

→ Negative wheal: Screen consecutively stronger to strongest negative wheal dilution on which no induced symptoms persist, and verify.

Figure 10-6. Testing the first foods—new brittle patients.

ment dilution is reached, 0.05 ml of this dilution is administered to verify that this is the actual treatment dilution. This is the only time 0.05 ml volumes are used in brittle patients. The same procedure is followed in testing any patient to highly allergenic foods such as peanut, egg, cottonseed, soy, mustard, nuts, shellfish, etc.

MEDICATIONS. Patients who are ill—for example, who are dyspneic and wheezing—should not be tested until their symptoms have been controlled adequately by medications such as epinephrine, beta agonists, aerosols, aminophylline, cromoglycate or, if necessary, steroids. These medications do not interfere with the development of test symptoms and characteristic wheals; therefore, treatment dilutions can be determined accurately.

SENSITIVITIES TO DILUENT, GLYCEROL, AND PHENOL. Some patients, particularly those who are very sensitive to chemicals, may also be sensitive to the diluent, to glycerol and/or to phenol. This can be determined easily by injecting 2 percent glycerol and/or 0.4 percent phenol intradermally. If, on testing, sensitivities to these chemicals are found, it may be necessary to use extracts free from them, or to treat these sensitivities.

Because only one antigen is injected at a time, testing may take two or more days. At the end of each days' testing, the patient should be given an injection that contains 0.05 ml of each of the treatment doses found thus far. This will help to ensure that there will be no delayed reactions from the extracts with which he has already been tested, and often starts providing protection from ingestion of these foods even while still testing. When testing has been completed, the patient should be started on immunotherapy, using 0.05 ml of all treatment dilutions subcutaneously twice weekly. Because this dose is both the maximum tolerated dose and the effective dose, it should *not* be increased.

In conclusion, it should be remembered that immunotherapy is only an adjunct to treatment. Environmental control, the avoidance of foods to which the patient is very sensitive and of chemicals to which he cannot be immunized, and a rotary diet composed of the better tolerated foods are all essential components of treatment.

REFERENCES

1. Aas, K. and Johansson, S.G.O.: The radioallergosorbent test in the *in vitro* diagnosis of multiple reaginic allergy. *J Allergy Clin Immunol, 48:*134, 1971.
2. Aas, K.: The diagnosis of hypersensitivity to ingested foods. Reliability of skin prick testing and the radioallergosorbent test with different materials. *Clin Allergy, 8:*39, 1978.
3. Alvarez, W.C.: Allergy-Caused Mental Ailments. *Mobile Press Register,* Aug. 20, 1970.
4. Berg, T.L.O. and Johansson, S.G.O.: Allergy diagnosis with the radioallergosorbent test. *J Allergy Clin Immunol, 54:*209, 1974.
5. Björkstén, F., Backman, A., Järvinen, K.A.J., Lehti, H., Savilahti, E., Syvänen, P., and Kärkkäinen, T.: Immunoglobulin E specific to wheat and rye flour proteins. *Clin Allergy, 7:*473, 1977.
6. Bock, S.A., Buckley, J., Holst, A., and May, C.D.: Proper use of skin tests with food extracts in diagnosis of hypersensitivity to food in children. *Clin Allergy, 7:*375, 1977.
7. Bock, S.A., Lee, W-Y., Remigio, L.K., Holst, A., and May, C.D.: Appraisal of skin tests with food extracts for diagnosis of food hypersensitivity. *Clin Allergy, 8:*559, 1978.
8. Bock, S.A., Lee, W-Y., Remigio, L.K., and May, C.D.: Studies of hypersensitivity reactions to foods in infants and children. *J Allergy Clin Immunol, 62:*327, 1978.
9. Chua, Y.Y., Bremner, K., Lakdawalla, N., Llobet, J.L., Kokubu, H.L., Orange, R., and Collins-Williams, C.: *In vivo* and *in vitro* correlates of food allergy. *J Allergy Clin Immunol, 58:*299, 1976.
10. Chua, Y.Y., Bremner, K., Llobet, J.L., Kokubu, H.L., and Collins-Williams, C.: Diagnosis of food allergy by the radioallergosorbent test. *J Allergy Clin Immunol, 58:*477, 1976.
11. Crook, W.G.: *Can Your Child Read? Is He Hyperactive?,* Jackson, Pedicenter Press, 1977, pp. 50-52 and 146-148.
12. Doeglas, H.M. and Nater, J.P.: Histamine in foods causing false pos-

itive scratch tests. *J Allergy, 42:*164, 1968.

13. Dow Chemical Company advertisement in *Food Technology, 29:*89, 1975.
14. Feingold, B.F.: *Introduction to Clinical Allergy.* Springfield: Thomas, 1973, pp. 148-150.
15. ———: *Why Your Child is Hyperactive.* New York: Random 1974, pp. 109-130.
16. Finn, R. and Cohen, H.N.: "Food allergy": fact or fiction? *Lancet, 1:*426, 1978.
17. Frankland, A.W.: Some observations on the RAST test (guest editorial). *Ann Allergy, 33:*105, 1974.
18. Frazier, C.A.: *Coping with Food Allergy.* New York: Quadrangle, 1974, p. 91.
19. *Ibid.,* pp. 91-92.
20. *Ibid.,* p. 83.
21. *Ibid.,* p. 304.
22. *Ibid.,* pp. 58-59 and 298.
23. *Ibid.,* p. 319.
24. Furia, T.E.: *Handbook of Food Additives.* Cleveland: The Chemical Rubber Company, 1968, p. 75.
25. *Ibid.,* p. 248.
26. *Ibid.,* p. 265.
27. *Ibid.,* pp. 377-378.
28. *Ibid.,* pp. 480-490.
29. *Ibid.,* p. 302.
30. *Ibid.,* pp. 149, 155, 161-162, 172, and 190.
31. *Ibid.,* p. 252.
32. *Ibid.,* p. 188.
33. *Ibid.,* p 358.
34. Gavani, U.D., Hyde, J.S., and Moore, B.S.: Hypersensitivity to milk and egg white. Skin tests, RAST results and clinical intolerance. *Ann Allergy, 40:*314, 1978.
35. Golos, N.: *Management of Complex Allergies.* Norwalk: New England Foundation of Allergic and Environmental Diseases, 1975, pp. R6-R19.
36. Hall, R.H.: *Food for Nought.* New York: Vintage Books, 1974, pp. 70-71.
37. Hollister-Stier Laboratories. Yeast—A brief description of common sources of contacts.
38. Hosen, H.: A program of comprehensive environmental control. In Dickey, L.D. (Ed.): *Clinical Ecology.* Springfield: Thomas, 1976, pp. 459-462.
39. Ingredient label (Louanna Oil).

40. Ingredient label (Morningstar Farm products).
41. Ingredient labels on nondairy creamers.
42. Ingredient labels on packages of described product types.
43. Ingredient labels on powdered artificial sweeteners.
44. Ingredient label (Wesson Oil).
45. Jenkins, G.H.: *Introduction to Cane Sugar Technology.* New York: Am Elsevier, 1966, pp. 172-174.
46. Knox, A.E.: Knox Gelatin Inc., December 9, 1966. Personal communication.
47. Larson, J., and Nugent, B.: *Very Basically Yours.* Chicago: Human Ecology Study Group, 1967, pp. 89-95.
48. Lichtenstein, L.M.: Allergy. In Bach, F.H. and Good, R.A. (Eds.): *Clinical Immunology,* vol. 1. New York: Acad Pr, 1972, p. 261.
49. Lockey, S.D.: Reactions to hidden agents in foods, beverages and drugs. *Ann Allergy, 29:*461, 1971.
50. Maclennan, J.G.: Some prerequisites for a total fasting investigation. In Dickey, L.D. (Ed.): *Clinical Ecology.* Springfield: Thomas, 1976, pp. 454-468.
51. Marine, G., and Van Allen, J.: *Food Pollution.* New York: HR & W, 1972, p. 180.
52. *Ibid.,* p. 9.
53. *Ibid.,* p. 197.
54. Meyer, W.H.: The Proctor and Gamble Company, September 19, 1966. Personal communication.
55. Miller, J.B.: A double-blind study of food extract injection therapy: A preliminary report. *Ann Allergy, 38:*185, 1977.
56. ———: *Food Allergy: Provocative Testing and Injection Therapy.* Springfield: Thomas, 1972.
57. ———: Food Allergy: Technique of intradermal testing and subcutaneous injection therapy. *Trans Am Soc Ophthalmol Otolaryngol Allergy, 16:*150, 1976.
58. Miyamoto, T., Johansson, S.G.O., Ito, K., and Horiuchi, Y.: Atopic Allergy in Japanese subjects: Studies primarily with radioallergosorbent test. *J Allergy Clin Immunol, 53:*9, 1974.
59. Morgan, J.T.: The water problem. In Dickey, L.D. (Ed.): *Clinical Ecology.* Springfield: Thomas, 1976, p. 306.
60. Nilsson, D.C.: Sources of allergenic gums. *Ann Allergy, 18:*518, 1960.
61. Norman, P.S., Lichtenstein, L.M., and Ishizaka, K.: Diagnostic tests in ragweed hay fever. *J Allergy Clin Immunol, 52:*210, 1973.
62. Randolph, T.G.: *Human Ecology and Susceptibility to the Chemical Environment.* Springfield: Thomas, 1962, pp. 91-99.
63. *Ibid.,* pp. 32-34.
64. *Ibid.,* pp. 73-75.
65. *Ibid.,* p. 93.

66. *Ibid.,* pp. 66-69.
67. *Ibid.,* pp. 115-116.
68. Randolph, T.G.: Adaptation to specific environmental exposures enhanced by individual susceptibility. In Dickey, L.D. (Ed.): *Clinical Ecology.* Springfield: Thomas, 1976, pp. 46-66.
69. *Ibid.,* p. 156.
70. Rapp, D.J.: *Questions and Answers About Allergies and Your Child.* New York. Drake Pubs, 1974, pp. 87-88.
71. *Ibid.,* pp. 148-154.
72. *Ibid.,* p. 157.
73. Rea, W.J.: Environmentally triggered cardiac disease. *Ann Allergy, 40*:243, 1978.
74. Reisman, R.: Data presented at the Thirty-First Annual Congress of the American College of Allergists, Bal Harbour, Florida, March 15-22, 1975.
75. Rinkel, H.J., Randolph, T.G., and Zeller, M.: *Food Allergy.* Springfield: Thomas, 1951, pp. 270-271.
76. *Ibid.,* p. 58.
77. *Ibid.,* p. 200.
78. Rowe, A.H.: *Food Allergy, Its Manifestations and Control and the Elimination Diets.* Springfield: Thomas, 1972, pp. 524-525.
79. *Ibid.,* pp. 41-75.
80. *Ibid.,* pp. 45-48.
81. *Ibid.,* p. 582.
82. Sheedy, C.B. and Keifetz, M.: *Cooking for Your Celiac Child.* New York: Dial, 1969, pp. 152-158.
83. Speer, F.: *Allergy of the Nervous System.* Springfield: Thomas, 1970, pp. 227-228.
84. Speer, F. and Dockhorn, R.J.: *Allergy and Immunology in Childhood.* Springfield: Thomas, 1973, p. 363.
85. Sullivan, G.: *Additives in Your Food.* New York: Cornerstone, 1976, p. 50.
86. Vaughn, W.T. and Black, H.J.: *Practice of Allergy.* St. Louis, Mosby, 1948, p. 414.
87. Walker, W.A., Wu, M., Isselbacher, K.J., and Bloch, K.J.: Intestinal uptake of macromolecules. III. Studies on the mechanism by which immunisation interferes with antigen uptake. *J Immunol, 115*:854, 1975.
88. Winter, R.: *Poisons in Your Foods.* USA. General Publishing Company, 1969, p. 41
89. *Ibid.,* pp. 42-43 and 46.

NAME INDEX

SUBJECT INDEX

E

G